To Lori Joy & Avery

Love
Mama
Christmas '97

Letitia Baldrige's Complete Guide to the New Manners for the '90s

OTHER BOOKS BY LETITIA BALDRIGE

Roman Candle
Tiffany Table Settings
Of Diamonds and Diplomats
Home
Juggling
Amy Vanderbilt's Everyday Etiquette
The Entertainers
The 1978 revision of *The Amy Vanderbilt Complete Book of Etiquette*
Letitia Baldrige's Complete Guide to Executive Manners
Letitia Baldrige's Complete Guide to a Great Social Life

Letitia Baldrige's Complete Guide to the New Manners for the '90s

LETITIA BALDRIGE

ILLUSTRATIONS BY
Denise Cavalieri Fike

Rawson Associates
NEW YORK

Library of Congress Cataloging-in-Publication Data

Baldrige, Letitia.
    [Complete guide to the new manners for the '90s]
    Letitia Baldrige's complete guide to the new manners for the '90s / Letitia
Baldrige.
    ISBN 0-89256-320-6
    1. Etiquette—United States. I. Title. II. Title: Complete
guide to the new manners for the '90s.
BJ1853.B35   1990
395—dc20   89-43052
                                               CIP

Rawson Associates
Macmillan Publishing Company
866 Third Avenue, New York, N.Y. 10022
Collier Macmillan Canada, Inc.

Macmillan books are available at special discounts for bulk purchases for sales
promotions, premiums, fund-raising, or educational use.
For details, contact:
    Special Sales Director
    Macmillan Publishing Company
    866 Third Avenue
    New York, N.Y. 10022

Packaged by Rapid Transcript, a division of March Tenth, Inc.

Designed by Stanley S. Drate/Folio Graphics Co. Inc.

Illustrations by Denise Cavalieri Fike

10

Printed in the United States of America

To my husband, Bob Hollensteiner—a wonderful man and the perfect antidote to a hyperactive writer. He is calm, quiet, and restrained—and the first to admit it's not easy living with a bookwriter spouse. He also has a perfect defense mechanism: He doesn't read what I write!

CONTENTS

5

6

7

16

PART V

DIFFICULT TIMES: HEALING YOURSELF AND OTHERS WHEN TROUBLE STRIKES

PART VI

KEEPING IN TOUCH 539

ACKNOWLEDGMENTS

I am greatly in debt to many people at Rawson Associates, without whom I would have jumped into a boiling sea long ago. What a production this opus turned out to be! Just one short year in which to write and publish—a year that my publisher and editor, Eleanor Rawson, her wonderful husband, Ken Rawson, and I will never forget.

Eleanor gave me free rein, swallowed hard more than once, but let me go. I call it faith and trust. She allowed this book to be a very personal statement, which books on manners traditionally are not. She guided and supported me with incredible stamina, pacing me as I rushed back and forth among subjects, generations, and lifestyles.

I am grateful to Grace Shaw, Eleanor's longtime friend and Executive Editor, who kept a calm, cool, and organized eye on the myriad details of this project, and to Ellen Ivens, Eleanor's young assistant ("The Danish Wonder," we call her), who conceived and produced her first child at the same time she helped us all to produce this book. If prenatal influence is important, how could that baby be anything other than well-mannered?

I owe a big vote of thanks to my talented illustrator, Denise Fike, a young Philadelphian on whose capable shoulders I would dump fifteen new drawing assignments at the same time she was nursing her small children with chicken pox and giving a dinner party for the couple's friends who had already had chicken pox. Ah, youth!

And, of course, I owe so much to Bob Oskam, my genius, brilliant copy editor, who managed to do the impossible: make order out of my chaos and words out of my hieroglyphics. He now knows far more than he ever wanted to know about the subjects covered in this book.

Manners from the Heart

Another book on manners?

Yes, another one—but this time one full of help in healing the woes of the previous tumultuous decade of the eighties and full of hope for the promising nineties ahead. Does our society need a change in its manners? A resounding "yes" is the answer from most of the educators, anthropologists, social scientists, and cultural leaders in this country with whom I have spoken informally during the past ten years.

This is an intensely personal book, with a strong point of view. Someone recently introduced me before a lecture as "a traditionalist and a realist who believes in good manners, kindness, having people over for dinner, chastity for the young, and condoms for the young who don't share her belief in chastity!"

I write the way I talk and feel—and I feel strongly about things. I care for the feelings of people who are lonely, but also for the young hostess whose guest of honor is a no-show. I empathize with the man who forgets his boss's name while introducing him to an associate, but I also agonize over the dilemma of a woman who wants to keep a new man in her life without having sex before she knows more about him. All people have problems that are real to them at any given moment in their lives. Solving those problems requires

- Stepping back to assess the situation
- Finding the most commonsensical and kind solution
- Taking action
- Keeping a sense of humor

I have lived a fast-paced, wonderful, and happy life, privileged not in wealth, but in the things that count—family, friends, and experiences. For decades I have walked through this busy, varied life of work and family, with eyes wide open, observing human behavior. (Perhaps I have used eyes on the sides and the back of my head, too.) As we change millennia, our mores and everyday lives are evolving so rapidly that a writer on social behavior must stay aboard a fast express to keep up.

And that is why this book is far removed in its outlook from the material that traditionally comprised a classic book of etiquette. Emily Post, who began writing in this field in the twenties, and Amy Vanderbilt, who entered the field in the early fifties, would probably be shocked

3

beyond belief at some of the subjects I have covered in this book—such as sexual manners, manners concerning homosexuality, questions women must ask of men that never had to be asked before, and problems faced by live-togethers who haven't been married, as well as problems faced by people who may have been married too often! Manners embrace every one of these New Lifestyle problems.

The tremendous upheaval in the roles of women, men, and children and the topics we now openly discuss that only a short time ago were taboo call for a new guide to the New Behavior that is demanded of us.

I have attempted to weave the advice in this book into the fabric of the nineties, to make it meaningful to our everyday lives. My editor has let me use my own voice—a rather breezy, slangy way of talking at times, but it's my way of talking. While I am introducing many new subjects that have never before appeared in books on manners, that does not mean I have not also updated some of the great old traditions of life, including how you get married (yes, I am a real traditionalist about that), how you wield your fork and knife (have you noticed how the young are misdoing that these days?), and conservative subjects such as how others should act when you are born—and yes, die, too.

Because of the chaos around us from broken homes, drugs, crime, sexually transmitted diseases, racism, homelessness, unemployment, pollution, and *more,* there really isn't any room in the nineties for "just an etiquette book." There's a need for something else—a manners book to teach us how to train our own children or somebody else's in this subject, so that we will have a strong nation and a healthy society in the future. There's a need for a manners book to help people just plain cope with the incredible social problems of today. There's a need to define manners in terms of our everyday lives, to give them a higher priority, to show others that good manners are much more than just a tool for success. (That phrase, "tool for success," may sound like the eighties, but the limited goals of financial and social success are not what I'm about or what this book is about.)

I always have believed that there is a difference between etiquette and manners—and never more so than now, as we enter the nineties. Etiquette is protocol, rules of behavior that you memorize and that rarely bend to encompass individual concerns and needs. Manners embrace socially acceptable behavior, of course, but also much more than that. They are an expression of how you treat others when you care about them, their self-esteem, and their feelings. Manners are under your control, because they come from your heart. In a chaotic world, they can make order out of disorder and give you the power to bring pleasure into other people's lives.

We've had enough of the deification of success and greed in the eighties. It is time for something else in the nineties—not just a *social* conscience, but a *people conscience*—an awareness of how nice it feels to be considerate of all those with whom we are in touch every day— our families, friends, the butcher, baker, and any stranger who could use a hand. It is urgent that rather than "I" and "me" we start to start to think about "you" and "they"—and about "us," all sharing this planet together.

We probably all agree that the primary purpose of any book on manners is to give you guidelines about *how, what, where, when, and why* in the social graces. Certainly, if learning about manners makes you feel secure in your movements, if it prevents you from feeling awkward or doing something silly that make people laugh at you, such a book has great value. I honestly think that reassurance is contained in the pages of this book. But what is much more important is that this book is about the rock on which manners are based: *good character,* which translates to kindness, compassion, thoughtfulness—yes, and *love,* too! This is also a book about *being happy,* which is not a contradiction in terms, because when you're nice to someone else (even just a stranger on the telephone), that someone else is nice back to you, and suddenly two people feel good about themselves and each other, and spread their good feeling. And that's what happiness is.

If the seventies and the eighties were the "strive, push, make lots of money, and show it all off decades," maybe the nineties some day will be described as the "helping, caring, asking forgiveness and being forgiven decade." Wouldn't that be nice? Let's call it a goal for the future!

Wait a minute. As yet, our times are far from being describable in such glowing terms. Have we not stopped communicating with one another in human terms during these tumultuous years of rapid techno-logical achievement? I don't know about your eyes, but mine are glazed over from sitting staring at the multi-rapid reflections in computer monitors all day and on television and VCR screens all night. (Good Lord, even little children are gazing at mini-screens all day as they push buttons and keys on their mini-computers, mini-calculators, and mini-everything else!) When was the last time you sat down and read a really great piece of literature? Wrote a newsy letter to a good friend? Called someone who is home alone and probably feeling lonely? When was the last time you took time out from a frantic schedule to chat with a friend face to face or to drop a congratulatory note to an office colleague who performed well in the conference room in front of the Big Brass?

Today's era is an uneasy one. Times are tough. And yet, there's great energy out there—a great capacity for good everywhere that human beings are. It's in the air. We just have to act positively, seize the initiative, and hold on tight. If we open our eyes wide and remove their fixation on the screen so we can see, if we remove our stereo earphones so we can hear, and if we look and talk to one another for a change, we'll find that energy. We'll be able to channel it toward the solution of human problems. We'll be nice to each other, even when we don't feel like it. We'll start getting along well with one another, even with strangers, even when we're being given the run-around in a crowded store or even when a driver who doesn't like the way we drive is honking and hurling strong epithets at us. (Instead of giving him or her the finger in return, we just might concentrate on being a better driver and hope that the other driver's obviously traumatized life eases up.)

If we channel the energy that's in the air, negatives can be willed into positives, and we can all move toward a solution of today's common problems.

Good manners in today's world are a larger part of that energy than you or I possibly realize. Remember, real manners are instinctive; they stem from your character and your heart. You don't turn them on and off like a light switch. They are genuine, because you *care* about others' dignity, welfare, and feelings.

You've heard it before—many times—that good manners are the lubricant of a smooth-working society. Today, they are much more than that. *Real manners are the very basis of wonderful human relationships.* Real manners govern the finest of our interactions at home, at work, and at leisure—in the supermarket, on the baseball field, in our place of worship, in an airport, and even in our government.

My definition of a really admired person—someone who has real class—is a person who has only one kind of manners: the caring kind. I remember hearing the late Ambassador Clare Boothe Luce (at that time my boss at our embassy in Rome, but at all times my role model and mentor) answer a reporter who had asked for a definition of "a really classy person." The reporter's notebook and pen were poised for a typically long Luce dissertation. "A person with class is someone you want to be around—all the time," she answered simply.

The reporter paused, and finally asked, "That's it?"

"There's no need for anything more," she replied.

Today's real manners, the kind that describe someone others want to be around, are those that:

- o Make you pick up a piece of litter someone left on your neighbor's sidewalk—or on anyone's sidewalk, for that matter
- o Cause you to rush to a friend's house to see what you can do when you hear a member of his or her family is in trouble
- o Inspire you to go up to the hired waiter at your dinner party who has just dropped a platter of sliced veal all over the floor in front of your guests, to help him clean up the mess, and then to pat his arm and tell him to forget about it—"It doesn't matter at all."
- o Make you realize that it's not worthwhile wondering who should go through the revolving door first, but it is worthwhile rushing to help an elderly or disabled person through the revolving door

- Help you notice some tiny garnet roses in a shop window, so you buy a small bouquet of them to bring home to your wife or your husband, or maybe to a child
- Motivate you to jump into a conversational lull when someone has just said something embarrassing, thus restarting everyone's conversation so that the one who made the gaffe can pull him- or herself together again
- Cause you to discover, when your laundryman delivers the shirts, that it's his twenty-fifth wedding anniversary, so you give him the bottle of champagne you were saving in the fridge for your own special occasion
- Have you bringing an entire supper over to a family on their moving day
- Remind you that a friend's car is being repaired, and he or she desperately needs it today, so you lend yours
- Make you rip an article out of one of your magazines, to send to a friend or colleague who would be greatly interested in it
- Motivate you to leave a big bunch of balloons in the office of a friend whose promotion will be announced that day
- Cause you to buy a special-interest self-help book for a young person who is just starting a job in that field
- Remind you to buy some concert tickets as a gift and arrange transportation for a lonely elderly friend whose great love is music

Today that person who's so nice to be around, as Clare Luce put it, is *not* Mr. Billionaire-Business-Whiz who yells obscenities at his driver when he makes a mistake, or Mrs. Nouveau-Riche who screams at her maid when she can't find her pantyhose.

That person who's so nice to be around:

- Is a consummate host
- Is a consummate guest
- Has good table manners
- Has a pleasant, well-modulated voice, uses good grammar, and has a graceful vocabulary
- Is someone who never mooches, but who returns others' hospitality, gifts, dinner invitations, and kindnesses of any kind— without ever demanding that anyone return his or her kindnesses
- Is a good communicator—someone who makes telephone calls and writes letters, who is in touch with people, instead of expecting everyone else to communicate with him or her
- Seeks out the wallflower at a social event and brings that person into the group
- Is a person who rises to defend anyone who is being unfairly criticized

o Is adept at making introductions and being introduced, saying hello or good-bye—and makes everyone feel good while it's happening

The crux of everything said above, and of everything in this book, of course, is the *home*. Home is where it *all* starts—manners, good character, values, ethics, social conscience. Home is where a child witnesses and can absorb the good example of caring parents or relatives. Home is where comfort and support can be found, where one person automatically makes an effort to help other members of the family and, in turn, is helped himself. Talk about success—a happy home is what real success is about, the proof positive of thinking about other people, of having their comfort and their happiness in mind. Home is where the discipline is, too—that wonderful magical chisel that sculpts the child into a beautiful work of art—a nice, in-control human being. Home is where the small child learns not just from his or her parents, but from his or her grandparents, too, so that he or she will be a shining mirror image of the best of both generations.

But wait a minute. Isn't that a picture just painted unrealistically rosy for these times? Where are all the homes today where the small child grows up in the constant company of both parents and grandparents? Isn't Mom off working? Are the parents divorced? Is there a confusion of stepparents and stepchildren around? Is the television going all the time so that no one has to talk—either about his or her own problems or someone else's? Are the family teenagers off on their own, out of the home, doing their own thing most of the time? Isn't anyone who happens to be home likely to be standing around the fridge or the microwave, eating with his or her fingers, while the nurturing dining table—the seat of conversation, manners, and the learning of human skills—stands there empty, unused, except as a storage surface?

And how about the delicious interchange of generations that used to be grouped around the dining table? Is the surviving grandparent in a retirement home? Is everyone too tired at night to sit down and just talk to one another? Where is the humanity is all this?

I believe in fighting. Since the development and polishing of manners is not a one-shot operation, but a continuous process that begins no place else but home, I think we can fight to put the home back in all of us again. And if we don't have children, then we can spend a lot of time with someone else's, who are perhaps neglected in this early training of manners, morals, ethics, and values. How about inviting a niece, nephew, grandchild, or godchild over for dinner by him- or herself? Every time you throw in a little lesson on how to act, making it fun and following it up with a hamburger and French fries or a hot fudge sundae, that child is going to love you and learn from you.

For happiness's sake, let's put the bodies back around the dinner table at home, and let's put the conversation back in the mouths of those bodies. It's a wondrous thing watching a child learn manners and consideration. First he or she learns how to do the right thing ("Don't scream at the table, and for heavens' sake, take your fingers out of the salad plate!"). Next, he or she learns how to do the nice thing—a big step up, by the way, from simply knowing not to do something wrong. (Suddenly you'll hear your child say, "Can I bring this present to Suzy's house, Mommy? I think she'd like it. Teacher says she's very sick and feels really bad.") Then you'll see the proof that your child has a heart, and you can pat yourself on the back and shout "Hallelujah! A giant step for mankind!" This is how manners are gradually built into a young person's character. This is how a beautiful human being is formed—one who will walk through life automatically reacting in a "you-they" way, instead of an "I-me" way.

Growing children aren't the only ones who need others to care about them. We all do. In a fast-moving, high-pressure age, the need *to be happy* is universal, but it's a subject that is seldom addressed. We've been so obsessed in the last decade with making money, getting icicle thin, staying healthy, and jazzing up our sex lives that happiness simply wasn't mentioned. People complained all the time about why they were *un*happy, but the affirmative state was rarely discussed. It is attainable, so let's head for it in this decade.

Late in the 1970s I updated and completely revised *The Amy Vanderbilt Complete Book of Etiquette,* the first of a series of books on manners. It addressed problems created by the social confusion of the sixties, a decade in which we survived the anti-establishment youth rebellion, the shock of women leaving home and going to work, and the blurring in definition of men's and women's roles. In the 1980s I wrote my *Complete Guide to Executive Manners,* to help that increasing population of families who spend most of their time at work to feel more secure in their relations in that environment. I followed that book with my *Complete Guide to a Great Social Life,* because so many young people in the workplace—and other singles, too—complained to me that they really didn't *have* a social life in this busy world. With each book addressing these human concerns, I have found people increasingly eager for information and thirsty for knowledge of what to do and when to do it, for information about how to show *their awareness* of other peoples' feelings.

As you read this book, you will not only find advice on what to buy as a christening gift, but also what to say to someone who has AIDS. You will learn how to manage a protocol-laden dinner party, but also how to help a person wracked with grief. It's important to know how to use your knife and fork properly, yes, but it's more important to know how to talk to someone whose child is in prison for dealing drugs. It's helpful if you have the reputation for being an expert on protocol, but it's even more helpful if you are able to stop a person from being falsely maligned. It's attractive for you to dress appropriately for social functions, but it's even more attractive for you to make someone who feels really down to feel up again.

I hope this book will impart knowledge, suggest solutions to dilemmas, answer tough questions, and spark your imagination—but also that it will *make you feel good.* I hope the pages will provide needed information, but also *give comfort,* because at this point in history, comfort is in short supply.

This is my eleventh published book—and the sixth on the subject of manners. Despite that fact, an important person in the Vassar English department once wrote me, "Tish, you are not a great writer—but you are a great communicator." I'll accept and be happy with that. If I understand and love people, and can communicate ideas to and from them, I will continue to be of service to my times, particularly, I hope, as we explore the new guidelines for our behavior toward one another in the new decade we are entering.

PART I
EVERYDAY MANNERS FOR OUR TIMES

Probably most of us would like to be thought of by others as moving through the world with grace and ease—no simple skill. There is no one-week, easy cram course for it. One of the great things about growing older—into your forties, fifties, sixties, and onward—is that the longer you live, the more you know about how to handle yourself—what to do and when to do it. You become like a computer with a multitude of bytes, able to call up answers by a flick of a key and a glance at the monitor screen.

It's a question of learning and using the proper mix of information and consideration—whether you're tipping someone, coping with grandmother when she comes to live with you or with an adult child who won't leave the nest, dealing with the plumber, or talking to the boss as you're waiting together in an airport for three hours. By the time you have an instinctive feel for what to do in all these situations, you could write this book—and I'd be the first to read it!

If you believe in the definition of happiness as having good relationships, and if you believe that good manners are essential to happiness, then you must also believe that one natural result of a person's good manners is his or her state of happiness.

Good relationships don't just happen in the everyday course of events. They are the result of someone's hard work and caring. They are constantly, dynamically changing, being refined and fine-tuned.

We can't escape a constant interaction with people (unless we choose to live as hermits). We interact all day long with family members, friends, and just plain people—the people at our place of work, the gas station, on the bus, at our house of worship. We react to the toll-road ticket taker, the doctor, barber, manicurist, and to the people who deliver our packages, collect our garbage, and read our utilities meters. They are, each and every one, individuals worthy of respect and consideration; when they behave as if they are not and are beastly to us, we must find a way to control our anger, so that we do not take it out on another human being. (When I am unjustly treated in a nasty manner, I immediately imagine myself sticking many pins into a pin cushion, and in my mind that takes care of the person who did me wrong. I recommend you find your own avenue of harmless revenge.)

When we graduate from the self-obsessed "I-I-Me-Me" school of philosophy, into a life of caring about other people, we begin to react automatically to those other people, whether they are close friends or not. We react in a uniform, decent, and considerate manner. It's not something we stop to think about. We just do it.

Manners at Home

The task of a writer on behavior is to remind the individual of the importance of his or her role in the world, the community, the family. We often spend so much time philosophizing about the big picture that we lose sight of the small details. But it's the small detail that is capable of making another person lose respect for us or, conversely, look upon us as a hero.

When you see my lists of things to remember in relationships—all those details—you might say, "Oh, but I know all that. I've always known that." The lists are there to jog your consciousness of what you have always known, to prompt you in applying that to your everyday encounters with others.

The home is where our most intimate relationships are formed, shaped, cemented, broken. As an adult, you interact with your spouse— and with your spouse's parents. You interact with your children and their friends. You are dealing with relations every step along the way—as your child leaves home, when that child comes back to live with you as an adult. Or with your parents—first as their child, and then as their guardians when one or both return to your home to live with you in their old age. Then there is the person with whom your child shares an apartment or house when he or she leaves home. It's *sharing* every day of the year, in all these situations—a call for sensitivity to feelings. For self-control. For learning to bite your tongue and swallow your resentment. For remaining kind. None of this is easy. But all of it can make life harmonious and pleasurable.

1

Your Manners with Those Close to You

It's only common sense. The people you are closest to warrant an extra measure of consideration. After all, they are part of your daily life, and you want your interactions with them to be as pleasant and smooth as possible. There's nothing that sours things quite so much as friction between family members or others sharing the same living space. It takes good manners to keep close relationships comfortable and warm, to sustain the love and mutual respect that make a house a home.

IN THE RELATIONSHIPS THAT GROW OUT OF MARRIAGE

Consideration and good manners cement many different family relationships, but it's the relationships that evolve out of marriage that particularly benefit by their presence—or suffer through their absence.

With Your Mate

In the good fight against taking someone for granted, a prime cause for unhappiness between couples, these are points to consider:

o A spouse needs building up, not putting down or being mocked in front of others.

o Help him or her through every major disappointment. Hopefully, he or she will do the same for you.

o It is important to be particularly nice to family members your spouse holds dear, such as his or her parents.

o Be nice to your spouse's friends, even the ones you don't like. (Maybe your spouse doesn't like some of *your* friends.)

o Be punctual for appointments he or she considers important.

o Compromise not only on big matters (the house to be purchased), but also on small ones (tonight's movie selection on television).

o When your mate faces a big problem, drop what you're doing and be there. There are times when you may have to put your spouse ahead of your children.

o Compliment your spouse often—and creatively, so that you don't sound metronome-predictable.

o Be imaginative and thoughtful with every gift for your spouse.

o Keep in constant touch when you are apart (with regular telephone calls, for example).

o If your mate is not feeling well or has a crash project to take care of, offer to do his or her chores as well as your own.

o Consult each other as equal partners on everything major concerning the children.

With Your Mother- and Father-in-Law

When you marry, your mate's parents become part of your inner family and should be treated as such. Treat them with love and respect from the outset, and you'll not only win their reciprocated love and respect—you'll strengthen the bonds of your relationship with your spouse.

o Make them feel their visits to your home are welcome, not an imposition.

o Arrange to have your children see them as often as possible.

o Don't take their baby-sitting help for granted; remember how pressured they may be by their own problems, so don't abuse their kindness.

o Never criticize them within earshot of your children; always refer to them with affection and respect.

o If they live in another town, telephone them regularly, and always on their birthdays and anniversary.

o If one of them becomes widowed, give much more of yourself than before to the remaining one.

o If one of them grossly oversteps the bounds of acceptable behavior, either in advising or criticizing you or your children, explain what he or she has done wrong with tact and kindness. Keep your voice calm and show you are in control of your emotions. (And no matter how poor your relationship may be at any given moment, never cut them off from their grandchildren.) Cool down; the situation will be better in a short while.

o Have your children write thank-you notes to their grandparents within a week of receiving any gifts from them.

o Welcome it when they give their grandchildren some lessons in table manners when they take them out for a meal (because your children probably can use them).

o Welcome their moments of reminiscing, but make them feel a part of your generation, too. (That means comments like this are never heard in your house: "You wouldn't understand, because you're of the older generation.")

o Never make fun of their forgetfulness or other signs of old age, and never allow your children to tease them either. Remember, some day you will be there, too.

With Your Son and Daughter-in-Law or Daughter and Son-in-Law

When you are the parents-in-law, be the best there are. The most important basis of a happy relationship with your children and their spouses is to accept that they must lead their own lives and raise their own children their way, not yours.

o Learn to sit on any criticism you might have of how they live or how they are raising your grandchildren—because, realistically, they will not be interested in your views.

o When your advice *is* sought, give it freely and lovingly, but don't expect to receive such a request very often.

o If you can't say something nice about their house and its decor, don't say anything at all.

o Don't push too aggressively for invitations; appreciate the fact that they may be very busy—too busy to entertain you.

o Ask them out to dinner more often than you make them ask you to their house. Be very sensitive to their voices when you suggest coming over—it may be the wrong time, in which case, back off.

o If you sense marital discord in the house, don't question anyone about it. Wait until one of them speaks to you—and never ever question their children about it.

o Remember your son- or daughter-in-law's birthday with the same enthusiasm you remember your child's.

o Offer to help with free baby-sitting chores, and don't act as though this puts them in your debt.

o If you're feeling neglected, call them, but just to check in, never to complain. A surefire way to cheer yourself up is to talk to your grandchildren on the telephone.

o Always pick up after yourself in their house; offer to help clean up after them, too. If they say no, don't argue!

o Help them out when they're going through a tough time financially. This may result in giving them a loan at no interest, in forgiving a debt, or in devising some creative way out of their problem. (As a daughter who had her hand in her father's pocket his entire life, this person can say with conviction that it takes a wonderful parent to remain generous for so many years!)

o Apologize when you've irked your son- or daughter-in-law, even if you feel innocent. Always take the first step to ask forgiveness, and keep those lines of communication open. In-laws become greatly upset with each other for the most insignificant of reasons. Deal with any negative at once, so that a small sore does not become a festering wound.

WITH ROOMMATES

If you share an apartment or house as an adult with a roommate of the same sex (and we are not talking here about a homosexual arrangement), getting on each other's nerves is almost inevitable. There are times when another person's habits or lack of courtesy grate on you, but if both roommates are well intentioned and prepared to share equal responsibilities, the relationship can be very successful, happy, and healthy.

• *Be up front with each other.* Don't allow some unspoken resentment to magnify in its importance. Don't sulk. Roommates who communicate well and speak frankly to each other have a successful household. Unaired problems are never solved—they just expand.

• *Share the work involving the household equally.* Discuss the division of responsibilities if one of you feels they are not fairly balanced. And if you have a chore, do it when you are supposed to. Sloppiness and procrastination on the part of one person can make the best relationship grow sour.

• *One roommate should help out the other when he or she has a guest*—either by getting out of the apartment, or by doing some extra chores or both.

• *Learn to entertain in tandem,* to get along with each other's friends, and to mix the two sets equally when you jointly entertain. It goes without saying that a primary rule in any shared housing is: Steal not thy roomate's boyfriend (or girlfriend).

• *Keep rigorous records of expenses*—everything from long distance calls to a shared bottle of wine, from cleaning supplies to newspaper subscriptions. Settle and pay up accounts quickly at the end or beginning of each month.

• *Take accurate telephone messages for your housemates,* and make sure you leave them where the person to whom they are directed can see them the minute he or she comes home.

• *Be neat.* Nothing gets on a person's nerves more than living with a slob, or having one's friends notice that he or she is living with a slob.

• *Don't be a "dinner guest hog,"* which means that your friends are the only ones regularly invited to have dinner at your house. Ask your roommates if they wouldn't like to have one or two of their friends at the next dinner party in your house. In other words, divide the opportunity for entertaining friends. But if your roommates don't seem to have anyone to suggest, just go ahead with your guests. Your roommates may prefer it that way. (Just be sure they do!)

• *Do not bring a third party into the apartment for purposes of sex.* This is important for people of the opposite as well as the same sex who are living together. It is unfair to your roommate or roommates. It is wrong and inconsiderate to bring someone in and to close your door to engage in sex while your roommates, who help pay the rent, are struggling to carry on their normal lives in the living room as though nothing were happening.

If you are planning on having sex on any particular evening, do it somewhere else. To do it in the shared apartment would be an invasion of your roommate's privacy. To have your lover move into the apartment, too, as some do, would only compound the insensitivity, arrogance, and rudeness on your part. People who are paying equal shares in the rent of a home should not have to put up with any roommate's visiting friend of either sex (including an overnight lover) sleeping in.

I remember a fascinating "crime of passion" trial when I was living in Italy: A young woman shot and killed her female roommate's male lover in the bedroom one night. The court acquitted her because, although she admitted she shot him, she also had been in love with the man herself, and to find him in bed, in her own bedroom, with her roommate, was more than she should have to bear.

With a Roommate of the Opposite Sex

After college graduation, some young people find that paying the expensive rent on a house or apartment in a big city is very difficult, particularly when they are just beginning their careers and are earning low salaries. Therefore, some young people of both sexes band together (sometimes it's only one young man and one young woman) to share the cost of an apartment or a house.

I have heard the following answers (all of them quite sensible) from offspring when parents (particularly a young woman's parents) protest this kind of living arrangement:

> "It's no different from what it was in our coed dorm. We live together like brothers and sisters, exactly as we did in college."

> *Young woman:* "I feel safer with a man in the house. This is not a good neighborhood, and I'd be scared if it weren't for Joe."

> *Young woman:* "You have no idea how useful George is to Betsy and me. He is a real handyman—does a hundred things a month to keep this place going. George is an important part of our lives!"

> *Young man:* "We like having Jenny living with us. Yes, she's one heck of a good cook. We do all the cleaning up, but she does the cooking, and we have such incredible gourmet meals! Besides, she's our friend. We confide in each other, help one another with emotional problems."

I think it's a good idea to accept a young person's explanation that the living arrangement is free from sexual innuendo. After all, if there was going to be any hanky-panky between two people, they would not have to rent a special house in which to do it.

However, a young person who chooses to live with one or more members of the opposite sex should realize that flying in the face of convention engenders certain problems to face. For example:

• *Others are going to think of you as having sexual relations with one or more of your roommates even when you are not.* It is just a natural jump to such a conclusion. Don't be defensive about it. If you are not sexually involved with your roommates, deny it matter-of-factly to anyone who insinuates it and then drop the subject: "We are living together as friends, not as lovers. It's a very ordinary, nonsexual relationship."

If you *are* having a sexual relationship with a roommate, my advice is to drop the pretext that you are just friends sharing the rent together. Two people who are sexually involved will have a difficult time concealing that from anyone else. (Three people involved in sex together have a three hundred percent more difficult time!)

If sex is part of the monthly rent arrangement, it might be a good idea for the two of you to make plans to file a joint income tax preparation next year. (In other words, get married!)

• *When you have a social life that appears more successful than that of your roommates, there is liable to be jealousy and resentment on their part.* When that is the case, it's wise to learn to be cool—in other words, keep quiet—about the parties you attend, the dates you have, the amusing and exciting experiences you have that your roommate or roommates do not share. There is no point engendering jealousy in them.

• *On the other hand, your roommates do not have the right to expect to be invited everywhere you go.* It's important to establish your independence the minute you begin your cohabitation arrangement. Make it clear to everyone that you will lead your own life at night and on weekends, that you will be a good citizen of the house, but that you do not expect to be cross-examined on a continuing basis about what you're doing and whom you're seeing.

• *Say nice things, rather than snide and critical things, about the dates your roommates bring to a meal or a party in your mutually shared house.* Part of getting along in life is to build people up, rather than bring them down, which is what criticizing a roommate's date or friend would amount to.

WITH THOSE WHO WORK IN YOUR HOUSE

The people you hire to work in or around your home are as worthy of your respect as anyone else. Don't think of or treat them as lesser individuals who should feel privileged to be working for you. Treat domestics like professionals who should have pride in their jobs.

o Make sure that you or someone else trains them thoroughly and that they understand their duties and the rules of the household. If you don't know how to train them, there is always a creative solution to be found. For example, ask a friend's domestic (with your friend's permission, of course) to train your domestic on her day off (for a fee, of course). An accomplished waitress in a local restaurant might come on a day off to train your helper. (The extra money earned is always welcome.) There are many possibilities.

o Write down and explain exactly what you expect this person to do each day. Make sure that every responsibility is carefully understood. (This is particularly important for *baby-sitters.* You should leave detailed instructions, even as to what they can eat in your kitchen.)

o Follow the rules of the Department of Labor as to the number of hours your employee works, and the amount of time off that is mandatory. Make the person's Social Security and Unemployment Insurance payments. Observe the minimum wage law (but if you exceed it, you will have a happier and more productive employee.)

o Don't lay too many responsibilities on a domestic employee. It is impossible for one employee to be in charge of a house—the cleaning, laundry, and cooking—and also take care of a baby or children, as well as the dog! Many women do this every day in their own houses, but their motivation in their own home is obviously much stronger than that of a paid outside person.

o Always give your domestic staff compensatory time off after a period of great effort, such as when you have gone through a schedule of constant entertaining or your house has been full of guests.

o Always praise and thank a domestic staff person after he or she has done a good job.

o Never criticize an employee in front of others, particularly in front of your children. Speak to him or her in private—and always right after he or she has done a poor job. Don't wait a couple of weeks, by which time the person will have forgotten what was done wrong.

o Give any member of your domestic staff a nice uniform—so that he or she will take pride in his or her personal appearance. If they are performing cleaning work in your house, they should not have to use their own clothes.

o Give a domestic a place to rest in your home—at least a comfortable chair—plus time to sit down and eat meals. Be sure that there is always sufficient food for this employee, including when you are away.

o If she or he smokes, you have a right to ask her or him not to when at work in your house.

o If you keep a cook, maid, or waitress very late for a party and she does not have a car, provide her transportation home, so that she won't have to take public transportation at an unsafe hour.

o If a maid lives with you, give her privacy in her living quarters. Don't let the children go into her room at will. Provide her with her own television set, and make sure her room is comfortable and attractive.

o Include her in family birthdays and other important family celebrations. She is, after all, a member of the family!

THE NEW FAMILY FORMATION: ADULTS LIVING TOGETHER HARMONIOUSLY

When the country got going, in the seventeenth and eighteenth centuries, entire families occupied small houses and managed to live together in very close quarters in what must have been a loving—but also sometimes combative—atmosphere. If three generations could live together in a small house in those days and manage to make this country great at the same time, two or three generations living together today should be able to do so, too. It's called *summoning self-control and cooperating for the sake of the family.*

An Adult Child Returns to the Nest

"I can't believe it," one of my college classmates said at our reunion, "in our one small block alone, we have five families with their children living home again—ages twenty-five to thirty-five! I thought we were unusual with both a son and a daughter camping with us again, but I feel so sorry for our neighbors next door. Their daughter, son-in-law, and two children have moved in on them. My husband and I are home free in comparison!"

Another classmate added in a tone that was meant to be funny but really wasn't, beneath the surface, "Our daughter has moved back, too. We think she is taking the tack that if she irritates us seriously long enough, we'll die from exasperation and then she'll have the house to herself!"

The skyrocketing costs of home purchases and apartment rentals have made it impossible for many young people who are in the early stages of their careers or studying for advanced degrees to live in their own homes. Usually the parents are initially delighted to have their young back in the nest again, but often that euphoria does not last for long. The occupants of the household begin to get on each others' nerves. Parents begin to find their privacy and their routines invaded; the adult children begin to wonder why their parents don't have the capacity, must less the desire, to understand their need for freedom and independence.

In the best of all worlds, when an adult child moves back into the parents' home, both generations will sit down at the bargaining table and lay out all the ifs, ands, and buts of the new living arrangements, so there will be no secrets or unpleasant surprises. The contract can always be renegotiated if one party feels unduly put upon! It's important that both generations understand every rule, responsibility, and financial obligation of the new living arrangement, and that each respects the lifestyle of the other—even though the parents rightly consider that their home is *their* home and not "the home of these unfeeling monsters we've raised," as one parent phrased it to me one day.

Details to Be Worked Out Beforehand

- What compensation or reimbursement is to be made to the parents for room and/or board?
- What work is to be done for the parents in the home (such as cleaning, marketing, cooking, driving) in addition to or in place of financial compensation for room and/or board?
- What kitchen privileges and responsibilities will your offspring have (including replacing popular fridge items when he or she uses them up)?
- The rules of privacy ("You don't go into my room, and I won't go into your room" . . . "You don't touch my mail, and I won't touch your mail").
- The entertaining privileges the child will have, and the rules on vacating the house to be respected by the parents when this entertaining occurs.
- Ordinary noise limitations in the household with respect to things like television, radio, and stereo system.
- What the rules are concerning the presence of guests in the offspring's room.
- The extent of the redecoration allowed (or perhaps urged by the parents) of the child's living quarters at the child's expense.
- Rules on the garaging and parking of his or her automobile, motorcycle, or bicycle.
- Rules of orderliness to be carefully observed in the household (examples: kitchen to be left in apple-pie condition before leaving it for one second; no dirty running shoes on the living room carpet; no dirty laundry piled on top of the washing machine and just left there).
- Rules governing the use of the washer and dryer, the hours in which the vacuum may be run, and who will answer the doorbells and telephones. (In some houses, even though the adult child has his own telephone in his room, part of the deal is that when he is home, he answers every telephone call and takes messages for his parents when they are out.)

I have seen a returned-home child make his parents furious and then watched his parents turn to mush when the reprobate returned with a dozen roses and a sentimental note of apology for "Mom." I witnessed a returned-home daughter make retribution to her father for taking his car unannounced and causing him to miss an important business appointment. (She had his car washed, greased, and filled with gas; she put a bagful of his favorite home-baked brownies on the car seat and left a note telling him that he was "the greatest father in the whole wide world and how could she have done such a terrible thing to such a wonderful person?")

In a re-established adult family home there will be moments of wonderful family togetherness, love, and support; there will probably also be moments of anguish and extreme irritation, but if each member of the household tries to make the living arrangements function smoothly, the re-established unit can be one of the greatest and happiest lifetime experiences of any of its members.

When a Parent Lives with You

Until the middle part of this century, grandparents lived with the families of the next two generations until they died. It was the accepted thing. Houses were bigger then, but also, it was the only humane thing to do—there was no alternative. In spite of the occasional bickering and sometimes strong disagreements, families grew closer and children greatly benefited from the extra measure of love and wisdom afforded by the different generations surrounding them. In those days you "put up with your parents until they died," because you loved them and they had loved you for a lot longer than you could remember.

After World War II, following the baby boom, living space was at a premium and people became increasingly jealous of their privacy and their rights. Rest homes, retirement communities, and housing for the elderly became part of our everyday social environment.

Now in the 1990s, just as there are many more postgraduate children who have returned to the nest, there are also more widowed grandparents once again living with an adult child and that child's spouse. It is often much less costly to the older people's children to have them at home than to pay for their independent housing and health care. It is usually much more compassionate to have them live with their children, but usually no one feels it to be the perfect solution for the aged parent or that person's family.

If an aged parent has come to live with you, look upon the strongly positive side of it. A grandparent (often the grandmother is the survivor, as women tend to outlive their husbands) may have an incredible potential for contributing to the development and education of her grandchildren. The new living arrangement tends to work if all generations exert self-control, give an extra measure, and learn to cooperate and sacrifice.

What the Children Should Be Taught

- *The children should be taught to show respect and deference to the grandparent.* For example:

  - At family meals (except breakfast), the children of the household stand by their chairs until Grandmother takes her seat. (This is the perfect time for a child to learn the meaning of deference and respect. Having learned it, the child will benefit later as an adult in the workplace because of it.)
  - Food should be offered first to any older person at table.
  - Grandmother's visitors should be treated politely as honored guests in the house.
  - The noise from a tape cassette, VCR, or "boom box" should be held down to a normal level when Grandmother is home.
  - Her rest hour should be respected.
  - Her telephone messages should be carefully taken, and her mail given to her unopened.
  - Her room should not be entered, except on her invitation.

- *Children should be encouraged to seek her advice and opinion on matters.* To ask Grandmother's opinion is important, not only as an act of kindness to make her feel an important member of the family, but also to gain her insight and wisdom on a particular subject.

- *They should be encouraged to confide in her without turning her into an adversary against one of the parents or against another sibling.* A grandparent often has experience and skills in handling troubling family disputes and can offer helpful advice to a young child in coping with his or her own problems. However, she should not allow herself to be lobbied by a child to help him more than his siblings, or to play favorites.

What You Might Do

- *Give a grandparent her own space.* Grandmother really needs her own room—hers to keep clean, but also hers in which to maintain her privacy. A son or daughter or son- or daughter-in-law really doesn't have the right to go through the older person's mail, personal effects, drawers, and closet—unless that person is incompetent. If there is some information that must be solicited for reasons of health, legal, or economic matters, *ask* Grandmother; don't go behind her back. Mutual trust is paramount to the success—even the survival—of a cross-generational living arrangement.

- *Remember not to take advantage of her presence by laying too much housework or too many baby-sitting responsibilities on her.* She it not, after all, a paid domestic employee, and although most likely she will want to work to repay your hospitality (and help out financially), she should not be treated like a domestic in terms of work responsibility, hours worked, and the like.

Of course she will watch the children while you are on vacation or out socially or at work, but hopefully you will not abuse this convenient presence in your house. Whether her financial contributions are helping pay household expenses, or whether she is unable to contribute any-thing toward household expenses, she should not be judged or treated according to her fiscal liabilities or assets. She should be treated as a parent deserving of your love and respect, without whom you or your spouse would not have been born. (If your aging parent has an unfortu-nate disposition and is entirely selfish and uncooperative, hopefully you will have made alternate arrangements and she won't be living with you anyway!)

• *Make her living quarters as pleasant as possible,* with a personal television set and radio, if possible. Her room should be attractive, freshly painted, and cheerful when she comes to live with you. Put in her room some cherished mementos, photographs, and perhaps a favorite piece or two of furniture from her former house. This will ease the difficult adjustment from a life of independence to one she will consider to be dependent on you. Having her own little space will give her a much-needed sense of dignity.

One couple I know invited a widowed grandmother to live with them. She had become increasingly crippled with arthritis and couldn't manage alone any more. They added on a small room and bath to their modest house, paid for by the grandmother from her savings. It was on the first floor, so that she would not have to manage stairs. The daughter had asked her mother several months before she came to live with them what her very favorite bedroom had looked like. When the mother walked into her new room in her daughter's home, she found it deco-rated with those same colors and fabric ideas (even a new carpet in the exact shade of green of a favorite old rug the mother had described to her daughter and her daughter had remembered). What could have been a traumatic experience for the mother became a happy one. She imme-diately felt comfortable in the new living arrangement.

• *Preserve her feelings of independence.* It is important that she have control of her own money—as long as she is capable of managing it. She should have her own bank account, checks, deposit slips, and if she cannot get to the bank alone, someone should take her regularly, so that she can maintain a semblance of financial independence. If she is a woman of means, she should have her own lawyer and financial adviser, so that you can never be accused of trying to manipulate her. If she is expected to (and, of course, is able to) contribute monthly to household and other expenses, those costs should be written down and carefully understood by all parties in advance, so that she will know her responsibilities and not feel her money is being taken for granted or wrested from her capriciously.

• *Allow her to receive her own friends.* On occasion, if she is up to it, the resident grandparent should be able to entertain without feeling she is upsetting everyone. She should know well beforehand what morning or afternoon—or even evening—the living room, kitchen, and dining room are hers for entertaining.

• *Make sure that the older member of the family gets taken to church, to the doctor, and takes her medication at the proper times.* You should be the eyes and ears of your senior resident, all the more so as the person grows older and becomes forgetful on occasion.

• *Refrain from criticizing the grandparent for occasional forgetfulness and other signs of growing older.* You and your children should keep reminding yourselves that some day you will be in the same situation. Therefore, never make fun of a grandparent or her friends. As the person living in the household ages, tolerance and patience will be required by everyone living there. (All you have to do is to keep remembering the Golden Rule: "Do unto others what you would have others do unto you"—because one day you will probably be old yourself!)

WHAT THE GRANDPARENT-IN-RESIDENCE SHOULD REMEMBER

• *Always respect the privacy of the younger generations in the house.* Do not enter their rooms uninvited, go through their drawers, or listen in on their telephone calls.

• *Refrain from "horning in" on the younger generations' social activities at home, unless specifically invited.* You should remain in your own room when your children or grandchildren are entertaining their friends. You might offer to help prepare the food or clean up, but do not be present when the guests arrive, tempting though it is to take a peek at what the younger generation is up to. (Perhaps it's just as well not to know.)

• *Refer to everyone's possessions as belonging to their specific owners, not to you.* For example, you should refer to the family automobile as "John and Barbara's car" not "our car." If the house belongs to your children and is not owned by you, refer to it as "my daughter and son's house," not "my house." In other words, as grandparent-in-residence, remember "to each his own."

• *Do not complain about the food that is served (unless, of course, it is insufficient, and then it's time to have a frank discussion with your children).* Perhaps they need more money for the food budget; perhaps your daughter needs more help with the cooking. It is not for you to criticize the condition of your daughter's or daughter-in-law's house, however. If you find it untidy in comparison with the house you used to keep, you can always ask if she would like you to help take care of it. If she refuses, then accept it the way it is.

• *Keep your own room wonderfully clean and neat,* regardless of how the rest of the house looks. This will influence your grandchildren. They will be able to discern the difference between a well-kept and a slovenly house.

• *Offer to help with housework, cooking, and baby-sitting chores as much as you are able to.* If you give more than is expected of you, you will probably find that the others give back more to you in return.

• *Handle your own financial affairs as long as you are able to.* Sometimes it's a question of consciously concentrating hard and thinking carefully when money matters are discussed, so that you will remain as independent as possible.

• *Provide surprises and treats once in a while,* when you are financially able to or if you have made a gift with your hands. I know a grandmother who always bakes a specially decorated cake for the birthday of each member of the family; she outdoes herself year after year in her creativity. I know a creative grandfather, too, who lives with one of his sons and his family and is full of surprises. One spring the garden suddenly burst forth into bloom with five new azalea bushes that no one had seen him plant the year before. In front of each bush was the name of a family member (painted on a small wooden stick). Even the family dog had a beautiful new bush named after him.

• *Avoid taking sides with your children in a marital dispute or in arguments over the grandchildren.* Be known as someone who offers wise counsel, even mediation services *when requested,* and as someone who is scrupulously fair, unprejudiced, and noninterfering.

The Family Forum

I used to marvel at a friend who had her father-in-law living with her family from the age of seventy-two to ninety-two. She and her husband built shelves on the walls of his room to house his many golf trophies. His room contained furniture from his old home, including the antique bed that he and his wife had shared until she had been killed in an automobile accident. I remember how much we all loved "Grandpa," as everyone called him, including his five grandchildren and all their friends. Family arguments and complaints were all handled in a "Family Forum" meeting, which was called when necessity warranted it. Matters were fully discussed, with all generations present, and remedial action to be taken was written in chalk on a blackboard hanging on the kitchen wall. Here is what was written on the blackboard one week in January of 1982:

FAMILY FORUM

Grandpa: Promises to stop clicking his loosened false teeth, because it drives *everyone*, repeat everyone, crazy.

Will make not one but two batches of his famous fudge, in repentance for not keeping his promise to Sarah to make it for her slumber party.

Father: Will get the car washed, as he promised to before Christmas, because his wife is furious.

Will fix the window in Jim's room, as he promised to last September, because Jim is furious.

Decrees that one night a week there will be NO rock music played in the house.

Mother: Will let Sarah wear makeup once a month, to all-girl parties.

Will get off Joey's back about his socks.

Won't let it happen again that there's no soda in the fridge.

Jim: Will keep, not cancel his appointment with the skin doctor next week.

Will remember to leave his boots in the mudroom, and not ruin the carpets.

Will put his jeans in the wash when they are dirty.

Will pick the rock music three nights a week without interference.

Sarah: Won't swipe Mom's makeup, and won't clean it off on a face towel.

Will pick the rock music three nights a week without interference.

Will not tie up the phone longer than fifteen minutes on any one call.

Joey: Will tie his socks together before they go in the wash.

Will pick the rock music no nights a week—until Jim goes away to school, and then he inherits his nights.

Will quit wiping his runny nose on his sleeve.

Annie: Will go quickly to the bathroom if she thinks she's going to throw up, instead of aiming for the rug.

Will not leave her doll on the living room floor when Mom and Dad have guests.

Will be nicer to the sitter.

Georgie: Knows he will not be smiled at in his high chair any longer if he puts the palm of his hand in the boiled egg and then puts his hand on the wall.

Promises he won't pull again so hard on Mom's pearl necklace that he breaks it. (Three times is enough, Georgie!)

This was one Family Forum that really worked!

*   *   *

Good relationships are the result of an affirmative attitude toward life. They are the result of someone stepping forward, making an effort—even making a sacrifice—and saying:

"I like what I see."

"I'll give him (or her) the benefit of the doubt, if I don't like what I see."

"This person could be important to me—now or in the future."

"This is a person I could help in some way."

"This is a member of my family—to be loved and supported, in spite of some bad chemistry between us."

We are like the dancers in an ancient French square dance—the *quadrille*—as we step in and out of each other's lives, back and forth, making fascinating patterns with family members, friends, co-workers and others who cross our paths in the course of a day. When we are the first to reach out with a smile, friendly bantering, and an emanation of warmth and good cheer, our relationships with others cannot help but be good. A flower tilts toward the sun; a human being turns toward another warm and kind human being. The similarity between good relationships and good manners is not only obvious—the two are one and the same!

2

Rearing Great Children: The Manners They Need to Know

Teaching your children manners is also teaching them values, ethics, and morals. The child's character develops and is shaped because of his or her own life experiences, but also in a major way through the influence and teaching of the people to whom he or she is close and whom he or she loves. In the best of all worlds, parents and children are politer to one another than to anyone else.

Since our children are our greatest national resource, and since in the opinion of many the moral fabric of this country is unravelling, a parent's responsibility in raising children today is monumental!

It's a heavy enough burden when there are two parents, but in today's society, with both parents working or with so many single, divorced, or remarried parents, the problems bearing down on the child seem to reproduce themselves like quickly dividing cells. Among current problem situations:

- Hostile stepparents and stepsiblings
- Hostile in-laws in a new marriage situation
- Latchkey children left on their own too much

- Victims of drug and alcohol abuse by parents in the home
- Children with undiagnosed learning difficulties
- The bad influence of peer pressure

That's a pretty heavy sackful of problems, but it does not take into account the resilience of children, particularly their native intelligence and their durability. Regardless of the problems both children and parents face in today's society, single parents can take heart. It takes only *one caring parent* (or relative or any loving adult close to the child) to shape and mold the child's character *for the good.*

Manner, together with ethics, values, and morals, are the basis of character, and these forces for good really cannot be separated. In the final analysis, we must do all we can to show children the right way—and then trust them. They are the leaders of tomorrow, and will have to deal with the mess today's adults are leaving them. They are our nation's hope and will most likely do far better than the present generation of adults, who have been watching rather helplessly the unravelling of the moral fiber of our country in an era of drugs, crime, and sexual excess.

Children need us to teach them *discipline,* for one thing, as well as *a firm sense of right and wrong.* If we are not a parent, we can be a terrific aunt or uncle, godparent, grandparent, cousin, stepfather, step-mother, stepbrother or -sister, nurse, baby-sitter, day-care center director, teacher, pastor, youth center director, coach, community volunteer, Big Brother, Big Sister, and office role model or mentor. Collectively and individually, we have enormous influence on a child with whom we spend time.

The ability to choose between the assistance offered by good people versus that offered by bad people is the moment of truth for a young person. The selection of peers and choice of leaders to follow means the success or failure of a young life.

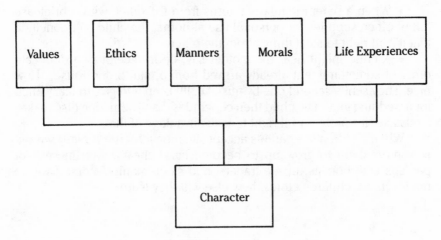

HOW A CHILD LEARNS TO DISTINGUISH BETWEEN RIGHT AND WRONG

The Example of His or Her Parents

Children learn from their parents' behavior. If parents do something a child feels is basically wrong, or if they accept behavior on the child's part that is basically wrong, "wrong" soon turns to "right." For example:

• A child who hears his or her parents talking to each other about new ways in which they can cheat on their income tax will conclude that it's all right to cheat the government.

• A child who watches a parent lying to a police officer, trying to get out of a ticket, will conclude that disrespect for the law and lying to a policeman are acceptable.

• When a child grabs a package of candy from the supermarket rack one day and a small packet of cookies the next, and his or her mother sees that but doesn't pay for the item, the child will conclude that it's all right to steal from the supermarket.

• When the child's mother puts coins in a slot to get a newspaper from a rack on the street and then takes three papers (one for herself and two for her neighbors) but only pays for one, the child will conclude that it's all right to pay for one thing but to help yourself to more if you can get away with that.

• When a child returns from a birthday party with a prize won in a game and tells his parents that he cheated in order to win it and then they don't say another word about it, he will conclude that it's all right to cheat. Since he doesn't have to return the prize, he concludes that it's all right if you're not caught.

• When a parent regularly returns from the office with a briefcase full of office supplies for personal use at home, the child will conclude that it's all right to steal things from the office.

• A child might hear his mother say, upon receipt of a duplicate order of something that already arrived from a mail order house, "How nice! They sent a second one by mistake. I'll keep it to give to Mary Ellen for a wedding gift." The child then concludes that if someone else makes a mistake, it's perfectly all right to take advantage of that.

When children see parents accept situations that are morally wrong, it inspires them to grow up to become liars, cheats, and thieves—or perhaps extortionists, inside traders, and stock manipulators. If we do not teach our children ethics, how else will they learn?

Moral Lessons a Small Child Gleans from Parents Through Reading and Conversation

A child learns to understand right from wrong at a very early age—with the help of his or her parents—through words spoken in a conversation and words read in a book. For example, when reading aloud a bedtime story—a fairy tale—with his little girl at night, a father might comment as he reads along, "Now, that's a bad person who would do a thing like that, isn't he?"

His daughter would say, "Yes, a very naughty person."

The father might say, "You'd *never* do a thing like that, now, would you, Suzy? It's mean to do something like that."

"Oh, nooo!" would be her reply, and they would continue happily along in their story.

As they go through all the stories, week after week, with her father emphasizing the *bad* things people do and the *good* things people do, with punishment meted out for the bad things, the little girl develops a growing sense of right and wrong, identifying herself always with the right.

Her father might explain to her once in a while how mean it is to do a cruel thing to someone else—in other words, "You don't do a bad thing because you'll be caught and punished, but more important, you don't do a bad thing because it hurts someone else." The little girl will begin to imitate her father when they come to a certain part of the story, reacting with sympathy for the victim of an injustice. Even at age three or four, she will be developing a social conscience.

A child sitting at the dinner table can absorb any number of little moral lessons from the way his or her parents talk about what has happened in the world today—in their city, in their small social circle, or in their respective work environments. A child can pick up the parents' reactions to someone who has been dealt an injustice, to someone who has done a bad thing and is being punished for it, or to someone who is suffering because of another person's bad deed. When a parent answers a child's questions with patience, the child will come to see through the parents' eyes the drama of good and evil and the need for one person to help another. A child might, for example:

- o Hear his or her parents discussing how to help a friend of theirs who is in financial need
- o Hear about a person who stole money from someone else but was caught and will pay for that crime
- o Listen to his or her parents' creative ideas of ways to extend a helping hand to a friend of theirs who is ill
- o Learn about heroism in the description of a fireman's or policeman's rescue of someone

o Overhear the parents' plans to help a family in which there has been a death
o Learn how to take action personally when something sad happens to a friend

Learning how to take action is particularly important. Take the example of a young boy who has learned that his friend's puppy recently died.

"Bobby," his mother might say, "Jimmy must feel very sad that his puppy died yesterday."

"He feels awful bad."

"Well, let's do something about that, don't you think?"

"What do you mean?"

"Well, how about doing something to make Jimmy feel better?"

"Let's do that. But . . . how?"

"Well, maybe you could bring him a present to cheer him up."

"Yes, a present! What will you get him as a present?"

"I thought I'd let you figure that out, Bobby."

"I don't know."

"What would *you* like to receive if your puppy had just died?"

"Well, maybe I'd like a new car to race."

"Do you want to go with me to the store this afternoon to see if there's a little car you think Jimmy would like?"

"Yes, let's go, Mommy. I'll make Jimmy feel better. I'll get him a nice car to race around and around."

These are important lessons to be learned.

WHEN YOUR CHILD IS CURIOUS ABOUT A DISABLED PERSON HE OR SHE SEES IN PUBLIC

When a child encounters a person on crutches, an unusually small person, someone with an unusual feature that stands out, or perhaps someone who is all bandaged up, often he or she will stare and then ask you in a loud voice, "What's wrong with that man?" or say, "Look at that funny-looking woman's face." You should, of course, tell your child to be quiet, not to stare, and that you will explain about that "very nice man" (or woman) when you both get home. A child might become frightened by seeing someone who is "different" in any way, so if necessary calm him or her in a low voice. If you are close by the person your child has asked about, whisper an apology as you leave—something like, "I'm very sorry my child said what he did. He just doesn't understand, and I apologize for any discomfort his remarks have given you."

The Help That Religious Faith Can Give

In my opinion—and as a result of observing the behavior of people through many decades—if you believe in God, one of the greatest gifts you can give to your children is a religious faith. Even if you don't have a faith yourself or attend church or temple services regularly, get your children to a service once a week. You might try different churches until you (they) find one you (they) like. By getting them to a house of worship regularly, you may be giving them the strongest and most effective help and support they will ever have in their lives, and you will certainly be giving them the opportunity to learn about right and wrong.

Parents who read Bible stories every night to their children, explaining the moral lessons contained in those pages, instill a respect not only for God but for other human beings in the hearts of their children. A respect for God and for other human beings is, after all, the foundation of manners, morals, ethics, and values.

BASIC BEHAVIOR RULES YOUR CHILD OF TEN OR OLDER SHOULD KNOW

By the time a boy and girl reach the age of ten, they should be reasonably well-socialized human beings, with good manners. In other words, they should be aware of almost all of the important tenets of good manners, lacking only the adult polish and the behavior nuances still to come—hopefully, by the end of their high school years.

• *As your children grow, from preschool age and onward, ask your public librarian about books on children's manners that you can read with them.* More come into the marketplace every year, including comic books featuring beloved cartoon figures and fairytale characters. They make the learning of manners a game.

• *Help your child make his or her own game out of manners.* For example, you can devise a multiple choice answers quiz for your eight-year-old, like a friend of mine did. She and her daughter worked on their quiz together, and once it was put in good English, it was run off on a duplicating machine. The third grader had great fun giving the quiz to her classmates at school. Here are some of their twenty-five questions:

You spill spaghetti sauce on the tablecloth at your friend's house. You:
1. Wipe it up with your fingers and then clean your fingers on your dress.
2. Run out to the kitchen to get more sauce, because your friend's Mom wants you to enjoy your dinner.

3. Apologize to your friend's Mom, and then ask your friend's Mom if you may get some wet paper towels in the kitchen to do a better job of cleaning it up.

You receive duplicate presents from guests at your birthday party. You:
1. Give one back to the friend you like least and ask her to exchange it for something else.
2. Thank both friends and tell them you will really have fun with the gift, and that you will exchange the other one yourself for something you would also like, and you will then be able to thank them for two wonderful presents instead of just one.
3. Tell them you are going to take both back and get a much bigger, nicer present in exchange.

A boy hits you during recess. You:
1. Go up to him in the next recess and hit him back—only harder.
2. Tell him that you are going to forget it this time, because he obviously didn't mean to do what he did, but if he does it again, you will make him very sorry that he did.
3. Go screaming to the school principal to get him punished.

Correct answers: 3, 2, 2

The Basics

By the time your child has reached the age of ten, he or she should have established a pattern of behavior that reflects a developing sense of manners.

- *The child should understand deference* and therefore

  o Stand whenever an adult from the outside enters the room—even if it is just your friend from next door popping in to borrow something, and even if the child is doing his or her own thing (listening to music, talking to pals, watching TV, or reading). Whenever an adult comes into the room, the child should rise automatically and say something in greeting, even if it is as brief as, "Hello, Mrs. Smith." The child doesn't need to keep popping up and down everytime Mrs. Smith comes through the room on her visit. Once is enough.

    If a parent introduces someone the child has never met before, a handshake should go along with the child's greeting of "Hello."
  o Stand by his or her chair at the dining table (or in the restaurant) until all adults are seated.
  o Pass the food first to the guests and his or her parents before

helping him- or herself; wait to begin eating until an adult has begun to do so.

o Defer to adults in conversation (which means simply that the child doesn't interrupt conversation in progress but waits until there is a pause to say what he or she wants to say).

• The child should be kind to and protective of younger brothers and sisters.

• He or she should have good table manners (see chapter 9, "The Right Thing to Do at Every Meal").

• He or she should know how to talk to an adult and help act as a parent's co-host.

For example, when the daughter of the household meets a visitor who has come to see her father in the hallway of her house, she would shake his hand and say with a smile, "Hello, Mr. Gray. I'm Amalia, nice to see you again. Here, I'll put your coat in the closet."

"Thank you, Amalia, nice to see *you* again."

"My father will be down right away. Would you like to sit down in the living room?" She then shows him into the living room and turns on some more lights in the room to make it more cheerful.

With this Amalia has done her duty and made the guest comfortable, so she may now leave, unless she wishes to stay and chat until her father arrives for his meeting with Mr. Gray.

• The child should realize that in public places it is rude to make a lot of noise with friends that upsets other people (on public transportation, at the beach, in a movie, on the street, or wherever).

• He or she should refrain from yelling at others in the house. (Hopefully, the parents don't yell, either!)

• He or she should show respect for elders at all times. That means no sassing, acting fresh, or defying authority. (Respect for parents, grandparents, teachers, the pastor, policemen, and anyone else *in a position of authority* should be instinctive.)

• He or she should answer when spoken to and not just maintain a sullen silence.

• The well-mannered child doesn't interrupt anyone else who is speaking.

• He or she respects the family home—and those of friends, too—which means not tracking in mud onto the floors, not putting feet up on a table or on the arms of the sofa, not eating on the floor and getting food on the carpet (particularly hard-to-clean items like popcorn, pizza, soda, and melted ice cream bars).

• The child should follow the house rules as to when and how the telephone is used and be able to take careful telephone messages for everyone else in the house.

• Children should keep their own rooms straightened on a routine basis by the age of ten.

- They should have good bathroom manners, including not staying in the bathroom so long that others don't have their allotted time. They should routinely pick up after themselves so that the bathroom remains tidy.

- A child should do any assigned household chores cheerfully, punctually, and efficiently—without wearing a long face.

- The child plays music at a low decibel rate so as to allow others in the house to go about their tasks in relative peace.

- He or she is mindful of the privacy of everyone else in the house, including that of siblings.

- He or she refrains from upsetting others with a loud cracking of chewing gum or an explosion of bubble gum.

- Well-mannered children do not push in ahead of anyone. They wait their proper turn in line and wait their turn to go through a door, into an elevator, or onto an escalator or bus. They do not jostle others while walking down a crowded passageway.

- They always say "Thank you" after anyone steps back to allow them through or holds a door for them.

- The well-mannered child is a good host and does what his or her guest wants to do, not what he or she wants to do. He or she does not desert a guest to go off to follow a personal agenda but offers a guest what the guest would like to eat, and lets the guest select the TV programs.

- He or she says "Excuse me" when inadvertently brushing against anyone or when hurrying by and obliging someone to make way for him.

- The well-mannered child has been taught to write a thank-you note for every gift (including any from grandparents, aunts, uncles, or friends of any age) or after every meal at a friend's house or as a friend's guest in a restaurant.

- He or she is punctual and doesn't hold up the family when they are going somewhere.

- He or she is respectful of the driver of a car and does not bother that person, knowing that is dangerous.

- The child is respectful of any laws governing the environment— discards litter properly and is careful of trees, lawns, flowers, and bushes when playing.

- He or she has learned—and scrupulously follows—the rules of safety (and good manners), whether crossing the street (at the light), rowing a boat on the lake (and observing the safety rules in the water), riding a bike (and following traffic rules), ice-skating (and being careful not to run into people), and the like.

- The well-mannered child is kind to animals and never mistreats them.

Teenagers Need a Few More Rules

Above and beyond the general rules that all children from ages ten to twenty should know, there are a few special ones that particularly apply for teenagers.

Even if their friends have no rules, your teenage children should be mindful of the following:

- o *Their noise level in the house* (from the radio, tapes, VCR, TV, or even a musical instrument they're learning to play—drums, for example).
- o *Their handling of your or their own car.* They should be clear about the unacceptability of using up your gas and not informing you, borrowing your car without your permission, eating with friends in your car without a thorough cleanup of the resulting mess, blocking the driveway with their own car, and the like.
- o *Not picking up after their parties in your house.* Make it clear you object to their leaving the sink full of dishes, the ashtrays full of broken potato chips, illegally consumed empty beer cans stashed beneath your slipcovered sofa and easy chairs, and the like.
- o *Drinking up all the cold sodas in the fridge and not replacing them with fresh bottles.* Leaving half-drunk cans of soda around is almost as irritating.
- o *Getting telephone calls from their friends late at night,* and tying up the house telephone all the time.
- o *Strewing athletic equipment and clothes all over the house*— such as a smelly basketball sneaker in the entrance foyer, a jockstrap on the radiator, a pair of running shorts draped on the back of the sofa, a sweaty sweatshirt and pair of athletic socks drying out over the big lampshade. The young, future Olympic contenders of America often make their home resemble a run-down gymnasium!
- o *Their behavior regarding drugs and alcohol.* Not only should they know that they may not use them, but that their friends may not use them in your house.

But with all of that, America's teenagers are still the sweetest kids in the world!

A Few Dating Manners

Whether it's a boy asking a girl for a date or vice versa, rejection is always feared, and when it comes, it's always worse than one ever imagined it could be!

- *When a boy asks a girl on a date:*

o He should ask her far enough ahead, so that she has time to prepare, and so that she doesn't think she was the fifth and last person he called.

o He should square with her as to all the details—where they are going, what they are going to do, who is going to do it with them. This gives her the chance to coordinate her wardrobe with any other girl who will be along (very important for a female's sense of security).

o He should be punctual. Every minute he is late is stressful for her. As the minutes tick by, she probably is wondering if she is being stood up.

o Upon returning her home he should see her to her door, not leave her fumbling for her key outside her house. It is no longer just good manners to see her safely inside, it is a question of security.

- *When a girl asks a boy,* unless she is a beauty, she often has to sell him on the idea of going out with her far more aggressively than he would have to sell her if he were doing the asking. Unless he's a total disaster, a boy can say, "Wanna do somethin' Saturday night?" and chances are the girl will quickly say yes. This unfair situation is just one of the sad facts of life in a society that still clings to the outdated notion of gallantry—that a man is always supposed to ask a woman for a date (even if it doesn't work that way).

A girl can successfully ask a boy for a date if she takes these steps in preparation. (The same suggestions will help a boy asking a girl for a date.)

o She gives him plenty of lead time, so he knows he isn't a last-minute substitute for someone else.

o She gets (or arranges to purchase) tickets to a really marvelous event in keeping with the boy's interests, whether it's a game, movie, concert, or to be in the audience for the "David Letterman Show."

o She extends the invitation by writing everything in a note, showing how well organized she is—including that she is providing transportation and paying for the tickets, dinner, and parking. If she were to invite him face to face, her nerves might get the better of her—she could botch the job of selling this beautifully planned evening. If she were to invite him to his face, she might also scare him into a quick regret to her invitation. A note gives a shy young man time to savor the proposal for all its plus attributes.

The girl should keep the date quiet in advance and not go talking all over about it so that they are both teased by their friends before the date even takes place. She should be prepared to let the boy appear to be paying for everything in front of his friends, if that's the only way he can feel comfortable about her contributing.

- *Out on the date, both should remember*

  o To be appropriately and nicely dressed for each other. It's unfair if a boy looks as though he's just finished a work shift in a mine or if the girl looks as though she just finished cleaning house when they meet for their date. Young people should make an effort to look clean and in fashion on a date—whether it's a dressy occasion or an informal get-together with just a bunch of friends. The theory is that the bigger the effort you make for a date, the more fun it will turn out to be (an old wives' tale that is mostly true!).

  o To have it completely understood by both who pays for what on the date, so that there are no embarrassing moments. They should be prepared to offer to help each other out with money if things cost more than the person who asked for the date figured. They can agree to "go dutch," if that is the best way to handle financial matters.

  o To let their respective parents know where they will be, and to follow the rules of the more stringent of the two sets of parents on the time the date is to end.

  o To give one another proper attention during the date and not flirt with other people present.

  o To be agreeable to the plans made, whatever they may be, and not to try to change everything around—and particularly not to complain and whine in disapproval as the date continues.

  o Never to speak pejoratively of the other—before, during, or after the date. The boy who moans to his friends, "I'm stuck with a real dog as a date tomorrow night," and the girl who describes her date to her friends as "a complete nerd—it shows you how desperate I must be to get out the door," do not sound cool to their friends; they sound mean and untrustworthy.

  o To thank the other person at the end of the date, even to write a thank-you note within the week to the date—or the date's parents if a meal or a weekend visit at their home was involved.

Making the Rules Easier to Take

- *When you give children the rules of citizenship for your household, make sure they adhere to them, but also that they understand the reason and logic behind them.* ("Johnny, one of your chores is to rinse the dishes, load the dishwasher, and clean up. You didn't do it—again. Each one of us has his or her own chores. Would you prefer to do your own job, or to have me have do it and thus miss preparing the next meal before I leave for my job? I think you might be very hungry if that happened.")

• *Instead of ordering them to act in a certain way, give them the humanity behind the rules of good manners toward others.* ("Jane, the reason I ask you to stand up when Mrs. Johnson comes into our house is because she is an older friend of mine, and she deserves a mark of respect from a young person. Some day, you'll be her age and you will be very pleased when a young person gets up to shake your hand and gives you a cheery 'Hello' when you enter her house.")

• *Criticize their friends only in private, and only fairly.* ("I know he's a good friend of yours, but I'm telling this to you without the others hearing me. He is disrespectful of this house. He puts his dirty boots up on the coffee table and mars the wood, he leaves his coat lying on the floor instead of hanging it up, and he uses bad language all the time. I think you ought to tell him quietly that he should respect this house— and us—more than he does when he comes here.")

• *Listen to your child when he or she feels passionate about something.* Check to see if you have laid down unfair rules in comparison to all the other parents whom you admire. ("I hate to bother you, Sue, but I'm just trying to find out if Jim and I are being unfair with Jim, Jr. We have always ordered him home on Saturday nights by eleven P.M., and he claims all the other kids don't have to be in until one A.M. What's the rule in your household, and do you know what it is in other classmates' families?")

• *Don't, however, go against your basic religious and philosophical convictions, just to please your children.* ("I don't care if the other kids are allowed to miss church this Sunday to go to the circus. In this family we go to church every Sunday. It's one of the things that makes us strong. We thank God for our blessings, and we don't abandon something so important just because something else conflicts that would be a lot more fun.")

• *Don't remove their last particle of self-esteem if your children fail at something.* Instead, fire them up with self-confidence to be able to face the next challenge. ("Hey, everyone has to lose at times. Not making the team does not mean you're a failure. You're a wonderful child, and you'll have other opportunities. You'll do better the next time. You're no less a person in this family's eyes, so buck up and forget it.")

• *Give them the opportunity to be present at dinner with your adult friends;* teach them to benefit from and to look forward to these experiences. ("Mr. and Mrs. Wellington are joining us for dinner tonight. He was a great tight end in his college football days and is now a lawyer who does a lot of volunteer work for our community. He's an inspiration. And his wife is very nice—she works in retailing and can tell you all about the fashion world. You're lucky to be able to listen to two such interesting people.")

• *Make it possible for them to spend as much time as possible with their grandparents on both sides, whether you are married or divorced.* Grandparents provide an important cross-generational influence, and a child's bonding with his or her grandparents will be one of the greatest affirmative influences on his or her life. Even if your feelings toward your ex-mate are bitter, never take it out on your ex-in-laws. Instead, keep them close to your children.

• *When a child has an important role* (playing in a piano concert, appearing in a class play, playing with the team in an important game), *be there.* No matter how important the business deal, you can take enough time off at least to appear, even if you have to leave early. No matter how demanding your employer is, you can always explain and work double compensatory time to repay your employer for your absences on these occasions. If you positively cannot attend an important occasion relating to your child, ask a favorite relative or friend of yours to stand in for you and make a full report afterward. (That is better than being a complete no-show.)

• *Make a game out of anything from a family physical fitness project to an intellectual exercise,* such as reading the daily newspaper thoroughly and then answering an informal quiz on its contents. When the family does things together, when conviviality and affection set the mood, children learn and grow in emotional stability. They receive love, and they learn how to give it back to others. Some day they will raise their own children in the same fashion.

• *Ask them at the end of each day how their day went,* so you can detect anything from a little problem to a real hurt. "All right, now it's Billy's turn. What happened today?" When Billy voices something that was "just terrible" that happened, his parents and siblings can all contribute advice on how to handle it. As his parents, you can remind him again of the best of those problem-solving ideas when he says good-night.

• *Describe your own day, too, to your children* in the evening hour. They should understand what you do, be able to describe it accurately to others, and feel proud of you. It helps them to know grown-ups have problems, too, which they also have to work to solve. ("I had a really bad day. The monthly figures came in, down again, and the boss told me to let three more people go in our department—at once. I had to tell them there were no more jobs for them, and it hurt. But, in answer to your question of what else I did, I sat them down and began calling other companies that might be able to use them. I wrote them enthusiastic letters of reference. I told them this job change might be a great opportunity for them. I'm spending this whole week helping them clear their desks, go through the Help Wanted ads, and write good résumés. I'm doing everything I can to help them.") Children feel more secure when they hear their parents talk about helping out other people; it teaches them to be unselfish and helpful to others.

• *When you buy young children clothing, they have no choice but to wear it.* When they develop a sense of fashion, which can occur even in grade school, allow them as much freedom as possible in making their own selections. From junior high school on, students want to be dressed according to the latest trends in their school, to which parents a generation away can't possibly be attuned. Within the limits of budget and propriety, let your children select what they want to wear.

YOUR ROLE IN YOUR CHILDREN'S RELATIONSHIPS

With Siblings

The forging of a closeness among brothers and sisters as they grow up is one of the greatest assets you can help them bank for their future happiness. Rivalry among siblings usually lessens by the time they go to college, but it is how the parents teach respect for each other in the early years that really helps solidify the sibling bonds that are so important in adult life. For example, when your children are small, it's the time to teach them:

- o A respect for the other person's possessions. ("You leave my things alone and I won't touch yours.")
- o A polite way of borrowing. (The child asks nicely and returns the item when it was promised and in perfect condition.)
- o A respect for his or her sibling's friends, whether referring to that friend in conversation or welcoming that friend to the family home.
- o The importance of acting as a support system for each other—to stand up for each other, to rise to the defense if one of them is maligned at school, and to be loyal to one another inside and outside the home.

THE SIBLING WITH A PHYSICAL OR MENTAL HANDICAP

It is truly inspirational to observe large families in which there is a handicapped child who is consequently the most loved and the most loving member of the family. Such a fortunate child will be watched over by his or her siblings all through life—long after the parents have died.

A child who is special deserves to be supported constantly within the family, but sometimes that child is teased or resented by siblings because he or she embarrasses them. This is yet another tough problem for the parents. There comes a time when they must help a sibling understand the responsibility toward the special child in the family.

Explain that although the brother or sister takes more of the parents' time, that does not mean that the others are loved any less. Resolve to make it up to the other children in other ways.

When there is only one sibling of a special child, parents naturally worry about what will happen to the child after their death. The parents should instill in their son or daughter that "you have been given an extra measure of strength and goodness, to enable you to take care of your brother (or sister) after we have gone."

With Adults

What do your children call your friends or the adult members of your family?

• Traditionally, children address adult family members with a name or title indicative of their position in the family.

o Parents are called "Mommy" or "Daddy," "Mama" or "Papa"— "Mom" or "Dad" when the children are older—or other nicknames derived from those names.

o Grandparents are called "Grandpa" and "Grandma," "Grandfather" and "Grandmother," or any number of nicknames, like "Gammy," "Gamma," "Gampops," "Grandaddy." When there are two sets of grandparents around, it sometimes confuses small children. One solution is for the children to use the grandparent title with the grandparent's given name, such as "Gamma Joan," "Grandpa George," "Grandma Cynthia," and "Grandpa Jim."

o Relatives are called by their title and given names: "Aunt Ginny," "Uncle Charlie," and so forth.

• Untraditionally, some people insist that their children call all their friends by their first names. I find this awkward, and it must be very difficult for a child to call his parents' friends by their first names and all other adults (such as teachers, the doctor, the minister, and the dance instructor) by their last names.

Some parents go to the extent of having their young children call them by their first names—all in the desire to show independence, perhaps hoping to be perceived as nonconformists. It is a free country. Parents can teach their children whatever they wish, but I believe that by encouraging nonconformist usage, the parents may be making it just that much more difficult for their children to learn deference and respect for older people.

• Your college-age children, if they are mature young people, might be urged by friends who feel they are young enough to be your children's peers to stop calling them "Mr. Brown" and "Mrs. Wentworth." If your friends specifically ask the children to address them by their first names, tell your children to do so—if they feel comfortable. It's always uncomfortable at first, but with time it becomes more automatic. However, if they feel it is improper at the age of twenty suddenly to address someone who is fifty by a first name, they should not be forced to.

• By the time children reach college age, if they are close to their aunts and uncles—and by mutual consent—they often drop the "Aunt" and "Uncle" and just use older adults' given names. It is a compliment to the aunt and uncle when it happens.

PARENTS SPEAK TO THEIR CHILDREN ABOUT SEX

A Mother Speaks to Her Daughter

Mothers and young daughters should have a special, private, and trusting relationship when it comes to matters of learning about sex. In this era of sexually transmitted diseases, learning how to say no to a boy who wants sex is one of the most important things a mother can teach her daughter. First, a mother should explain *why "no" has to be said*— whether the mother's reasons are based on morality and religious conviction or on concern for her daughter's health and safety. Second, there is a well-mannered way of saying no to a man—without making him feel he repulses the woman, making him think she is cold and frigid, or making him feel badly rejected for even having made the suggestion. (If he tries to use force, of course, there is no reason to be nice or to think of his feelings; the only importance in this situation is to escape or to get help—and fast.)

This advice is offered to help a mother put into words the caution that is so necessary today in approaching the concept of sex among young people. The advice is obvious, but the obvious is often difficult for a mother to articulate to a young daughter.

I think that a mother today should bring back a caution that meant a lot to the women of my day and before me: the question of a young woman's reputation. After 1965, concern for one's reputation went out of style, and moral standards came to be regarded as archaic and irrelevant. However, the more the words "ethics" and "morality" float through the air today, the more caution will be practiced in sexual activity. The danger of AIDS and other sexually transmitted diseases has lessened the pressure on everyone to be held in their peers' esteem as sexual athletes. There are strong reasons for *not* engaging in sex these days; the logical result is that the word "reputation" will once again become something of importance to a young woman. Young women of the seventies used to brag about being "available." Young women of the nineties are very possibly going to brag about being "unavailable."

A mother talking to her young daughter might explain, after pointing out the reasons why a girl should say no to sex, that a turn-down should be made in a pleasant way, not an abrupt or even mean way. For example:

"If a man makes a move on you, don't react with great disdain— 'What? Sex with *you?* You must be kidding!'—which guarantees that you will never see that man again. Remember, men who have been turned down in a nice way often become great friends and beaux—and have even turned into great husband material at a later date. Therefore, say no firmly, but couch the rejection with some kind words—for example, 'I'm sorry, I can't do that. I'm not ready for that kind of relationship, even if you're a really nice person.' Or, 'We know each other so little. I would like to continue seeing you very much, but you will have to understand that I'm not ready to sleep with you.' "

The mother might continue, "If he says, 'But why?'—which he might say very persistently—be prepared with your answers. Don't be afraid to come out with any of these reasons:

" 'Because I have strong moral and religious feelings about this subject. You can laugh all you want, but I am saving myself for the man I marry.' (Most young men are stopped cold with that one. It's an old-fashioned argument that a modern macho type has difficulty handling.)

" 'Because of AIDS, herpes—all of that. And don't give me that condom jazz either, because I happen to know there are a lot of mistakes made, even with condoms. I don't know you well enough. Therefore, I am not ready for a sexual relationship at this point in our friendship.'

"Flattery helps soothe a rejected soul. For example, you might sugar-coat your rejection with something like this:

" 'I have a *really* good time with you, and I think you're a terrific guy. If you can't have an equally good time with me without the sex, then I guess we had better not see each other again. I guess the real truth is that I like to be with you more than you like to be with me.'

"His response will be—inevitably—'Then show how much you like me.' Your next move is to repeat what you said before, that you are not going to have sex with him, that you are not ready, and that the two of you had better not see each other again."

The majority of today's young men respect a young woman of moral integrity—call it virtue, or self-control and self-discipline—call it anything you want. A man who has been rejected in his quest for sex, if he has character and if he is really attracted to the woman, will keep coming back. And a long period of getting to know each other and having fun together, without the pressures of sleeping together, might logically lead to love, marriage, and all the sex that goes with it.

I have put this discussion of a mother's advice to her daughter in my own words. Hopefully, it can be put into others' own words. Once again, it is time for mothers and daughters to talk to each other about sex; in past generations they almost always did before a girl married.

A Father Speaks to His Son

Much that I have said in the preceding section of advice from a mother to her daughter holds true also for a father speaking to his son.

Values are not something that are popped like bubble gum into a teenager's mouth. The groundwork for a set of values is laid in childhood. If a boy grows up hearing his father constantly "talk macho," jokingly referring to girls as "broads," sharing laughs with his son as to which woman on TV has the sexiest body, and in general making a joke out of sexual stereotypes of women, there is no way that his boy, upon entering his teens, will understand the meaning of respect for women. There is no way under those circumstances that a father will be able to advise his son on self-control and good manners when he is on a date.

A father first teaches his son to respect women by respecting his own wife, and by referring to women in general in dignified terms in the presence of his children. It is his example that instills in his son the attitude that women are to be treated as equal human beings—emotional and intellectual partners—and not as objects created for his pleasure.

In the matter of sex, a father is wise to help his son understand his own sexual appetite and how important self-control is in his relationships with girls. Hopefully, they have discussed just how you get sexually transmitted diseases, and if the father believes in his son's using condoms, he has carefully explained when and how to use them.

GUARDING YOUR CHILD AGAINST THE PERILS OF DRUGS AND ALCOHOL

There Is No "Socially Acceptable" Use of Drugs

"Socially acceptable drugs" has to be one of the most ironic phrases ever coined in modern-day use. *There really is no socially acceptable nonmedicinal drug.* All are abused for the most part, even though people may start out using small amounts. Every second or third glass of liquor or beer begins to be dangerous, not socially acceptable. Every puff of a marijuana cigarette is against the law and potentially harmful—it's like lighting matches in a dry forest. It's a quick step up from a drag on a marijuana cigarette to speed, crack, cocaine, heroin, PCP, opium—through the entire spectrum of mind-altering drugs.

• *Attack the subject of drug use as early in a child's development as you can make him or her understand it.* Teach your son and daughter to like and respect their minds, so they won't feel the need for altering them, and to love and respect their bodies, so they won't willfully harm them. Five-year-olds watching violence on television that is associated with drugs quickly come to know the lingo. They don't really understand drug use, but they know it's there and that it's dark and dangerous. Often they find it fascinating—another glamorous vestige of being grown-up, in the same category as getting a driver's license to be able to have wheels and hang out with one's friends.

Make drug-taking *un*fascinating to your small children. Make it *un*glamorous. Please don't claim your child of five never sees "bad" things on television. This may be true in a few rare cases, but most children, even if TV is regulated in their own homes, find it is not regulated in their friends' homes. And show me a five-year-old with older brothers and sisters who docsn't watch violence on television right along with them—and I'll show you an unusual (but amazingly caring and wonderful) family.

When you see people selling drugs on the street, point them out to your child. Let the child see the seediness of that scene. Point out people reeling around high on drugs, which you can see in any large city of the world. Maybe the pathetic and sordid effects of drug and alcohol abuse will sink in. Do not protect your child by keeping him or her ignorant on this subject. Educate your child forthrightly when you see the horror of it around you.

• *The most important weapon of all in teaching a child to refuse drugs is the example set by you, the parents!* You cannot teach a child to renounce addictive drugs (including alcohol and tobacco) if you, a parent, indulge in them. You cannot say to a child, "Do as I say, not as I do."

• *Comment on the day's news about drug dealers being appre-hended.* When children eat their meals, their ears are usually innocently wide open, even if you don't think they are paying any attention to what you're saying about the news in today's papers or on the evening telecast. As adults talk to each other, the children usually take it all in, particularly if the subject is something as dangerous as drugs, which their parents always seem to discuss in alarmed tones. Children can detect the importance of the subject in their parents' tone of voice and emphatic way of speaking. Let them eavesdrop on your discussion of this subject. Speak in simple terms that they can understand.

When you mention "the bad, terrible men and women who sell those drugs," and how drugs ruin people's lives, and how people must be punished for selling, buying, *or* using the stuff, a child begins to look at the subject as a real-life example of evil and the need to punish those forces of evil. A child may or may not question you further at the dinner table after you switch to another subject. But then again, he or she might open up and tell you something you had no idea of—about drug-selling going on close to or in school, for example.

● *Every so often reinforce in the mind even of a kindergarten child the evil connotation of drugs*—that they are like a wicked witch or a bad dragon. Don't do an overkill, just give them a gentle reminder that *they have the power to refuse taking something that will always hurt them in the end.* (If your teenager is in fast company, it isn't a bad idea to arrange with the school and a state prison or city jail for a class tour of the facilities. It's a very sobering experience!)

One night a friend of mine, a young father, wrote in his journal, word for word as well as he could remember it, the conversation he had just had with his six-year-old son while the latter was getting ready for bed. He later showed it to me.

His son told him something that had greatly impressed him and their class—that two fourteen-year-olds in the upper school had been arrested on the school grounds at noon that day for selling drugs to other students. The father said he hoped his little boy would never touch the stuff.

Billie, the son, asked him, "What do drugs taste like? Yummy, like candy or soda?"

"No, sometimes they don't taste at all. People swallow them by mouth or take them by sticking a needle into a vein in their arm." The little boy grabbed his arm as if in pain at this thought. "Or they smoke drugs like in a pipe or a cigarette."

"Sounds dumb. And it hurts. Why?" asked Billie.

"Because it makes them feel good for a very little while."

"Well, what's bad about that?"

"Because then later they feel awful, and they get weak and sick and can't play games or do their homework."

"It's easy. The bad will go away when they just stop."

"No, they can't stop."

"Why can't they?"

"Because when they keep doing it, they can't stop. They're trapped, like an animal caught in a forest trap. They just keep taking it and wanting more and taking it—and poisoning themselves more each time."

"Sounds stupid. Just how bad do the drugs make them feel after a while, Daddy?" The little boy continued to pepper his father with questions, obsessed with the desire to know about how bad drugs make you feel and, if they did that, why people took them.

"Well," his father said, "remember when you had that really bad sore throat last month?" The little boy nodded his head affirmatively. "And how you felt when you had that last bad cold at Christmas and were all stuffed up, feverish, and hot?"

Billie nodded yes again.

"And how you felt when you had your appendix out?"

Billie said, "Yeah. It really hurt."

"Well, that's how people who take illegal drugs eventually feel. The medicine the doctor tells you to take when you're sick doesn't make you feel bad. That kind of drug makes you feel well. We're talking about *illegal drugs*—bad stuff, the kind those boys were selling near your school."

"I'll never do that!" Billie said very firmly.

"I hope you don't, son."

Billie received an excellent lesson that night. Three years later, I asked his father if Billie had ever again mentioned the "Don't take drugs" lesson his father once taught him. "Yes," Bill, Sr., smiled. "It took, like a vaccination. He brought home his class paper from school last week, with an 'A' on it. His paper was titled 'Drugs Are Bad. Don't Take Them.' "

Drugs and the Vulnerable Teenager

When your child enters the teens, the lure of drugs, alcohol, and tobacco is much more intense, particularly when the cool kids in school are experimenting with these dangerous substances. Now is the time to watch your child's friends, to help him or her entertain often in your home rather than in someone else's, where you don't know the parents or even know if they are home. (It is also imperative that your child does not go to someone's home where parents are present but are doing drugs or drinking to excess.)

One way to keep children off drugs is to know what they are doing in their free time, where and with whom they are spending free time. If you urge your children to hold their parties in your house and get college students to serve as paid chaperones, then you, the parents, can be out of the house, but the children will be under the watchful eyes of those "really grown-up college guys" (of either sex).

It's the parents who don't care, who are too busy with their own lives and don't know what's going on in their children's lives, who let these young people slip away from them. It's a selfish, unthinking parent who won't go to the effort of helping a child have friends over rather than forcing him or her to seek entertainment elsewhere, and possibly under dangerous circumstances.

When you hold a newborn in your arms, you promise to do everything in the world for that child, to love and protect him or her forever. I guess it's a promise we all make, but it's more important to keep it than to make it. And the teen years are when it's particularly important to be alert to your child's development.

The Kinds of Drugs Around Us

If a child is curious about drugs, be ready to answer the questions as to what they are and what they are called.

• *Alcohol and tobacco,* the gateway drugs, can become addictive and introduce a person to the drug culture.

• *Inhalants* can be poisonous and dangerous, and young children often fall prey to them. Inhaling anything from hairspray and gasoline to airplane glue can give a person—particularly a child—a dizzy kind of high. One of the most popular inhalants is butyl nitrite, which causes blood vessels to expand and can have serious consequences.

• *Marijuana and hashish.* Smoking the chopped-up leaves or the dark brown resin from the tops of the *Cannabis sativa* plant may give the smokers pleasure, but it also impairs their performance in anything from driving a car to working on a machine. The smoker may suffer disorientation, but most important of all, it's an easy jump from marijuana or hashish up to another illegal, more powerfully addictive drug.

• *Depressants* (or "downers") are drugs that calm the central nervous system. People take these when they're feeling hyper, nervous, or too agitated. The sedative Quaalude (the brand name for methaqualone), also known as "ludes" or "sopors," is one of the very hazardous drugs young people are attracted to because of its reputation for enhancing sexual experience. It is also sold in counterfeit tablets containing other substances that can produce unexpected, dangerous reactions.

• *Stimulants* do the opposite of what a depressant does to you. They wake you up, fight drowsiness. The most popular stimulant is caffeine (found in coffee, tea, and cola). Taken often and for a long time, they become addictive. Amphetamines (speed), methamphetamines, crack, and cocaine (coke) are in this category. The drug world has its own terminology for the terrible pursuit of pleasure through stimulants. "Chasing the dragon," for example, is smoking cocaine and heroin at the same time.

• *Narcotics*—the painkillers in medicine that are derived from opium or made synthetically, such as codeine, morphine, and Demerol, are all narcotics—are very addictive. The illegal drug heroin is in this category, too.

• *Hallucinogens.* These are called perceptual drugs because a person who takes them changes his or her perception of the reality of the world around him. PCP ("angel dust") and LSD are the best known. (PCP is very dangerous and can cause temporary psychosis.) There are also natural hallucinogens growing in nature—for example, the psyloci-bin ("magic mushrooms") of Mexico and mescaline.

Teaching Your Young Child About Alcohol

In some schools in this country, sixth-graders now have access to alcohol. It's no longer a worry to face when the kids are in high school. It's a worry to face in grade school! It's a very big worry by the time a child is in the eighth grade in many parts of the country.

When you first smell alcohol on your child's breath—or when he or she first tells you about classmates' drinking in school (which seems to be done in lower and lower grades every decade)—it's time to teach him or her about the dangers and addictiveness of alcohol. (If you have a drink in your hand when you wish to start this little talk, forget it. In that case, let someone else teach your child about alcohol.)

If you smell alcohol on your young child three or four times, don't just punish him. Go to work on him or her quickly, as a family unit (almost as though you were doing a family confrontation with a con-firmed adult alcoholic to force that person into treatment). You want to save this child from becoming an alcoholic. The danger signals are flashing all over the place. Talk to your family doctor. Get older brothers and sisters and favorite aunts and uncles to sit down in a group to explain to the child the seriousness of his or her actions and the almost certain outcome of the child's becoming an alcoholic if he or she continues. Talk to Alcoholics Anonymous and find out about its excellent children's programs. Talk to the local alcoholic rehabilitation clinic in your town in order to collect some ammunition and advice. In other words, get ready to scare the pants off the child in your family who is drinking.

He or she probably regards drinking as macho or sophisticated, glamorous, bigtime movie hero stuff. Dispel those notions, even if in the great old movies chic heroes are always drinking and smoking.

Teenage Drinking

If your child is in high school and tells you there is lots of drinking among classmates:

• Tell your child that if he or she just has to try a drink or a special cocktail, you will let him or her try it home *with you.*

• Show your child how drinkers, all of whom started out taking just an occasional drink but then became hooked on alcohol, ruin their bodies, get bloated and red in the face, become nutritionally starved, have liver problems, and seriously damage their hearts. Most serious of all, alcohol abuse results in brain damage, and you have only to point out a homeless alcoholic lying in the street in any large city to make that point to your child. Alcohol is debilitating to the system, yes, but it also damages a young person's looks and, ultimately, his or her ability to stay alive.

• Agree with your child that, yes, a drink might make a shy young person less shy and more at ease at a party, but it's a temporary, phony kind of comfort. The life of the party, high on alcohol, very quickly becomes the bore of the party. The only real party high is one you make yourself, with your own wonderful contribution to the group—giving of yourself and making an effort to make others feel good.

• Impress upon your child that even mild social drinking will dull one's reflexes. Tell your child about the thousands of fatal automobile accidents every year in which merely social drinking is involved. Make him or her understand the devastating penalties underaged youths pay who are involved in an accident and found to be drinking.

• Your child can't really know how quickly alcohol will take effect in his or her system. It hits some people faster than others. The effect depends upon a person's weight—and on other factors, such as heredity and how much food a person has eaten recently. Don't let your child get away with bragging about being able to drink anyone under the table, about having an amazing capacity for alcohol—no one does.

• If your son's or daughter's peers are all drinking in college and you know he or she will, too, warn him or her to sip a drink slowly and to eat as often as possible along with it to provide a kind of blotter for the alcohol.

• If your young daughter is a drinker, share an occasional article with her on what alcohol does to babies carried in the womb. The evidence is compelling, and it is enough to stop many young women from ever taking a drink.

Where to Get Help

The National Clearing House for Alcohol and Drug Information publishes a free "National Directory of Drug Abuse and Alcoholism Treatment and Prevention Programs," which lists alphabetically all of the many resources by state and then by city. In order to obtain a copy of this directory, write to:

National Clearing House for Alcohol and Drug Information
P.O. Box 2345
Rockville, MD 20852

In all middle-size to large cities, ask Directory Assistance for the telephone number of the local chapter of these national support groups:

o Narcotics Anonymous
o Alcoholics Anonymous

The local chapter will refer you to the local:

o Adult Children of Alcoholics (ACA)
o Alateen (Children of Alcoholics)
o Alanon (Spouses of Alcoholics)

You may also call the National Institute on Drug Abuse (NIDA) hotline to ask for the names of free drug treatment centers in your area: 1-800-662-HELP. Call this hotline weekdays between nine A.M. and three A.M.; on weekends call between noon and three A.M.

WHEN YOUR CHILDREN BECOME ADULTS: KEEPING YOUR FAMILY TOGETHER

• Arrange family reunions as often as possible. Check ahead with the children on all their schedules, so that no one is left out.

• Urge your offspring to support a sibling's choice of mate; have everyone contribute to a warm welcoming of the new member of the family.

• Help them all keep in touch with one another. (One of my favorite mothers has always paid for all the long distance telephone calls her five adult children make to each other. She claims that although the reimbursements are extensive, she has never enjoyed paying for anything so much.)

• When someone needs help, subtly suggest to the other siblings the ways in which they can help—whether it's to buck up a failing marriage or to lend a little money to someone who has a sudden financial need. Encourage them to act as surrogate parents for their brothers and sisters in times of family distress (for example, standing in for the bride's mother or father if one's sister or brother is seriously ill at the time of a daughter's wedding).

• Keep them all aware of their various successes, too, even if it means sending a regular family newsletter to the younger generation, bearing only happy news of each sibling and his or her family.

* * *

Keeping a family together is a job. There isn't a more important one in this world. The more a child is helped to grow up by siblings, parents, grandparents, and other adults, the more likely he or she is to do the very same thing as an adult with the generations to come. Once you're a parent, you remain one, even when your children are in their forties. And since you were once a child, there's always a little of that in you, too.

That's what families are all about.

Everyday Manners
Out in the World

A person who is loved and popular—a person with naturally good relationships—does not turn his or her behavior on and off like a spigot, according to the person he or she is with at any given time. The person who has a smile and a good word for a member of the family also has it for the postman passing by, the man in the city garage who brings his or her car up from the lower levels, the receptionist in the executive's office where he or she has an appointment, and the person in the newspaper stand who sells him or her the morning paper.

Our relationships with *everyone* are important. I remember asking a question of a simply wonderful woman who was greatly loved by every single person who came to know her: "Don't you get tired being nice to *everyone?*"

Her answer: "It's much more exhausting going back and forth—being nice to some people and not nice to others." In thinking over her words, I had to agree. It is a lot easier, for example, to thank a salesperson for her help and not complain about her inefficiency than it is to pick a fight with her and not carry the resulting bad feelings into a next encounter. It's a negative reason for being nice perhaps, but, come to think of it, any reason for being nice has value in this world of ours!

With good manners, attitude is as important as the act. You might give the world's biggest tip but do it in a way that insults the person who earned it; on the other hand, you might make the slightest of thoughtful gestures that means *so much* to the recipient. The ultimate success of anything you do depends on how nicely you do it.

3

Making Friends in a Busy World

I will never forget my first celebrity interview experience—at age twelve. I had arranged to interview the late actor Henry Fonda at the Omaha Playhouse for my school newspaper. He had grown up in Omaha and knew my parents, so he agreed to let me speak with him for *exactly* two minutes. Racking my brain for a single *big* question, I came up with one that was enough to make any intelligent celebrity feel a bit queasy: "What is the key to happiness?"

The actor grimaced, thought for a few seconds, and replied, "Knowing how to cook well, knowing the name of a good doctor who makes house calls, and making good friends." And then the interview was over. I have never forgotten his reply.

Lots of people have mastered the first two requisites of Henry Fonda's philosophy, but many have trouble with the last part—making good friends.

It's very wise to be nice to every person you meet, because you can't possibly judge people by snap first impressions. The person whom you like least when you first meet in a large gathering may turn out to be your best friend later. (I know this from experience. If I had a quarter for every person I have misjudged upon the first meeting, I would be a rich woman today!)

THE FIRST STEP:
MEETING PEOPLE WHO MAY BECOME FRIENDS

*I*n order to have good friends, you have to meet them first. But even before
worrying about meeting people, you must be "meetable" yourself, or it
just won't happen. Being "meetable" means that you:

- Walk down the street with a deliberately pleasant expression on
  your face (not a suffering frown, such as many of us have when
  we're trying to remember, "What were those six things I set out
  to buy that were so desperately needed?")
- Look as if you're having a great time at every party you attend,
  even if you're miserable. A smiling face, symptomatic of an
  upbeat personality, is like the flame that fascinates and draws the
  moths.
- Don't complain to others, even if your feet are hurting or you are
  exhausted from a hard day. Whether people know you well or
  have just met you, they do not wish to hear how awful you feel.
  (That may only motivate them to convince you that they feel a lot
  worse.)
- Act fascinated by the new people you meet, even if they look very
  boring indeed. You never know until you have really had time to
  know someone whether or not a real pearl might be lying hidden
  in that unopened oyster shell.

Become Creative in Your Leisure Time

You will meet people by getting out of your home, away from your
hum-drum schedule, and into a new routine of extracurricular activities.

- Maybe you will meet the person of your dreams at the next
  cocktail party you attend. You should never turn down an invitation to a party. Go! You can never be sure that something
  delightful will *not* happen on any given evening—how are you
  going to know unless you go out? Don't turn down a blind date,
  either. He or she may be a dud but may have knockout friends.
  How will you know unless you go out with that person and meet
  those friends?
- Maybe you were destined to meet a special friend by joining a
  new association—for example, a miniature sailboat racing club.
  I know a divorced woman who found a new husband—a divorced
  man—as he was sailing boats with his little boy on a Saturday in
  the park. She and her little girl were sailing enthusiasts, too, so it
  was quite natural that the two single parents began chatting. Now

this couple and their children can stage their own private regattas!

My daughter Clare and her husband, Jim, found each other poking around on a Saturday in an Irish bookstore in lower Manhattan. Since they were the only customers in the bookstore, they had plenty of time to talk. A shared interest in books on Ireland led to their engagement just a few months later. (Clare's unmarried women friends, all in their mid-twenties, have been spending more time in bookstores on Saturdays ever since.)

o Perhaps you were meant to make friends working on a nonprofit project. There is a powerful need for volunteers in all cities today. And it's quite apparent that some of the nicest people in any community are those who give of themselves to help others and to make this a better world. A newcomer anywhere can volunteer for a worthy cause and make close new friends through sharing worthwhile activities undertaken in a spirit of concern.

I know a senior citizen who pushes the book and magazine cart around one of New York's biggest hospitals. She is always smiling and cheering up patients and is much loved by them. Many of them remain her good friends when they leave the hospital. "I have such a busy social life," she told us. "I have a very difficult time fitting it all in!" She added that she "is the happiest septuagenarian you'll probably ever see—between my volunteer work and the friends it brings me."

o Perhaps in sampling your city's cultural activities, you will meet a person who shares your interests. If you are a season ticket holder at the theater, concert hall, or ballet, for example, inevitably you will begin to make friends with others who hold tickets to the same performances. During the intermission, you will find yourself talking to other subscribers whom you see each time. You can discuss the performance, chat about other things, and then suggest going to have a cup of coffee or tea.

o Look for the nearest place where you can engage in a sport in which you excel. If you are a passably good tennis player, skier, softball player, ice-skater, or croquet player, don't be shy. Start playing *better*. Pick up games; ask someone to be your partner or opponent—anything to let the world see how good you are. Others will want to play with you, and having "a bite to eat" afterward is a natural outcome of playing a good game. The friendship solidifies if, after you play a game, you break bread together.

o It may be helpful to join a church or temple group. So many activities are sponsored by houses of worship that a person participating in these activities inevitably meets a wide variety of people.

o Perhaps you should become active in your child's school. If you work hard to make the school better, you'll meet a sizable group of parents who will appreciate your ideas, time, and effort and will want to support you in your projects.

o You might try to learn a new skill. While you are working hard at it, you'll meet and make friends with others who have the same goals. Whether it's learning a foreign language, Japanese flower arranging, sculpting, belly dancing, the history of art, ice-boating, or Thai cooking, you will enjoy the company of others doing the same thing.

o Maybe, if you love the outdoors, you would enjoy joining groups that take overnight hikes on weekends. Sometimes these expeditions are for singles, sometimes they are for entire families, and other times they are for single parents with children. The newspapers generally list these outings (the listings may be more complete in suburban papers). By the time you have spent forty-eight hours huddled together in a cave for shelter during an endless rainstorm, there is no question but that you will emerge from it as good friends—or ardent enemies, but hopefully the former!

o Go where the action is in your field of interest. You will meet people there who are enthusiasts of your sport, hobby, or intellectual pursuit. Join a bird-watching group or computer club, or attend old film festivals. Take a history course, or attend all the philosophy lectures sponsored by your local university. Go to a gourmet cooking school, and then share the fruit of your efforts with new friends.

o *Whatever you do, keep your eyes open and be alert.* Is that person who's buying his or her single-portion dinner every night at the grocery store (when you're there) an eligible single person? Pay attention to the people around you in your neighborhood— whether you're looking for a friend or a lover. He or she might be standing right next to you in the checkout line at the supermarket! People who are cynical and pessimistic in a city like New York might think that the person standing next to them in a checkout line could be dangerous, but there's another point of view: That person might be your next date!

It's a question of philosophy. There are those who look out the window and say, "There's sunshine with just a bit of clouds out there." Others say, "It's all cloudy out there, with just a bit of sunshine." Take your pick.

SOLIDIFYING A NEW FRIENDSHIP

Once you have made a real friend, keep that person. An established friendship should be viewed as a treasured relationship, requiring not only loyalty, but also time and attention.

• *The best way to solidify that friendship is to invite that person to a meal.*

Once you meet someone who is *simpatico* and with whom you share good chemistry, don't let him (or her or them) evaporate into thin air just because everyone is too busy. *You* take the initiative. Use that person's telephone number. Invite him (or her or that couple) out to dinner—or to a Saturday or Sunday lunch. When you ask someone to share a meal, it is the ultimate compliment.

If you think your new friend or friends would feel more comfortable with others present, invite one or two other people as well. If you don't know one or two other people to ask, don't worry about it.

Plan a short cocktail hour and a delicious meal. Make your home look as attractive as possible. Put some flowers around, have good music playing softly in the background, and show what a relaxed, caring host you are. The art of entertaining well is one of the greatest people assets there is, and it should be used as part of your repertoire for making friends.

• *You should also be on the giving, not always on the receiving end.* This means that you repay your friends' hospitality and kindnesses. Sometimes repayment takes a different form, but it's a repayment nevertheless. For example, John and Agnes may invite the Masons to dinner quite often, but if the Masons work hard to get John and Agnes's children into a college where the Masons have a lot of clout, John and Agnes are not going to count the number of times the Masons come to dinner without a return dinner invitation.

• *You should rise in defense of good friends when they are criticized.* When you hear a mutual friend criticizing your friend, intervene. You don't have to mince any words: "That's an untrue accusation; I know it is. And even if it were true, it's disloyal to talk about him that way."

• *Check in with a real friend on a regular basis, no matter how busy you may be and how unbusy he or she may be.* Friends are to be enjoyed when it suits your schedule, but their needs also should be respected when it doesn't suit your schedule. You may be exhausted after working particularly hard at your office all week, but when a close friend who complains she "never sees you any more" calls to ask your help with a project on your one free Saturday afternoon, extend yourself.

• *Be ready to help in an emergency—short- or long-term.* If a single-parent woman friend suddenly has to go to the hospital for a few days, offer to take care of her children in your own home during that time, or find another good solution. If a friend is moving, do everything from helping him pack to bringing him dinner and a bottle of wine on the evening of his move. If a friend's car is in the shop for a week, lend him your extra car, or pick him up and take him home every day from work.

• *Be sensitive to a friend's emotions.* When you sense that a married friend feels down, for example, be ready to help. Perhaps what she needs is just an invitation to dinner and a pep talk; perhaps what he needs is just a sympathetic ear; perhaps what they both need is the name of a good marriage counselor!

• Remember that good friends

o *Never ask too much of each other.* They never step over the bounds of good taste and into excess. They never take one another for granted.

o *Compromise on what they do together; one person's wish is not the only deciding factor.* ("Look, since you're nice about going to Shakespeare this Saturday with me, I'll be glad to go to the baseball game with you next Saturday, okay?")

o *Remember what's important to the other person and respect it,* whether it's a birthday celebration, free time to concentrate on a hobby, or simply lending shopping expertise (to keep the other one from making any more wardrobe mistakes).

o *Enjoy surprising each other with creative acts of kindness*—for example, with

An unexpected telephone call. ("I just called, because I happened to hear some Scottish music and it reminded me of our trip to Scotland.")

A timely unexpected visit. ("I know I'm not expected, but you didn't sound too chipper the last time I talked to you with that cold of yours, so I brought you some hot homemade soup.")

An unexpected gift (with a card that reads: "With love, from Aggie, just because it feels like spring outside today, and I wanted you to have some of the first daffodils to brighten up your office desk!").

Helping out when some assistance would really be needed (anything from taking over a friend's car-pooling duties when she isn't feeling well to lending a couple your lakeside cabin when they can obviously use a weekend of quiet and rest).

MAKING FRIENDS AT WORK

The best way to make friends at work is to be a bright, sunny person, so that you lift up the spirits of others. Co-workers will want to be around you because you're the one with the sunny disposition.

Be a good citizen around the office. Don't welch on your responsibilities (including getting coffee on a certain day, turning off the lights before going home, returning everything you borrowed from a colleague—on time and in good shape). Lend a helping hand, even when it's not your responsibility. If someone is stuck late on an emergency job, stay late once in a while to help out. That's what friends are for.

Stick up for a friend who is being wrongfully criticized at the office, praise a friend who is doing a good job, and pass on helpful advice and information when that friend would find it useful.

• *When you're new, take people to lunch!* Invite your peers, even those higher up the corporate ladder, to a nice (not luxurious, just nice) restaurant for lunch. It's an investment. However, don't talk around the office about any of your lunch appointments, or people will think you're apple-polishing. These lunches will help you learn office procedures and politics—and allow you to show how personable, intelligent, and attractive you are in a relaxed situation. They allow you and the other person to get to know each other. You spend so many hours at work that it really is important to have friends there. They are a necessary support system in helping you get through the day. However, don't come on too strong with these invitations. Don't look overeager and aggressive. Be subtle and discreet about those lunch invitations.

WIDENING YOUR HORIZONS
THROUGH VOLUNTEER WORK

The nonprofit world has always involved charity, generosity, love, and caring for others. But in today's mobile world it may also serve as the most efficient vehicle for newcomers in a community to form friendships and establish new business contacts. Volunteer service also provides people who serve on the boards of nonprofit institutions—women, in particular—invaluable management training for the business world.

The most important part of serving the nonprofit community is that whether you give your time or your money or both, you will receive enormous personal satisfaction. Knowing you have helped is one of the pleasantest of all experiences.

Choosing a Volunteer Activity

The best philanthropic work for you may be one in which you have a personal interest. You may be faced with a bewildering array of organizations needing your free time, your ideas, your hands, your present or future clout, and your money (however little that may be). If you have a personal reason for working for a nonprofit institution, you have the best kind of inbuilt motivation there is. Princess Yasmin Khan, for example, the daughter of the late film star Rita Hayworth, devotes her efforts to raising money to fight Alzheimer's—the disease that afflicted her mother through much of her later life. In fact, if it were not for Rita Hayworth, many Americans would not have been aware of the nature of this disease or of the need for research in fighting it. Betty Ford, wife of former President Gerald Ford, a victim of cross addiction to alcohol and drugs, works tirelessly to combat such addictions, and the successful Betty Ford Clinic in California is a testimonial to her efforts. A well-known businessman whose daughter is blind works nonstop to raise money for training the dogs that help the blind. Famous people who have had cancer always seem ready to make appearances and write articles to help the fight against this dreaded disease.

But for every celebrity out in front, there are hundreds of thousands of noncelebrities who have personally suffered with a disease or seen it touch a member of their family or a friend. That is motivation enough.

The health field is by no means the only one in serious need of volunteer time and money. Feeding and clothing the poor and the homeless . . . working with churches and temples to assist the very young or the very old . . . acting as surrogate parents to underprivileged children to keep them from becoming dropouts . . . women serving as role models to help economically deprived women work and support their families . . . couples laboring to solve the disastrous financial problems of the arts and to stimulate their growth in small communities . . . parents going far beyond their usual responsibilities to help make their children's schools better—these are just a sampling of what is out there that needs doing.

First Lady Barbara Bush, who comes from a family of readers, has long been a leader in the literacy movement, since even before her White House days. Her advocacy has directed attention to this serious problem in our country—and to its solutions. Jimmy and Rosalynn Carter have worked long and hard for better housing for the poor. Jacqueline Onassis is a leader in the fight for historic preservation in our cities. However, you don't need to be a member of a president's family to be effective.

You don't have to look far for suggestions on what you personally can do and where you can do it. You may only have to look around your neighborhood, listen to and read the local news. There is always enough time in a week to wring out a few more hours of service dedicated to others, even if you work hard at a job. The rewards are tremendous in terms of personal satisfaction. A New York woman made famous by the gossip columnists because of her lavish parties, French designer clothes, and incredible jewels works secretly in one of the toughest sections of New York in a special program for gifted black students. She goes there three times a week in a cab (not in her chauffeured Jaguar), dressed in the simplest clothes. When I saw her recently, we discussed her volunteer work. Her reputation around town is mainly that of a vapid, spoiled woman. Yet she looked at me with eyes full of pure joy as she confided, "You know, I have really made a difference there. I've been working with three kids in particular who are deep into the sciences, and I've found someone to pay scholarships for them to the top colleges of their choice. Now the others want to excel in their own things and have me help them find scholarships, too. It's making a difference!"

• *If you are fortunate enough to be able to donate a sizeable amount of money to something, make it a quiet, anonymous gift.* Word of your generosity will get around anyway, and you have no idea in this world of self-promotion how much people will admire you for your discretion and self-effacement in making your gift quietly, without fanfare. In other words, let others publicize and praise you. They will do it far more effectively than you could.

The Way to Get on a Nonprofit Agency Board

There are two ways to get on this kind of a board—through very generous donations that look as though they will never stop or through hard work and energy. Most people have to use the second route.

If you're new in town, decide on the field in which you wish to work, then go right to the main office at that organization and volunteer. If you know someone who is already there as a volunteer, then you can be introduced to the director of the organization, and the contacts are easily made. If you know no one within the organization, just go and present yourself. The question "What can I do to help?" is beautiful music to almost every pair of ears in the volunteer management world. It's the quality of your volunteer work that is going to make you a star. When you do the dirty jobs cheerfully, when you show an ability to follow someone's direction, and when you also show your own creativity, you will rise very naturally to important new positions of responsibility within the volunteer structure.

Here are the characteristics of what a director of volunteers at a hospital told me makes an outstanding volunteer, who then may become a candidate for an advisory board position. The volunteer

- o Takes direction with intelligence, obedience, and loyalty
- o Is punctilious about arrival time
- o Will remain longer than the required hours in case of an emergency
- o Doesn't accept a job and then announce that he or she is going on vacation for two months
- o When other obligations intrude so that volunteer hours must be temporarily curtailed, she reports it far in advance to allow time for a qualified substitute to be located
- o Dresses appropriately for the job—not flashily or ostentatiously, but professionally
- o Keeps meticulously accurate records when they are called for, such as in fund-raising
- o Respects the confidentiality of the institution and does not spread gossip about the people served there or the other volunteers; acts as a source of good public relations for the institution when talking about it in her family, work, or social milieu
- o Does not make personal telephone calls during volunteer hours
- o If her primary work is interaction with the people served by the institution, learns to polish her interpersonal skills, becomes even more sensitive to others' problems, and practices kindness and self-control, even when the people she is serving do not
- o Remains in a creative mode, so that she can suggest to management ways of doing things better and at less cost

If Your Volunteer Motives Are Partly Social

Some people, men and women both, are primarily interested in helping organize benefits to widen their social lives. The way to work your way up in the social strata of a benefit committee is to offer to do any dirty work that needs to be done (such as helping to hand-address 2000 invitations). One woman I know did just that. She sat and wrote for days, listening to what her fellow addressers were saying about the people on the master list. "I learned more about the local scene while doing those invitations than I could have in fifty years under any other circumstances," she told me. She said it was the best orientation to the social scene in that community she could have received as a newcomer in that town.

A person who is a tireless worker in helping organize a benefit becomes admired and befriended by the other members of an organization. It is one of the best ways to widen the circle of friends who share your interests.

But the best motivation of all is to become involved in an organization that *truly* interests you and needs your help, whether it is in the area of fund-raising, giving volunteer hours, lending administrative expertise, or doing whatever you do well.

"I have a good volunteer job" means that you're useful, you enjoy what you're doing, you're in the mainstream, you give the gift of yourself, and you make good friends while you're doing it. Any one of those benefits makes volunteer effort well worth it.

*　*　*

Like anything of value, friends require loving care, whatever their age, sex, or socio-economic level, and that attention should be consistent. No matter how busy you may be, you can always check in with a quick telephone call or note. You can't quantify your relationship with friends. The pleasure they give you in return for your acts of kindness toward them is immeasurable.

Making friends really does take a great deal of effort, and it seems you are always required to give more to them than they give to you. What is ironic is that your friends are probably saying the very same thing about you!

4

Manners That Succeed at Work

I have already written an entire work on this subject, a book that I will immodestly describe as the standard reference text in the corporate, professional, and entrepreneurial worlds (*Letitia Baldrige's Complete Guide to Executive Manners,* Rawson Associates, publishers). But it never hurts to take a fresh look at such an important topic. I have encapsulated some of the advice from that book into this short chapter. Reading it will be a refresher course for some, but uncharted territory for others just entering the business world. One can also safely say that anyone comfortably settled in the business world—or aspiring to be— should find the material in all the other chapters of this *New Manners for the Nineties* book useful, too. It is illogical to define business manners as the *only* kind a person in business needs to possess.

I firmly believe that, along with talent and business acumen, the magic a person needs in order to cut a graceful path through the business world (which means being admired, respected, and liked) consists of these assets:

- ○ A kind heart
- ○ An awareness of others
- ○ A sense of humor

If you have all three (all relating to your character and your manners), you will get ahead. The kind heart and awareness of others mean that you are sensitive to people—a requirement of leadership. It means you are popular with your cohorts. People will want to work with you—follow you—and help you get ahead. They will be pulling for you. Promotions always seem to follow that kind of peer loyalty.

• *Never underestimate the importance of a sense of humor.* A sense of humor can be a swing factor in many difficult, embarrassing, or awkward situations. If you can laugh at yourself when you make a mistake, people will laugh with you, not at you. They will be smiling instead of suffering inside with empathy for you. And if you can glide over someone else's mistake with a quick change of subject, you will relieve the tension in the room, everyone will relax, and the person who made the mistake will have time to compose him- or herself and recover.

WHETHER YOU'RE A BOSS OR DOWN IN THE RANKS

Commonsense Business Behavior
That Can Advance Your Career

Whatever your position in business—whether you're an executive or someone who's just stepped onto the bottom rung of the corporate ladder—simple commonsense consideration for others is always appropriate. It wins respect from others and marks you as a team player who is a real asset to the company.

o Be as nice to the people on the bottom of the job scale in your office as you are to the boss. Quite apart from the factors of kindness and respect involved, these people will become your friends and valuable supporters, which will probably prove to be the greatest asset of your career.

o Be loyal to and defend the boss inside or out of the office.

o Don't "rat" on anyone, unless that person is committing a serious offense (drug-dealing, stealing, or the like).

o Unless you are a person's supervisor, don't criticize him or her directly, and especially not behind his or her back. After all, that person could be your boss one day.

o Be nice to newcomers. Show them around, make them feel welcome and part of the team. Give them a feel for the politics of the office. In other words, follow the Golden Rule, because you would certainly want someone to do the same for you if you were the newcomer.

o Always keep your promises. Establish—and keep—your reputation as that of a person of good faith.

o Pay back your lunch obligations. Don't become known as the person who never picks up the check.

o Don't put down and interrupt someone with whom you disagree when that person is making a presentation in the office. Voice your objections in private. To humiliate someone in public will not advance your career.

When You're New in the Office

● You need information—on how things work, on what everyone does, on the politics of the office. You find out the answers to all those questions by

o *Asking intelligent questions of intelligent people when they have the time to talk to you.* Timing is everything in the business world, and you must learn to be sensitive to it. Never try to take up someone's time when he or she is obviously late, on a deadline, or overloaded with work.

o *Going through the files,* which reveals how the people in the company write their letters, talk to their customers or clients, and communicate among themselves.

o Most important of all, *listening!* What you hear all around you is the best education of all. Some people when they are new in an office are so entranced with their own conversations that they hear nothing else. They are not listeners and thereby often lose the forest just to save a couple of trees.

● *Be nice to absolutely everyone,* from the messenger to the CEO. If you want to look at it clinically, every person in that office environment may be key to the advancement of your career. But more important, when you are genuinely nice to everyone, you greatly improve the atmosphere and the general office morale. I learned long ago, by the way, that my best friends and supporters in *any* office are the secretaries and receptionists.

● *Ask your peers to lunch, one by one,* so that you will get to know each one on a personal, relaxed basis (as well as obtain valuable information about the company or firm from each one).

● *Be very modest about your past jobs and your qualifications for this job.* People are immediately attracted to someone who downplays his or her importance and usually think of that person as more important than he or she actually is.

TO BE A WELL-LIKED, SUCCESSFUL EXECUTIVE

• *Do not gossip.* Senior management views the office gossip as a mean-spirited person who thinks he or she has more time to spend on nonwork-related conversation than he or she actually has!

• *Do not put down anyone in front of others.* The person who puts someone else down may think he or she looks very clever and witty, but the perception of others is just the opposite.

• *Always give credit where credit is due,* which means not trying to accept praise for something not really of his doing.

• *Always make reference to the team effort—i.e., "We did this" or "We did that," not* "I then did this, and then I did that." This also implies taking the rap for the team when something goes wrong. The person who whines to senior management, "Of course, this wasn't my doing; it was John's and Mary's idea—I had nothing to do with it," shows a total lack of leadership, even if he did have nothing to do with it.

• *Keep your promises*—for example, when promising to stay late and help put a project to bed, making promised telephone calls, or putting in a good word for someone as promised.

• *Return telephone calls within twenty-four hours,* or at least have someone else handle the matter. It is good manners, but also good business to do this.

• *Answer important letters within the week,* unimportant mail within two to three weeks.

• *Be punctual for all appointments*—again, the nice thing to do, but also essential to the efficiency of operations. I'll never forget waiting in a CEO's office one day for the son of one of that company's directors to appear. He was thirty minutes late and made the CEO miss his train. When the CEO asked him what the purpose of his visit was, the young man replied that he wanted help in finding a job. The CEO, by now absolutely furious, told him, "There is definitely one company where you will never find a job, and that's this one." The young man's father later called the CEO and thanked him for teaching his overly casual son a good lesson.

• *Inform everyone who should be informed* with information on the developments of a project of mutual interest. In other words, don't hold a project "close to the vest."

• *If you are a senior manager, make sure your employees have a proper working environment,* such as efficient desks, comfortable chairs, and good lighting.

• *Help the younger staff members with their training*—by giving suggestions, answering their questions patiently, and in general serving as a friendly guiding hand while they learn the ropes. A thirty-year-old person can serve as a mentor for a twenty-five-year-old person. All that is required is more experience and a good amount of patience.

• *Answer all invitations within a week's time,* and attend the event if you accepted the invitation. The well-mannered executive respects an RSVP on an invitation and is never an unexplained no-show. When an executive is a no-show at a corporate or private social affair, it reflects badly on him or her and the company.

• *Promptly return anything borrowed from a colleague, in perfect condition,* and with a spoken or written word of thanks. I recently lent my personal computer for an entire afternoon to someone who claimed she desperately needed it. I remained irritated and resentful until I went back to my computer, found it with its cover neatly on (which I always forget), the keyboard cleaned with a special solution (it badly needed it), and a lovely note expressing how my loan of the computer had saved her from a fate worse than death. A good bottle of wine, tied with a ribbon, accompanied the note. All of a sudden, I didn't mind at all that she had tied up my PC.

• *Err on the side of generosity, rather than cheapness,* in matters such as picking up the check for a meal.

• *Be rigorous about repaying hospitality and acknowledging favors.* You may be a dazzler at any party, but no host in the world is going to want to continue to invite you forever to functions at which you can shine and show your stuff if you never reciprocate or are never properly grateful.

• *Be quick to drop a line (and go on record) to congratulate someone who has performed well.* It's those words on a piece of paper that the recipient can read, reread, and show around to friends and family that make him or her feel proud and love the job.

• *Enthusiastically defend at any level of management a colleague who has been wronged.* It might be something as major as telling the big boss that the person in the office next to you was not the last person to leave the other night, and therefore could not have been the one who committed the security violation of leaving the door unlatched. It might be something as minor as defending the way a colleague who is being blamed for being a sloppy manager explained to the messenger where to take a certain envelope, which was brought to the wrong address.

• *Know how to dress on business or social occasions,* so that the company or firm is proud, not embarrassed, to have you representing them. (The executive who shows up for dinner without a jacket and tie in the dining room of a fancy resort like the Greenbriar, in West Virginia, does not cast a good reflection on his company name.)

• *Show deference to people who are senior,* rather than treating them with the same "first-name, slap-on-the-back, we're-all-equal" attitude. I have seen many a senior executive in his sixties wince upon meeting a young executive from another company who immediately calls him by his first name.

• *Don't boast about your past—or present, for that matter.* Someone who, because of family connections, is friendly with the CEO, doesn't talk about it in the presence of colleagues. Nor does that person talk about parties he or she has been invited to and opportunities enjoyed that the others have not shared.

• *Show compassion to a colleague who has had bad news.* This means taking the person aside, with an arm around his or her shoulders, to say how sorry you are, and to ask if you may be of assistance in any way.

• *Don't treat hot new information as your personal property, not to be shared with others.* Someone who finds out something and then keeps it a secret until it can be presented to senior management is no team player. He or she should share it with colleagues—you can still get the credit for uncovering.

• *Don't waste company time with idle chit-chat or with personal telephone calls.* Never bother someone by insisting on talking when that person is obviously trying to concentrate and finish a project.

• *Talk lovingly about your spouse and children, but only minimally,* so as not to distract the work in progress of others. (The same can be said for discussion of your sex or love life.)

• *Write a personal letter to thank for a meal, gift, or favor.* There is no question but that a person who writes personal notes (President and Mrs. Bush are inveterate note-writers, for example) is remembered fondly and gets ahead in life!

• *Buck up a colleague who is feeling discouraged.* Sometimes it takes as little as sticking your head in someone's office door and saying, "Hey, cheer up! This mess will be over soon, the sun will shine again, and you'll be on top of the world. A little patience! A little courage!" Sometimes it takes several meetings to persuade a friend who needs help to seek psychological counseling. No matter how hard you are working at the office, think about your friends, and help them when they need it. You might need help of this kind yourself some day.

• *Organize a continuing show of office support for someone who is hospitalized, injured, or ill.* This means, not just one bunch of flowers or one card signed by everyone in the office, but a message of affection—and office news—going out once a week to that person.

• *Introduce people so as to make each person sound—and feel— important and wonderful.* At lunch in the Executive Dining Room you can introduce Elmer Snowden as "Elmer Snowden from Deloitte and Touche," or you can introduce him with exaggerated humor: "This is Elmer Snowden, one of the best accountants Deloitte and Touche has ever had in their firm since it was founded. Elmer is absolutely top drawer—and a nice guy in spite of it!"

• *Remember to thank the little people who do all the work on a major event*—such as arranging the travel, making the audio-visuals for a presentation, copying necessary materials, organizing large conferences or corporate parties, and the like. This kind of recognition should be on the record—via personal letters to the people involved, in a verbal salute in front of the group, or in a tribute published in the company magazine.

• *Work the entire time at a company party,* instead of standing in a corner, chatting with office pals, enjoying the food and drinks. Every person in the host company should be out there, introducing guests around, making sure that everyone has a drink and someone to talk to— and that everyone has met the corporate hosts. Members of the staff should remember they are hosts, not guests!

• *Cultivate beautiful telephone manners.*

○ Place your own calls.
○ Do not put people on endless hold.
○ Do not take telephone calls when someone with an appointment is sitting in your office.
○ When you have called a busy person, be sensitive about that person's time pressures.
○ Do not have your calls screened, and do not blow your stack when someone else does.
○ Apologize for dialing a wrong number.

• *Rise and stand every time someone from the outside—a peer or someone more senior—enters the room.* Men and women alike, of any age, should rise at their desks and step forward to greet their callers, just as you should rise and step forward to greet a new guest when he or she arrives at your or anyone else's party.

• *Know how to introduce people properly—a younger person to a more senior one,* a nonofficial person *to* a person with rank or a title, and so forth.

• *Use a firm, practiced, but not bone-crushing handshake,* and shake hands outside the office every time you meet someone or tell a person good-bye.

• *Know how to make small talk with people senior to you or who are strangers.* The art of making good business conversation includes the ability to pass the time of day in agreeable conversation, talking about unimportant subjects while waiting for more substantial discussions to begin.

• *Never expect anyone who answers to you to follow a rule you do not yourself obey.*

Traveling with the Boss

When traveling with the boss, a young executive should always

- o Give the boss the best seat—in a restaurant, taxi, or limo (never let the boss sit on a jumpseat!) or on the plane, bus, or train.
- o Unless instructed not to, take care of all baggage matters, checking into hotels, ordering of cars, tipping, and paying the bills for lodging, meals, and transportation.
- o Carry all of the heavy paraphernalia when the two are in transit.
- o Remain silent when the boss opens his or her briefcase or files and is studying them.
- o Speak frankly if the boss asks direct questions, such as, "How are things coming along in your section?" or "Any particular complaints in your division?" (This is an opportunity to score some points for your section; it should not be looked upon as a chance to derail the career of someone you personally dislike.)
- o Make it a top priority to make life easy and comfortable for the boss en route to any destination.

The number is legion of today's very successful chief executive officers who began their careers as young assistants to other CEOs. A brash MBA graduate commented to me, "Think of what I'd learn if I were the right arm and the aide-de-camp of the big boss. What an opportunity it would be for me to learn the corporation!"

I reminded him that he wouldn't get the job of a CEO's right arm, unless he had the skills and the polish necessary. "What kind of polish?" he asked quizzically.

"Manners," I replied.

"Oh, those," he said disdainfully. "I can learn those overnight."

"No, you can't," I replied.

"Well, how long does it take?"

"As long as it takes you to start thinking about someone other than yourself." End of conversation!

*   *   *

I love the zest with which young people in the corporate world seize every bit of information they can get their hands on in the field of manners. They're signing out etiquette books from the public library and buying them in bookstores. They're lining up to gain entrance to the lecture hall when people like myself lecture on business manners. They are in search of information they know they will need but which was never made available at business school. Today's young executives and professionals feel very at ease working with computers and spread sheets but often ill at ease in certain social situations. One young woman remarked to me at the Wharton School in Philadelphia, "I'm embarrassed about being so embarrassed!"

Many parents assumed that they knew everything about appropriate and proper ways of relating to others even when they knew very little about manners either in the home or on the job. Their children, now beginning to move up in today's workplace, know they know very little and want to learn much more. That makes one feel great hope for the future!

5

The Manners That Make Travel Easier

The opportunity to travel is precious. Yes, there *are* inconveniences and moments of great discomfort, but even people such as I, who must travel constantly and who complain about it constantly, know that we would be bereft without it.

To go *somewhere else*—to see what *other* people are doing, how they look and how they are dressed, to hear what they are saying, and to be exposed to their culture, sports, and politics—is a fantastic plus. This stimulus holds true for travel to Smalltown America, as well as to a great cosmopolitan city. For both the traveler and the people who live in the destination city or country, manners are key to successful interaction. The well-mannered traveler is the best kind there is.

ENSURING A PLEASURABLE TRIP

Having a Good Time with a Traveling Companion

Two people may be very good friends to begin with, but it's amazing how much better they will know each other after having traveled together.

81

Being together day in and day out; many times having to share the same hotel, motel, or bed-and-breakfast room and bathroom; being forced to adjust to each other's preferences in restaurants; agreeing on activities according to separate likes and dislikes; being able to cope either with contracting stomach flu in a foreign city or taking care of your traveling companion who has it—these are all part of the pleasures of living and traveling together. The way you and your traveling companion handle them together will make the trip a great success or an unmitigated failure. Willpower, compromise, and unselfishness are the keys to a favorable outcome.

Any trip can be a success—if the people taking it *will* its success. That old cliché of having a positive attitude really works when you're traveling. If you arrive hot, tired, and dirty in a little Austrian hotel (with less than comfortable appointments in your room), you might look out the window and say to your traveling companion, "Isn't this a beautiful little town? Isn't it charming and quaint? Listen to the bells in the old belltower. Come here and look!" Or you might look out the window and say to your traveling companion, "Come here and look at this dirty old place. What a dump this town is!" Needless to say, the first reaction will help make your traveling companion glad he or she accompanied you and eager to put on the same pair of rosy glasses you did when you looked out that window. One person in a group can pull all the others down, but one person can also pull all the others up.

If you insist on having a great time on your travels, you *will.*

Actions You Might Take to Ensure Your Trip's Success

• *Have every aspect of the financial arrangements worked out well ahead of time.* Make sure that each pays an equal share during the trip. (One way of organizing this is to have a cash kitty, from which each day's expenses are paid and into which each person puts an equal amount of money each day.)

• It is advisable to keep a daily log of lodging expenses, with each person's personal expenses (pressing and laundry, room service, long distance calls, wine ordered with meals), so that each person will be paying a fair share of the hotel bill.

• *Reach a consensus on the next day's plans the night before.* Alternate the wishes of each person, so that everyone has his or her own turn in deciding what the pair or group will do that day. If an agreement is impossible to reach, each should go off and do his or her own thing, which is healthy and often rewarding if you have been suffering from too much togetherness.

- In the preplanning stages, an agreement should be reached on

  o The election of the person who will handle the trip arrangements, including dealing with the travel agent or making the reservations directly.
  o The budget to be followed (for example, what kind of hotels will be booked—luxury, middle-priced, modest).
  o The major tours to be taken in each country. Some people are beach-sitters, others cafe-sitters, others inveterate sightseers. A compromise should be reached before taking off on the trip.
  o The method of transport to be used—bus, train, airplane, boat, rented car, or car with driver.

- Compromise again on the sports you wish to play or watch, including those games for which you will purchase tickets.
- If your companion is feeling under the weather, the best thing you can do—after he or she has seen a doctor, been given the proper medication, and declared capable of being left alone—is to take off and have an interesting day by yourself. But bring a little present back to your friend, for he or she probably will be feeling very depressed at missing the day's planned activities.
- *Always pack a couple of good books* in your suitcase—an excellent antidote to boredom, insomnia, or a disagreement with your traveling companion.
- If one of you is unduly irritated with the other, have an open discussion of what caused the irritation. Travelers in close quarters often become temporarily out of sorts, for one reason or another. The hostility can be defused by a frank and calm talk—and a little time spent apart (maybe only two or three hours), to regain some perspective on the friendship. I remember a talk I had on one trip after a friend and I had begun to get on each other's nerves. She finally revealed that my constant chatting on the telephone with old school friends wherever we went was getting her down; I confessed that her hanging her underwear to dry out the window of whatever hotel we were staying in was getting to me. We laughed, shook hands, and did not repeat those annoying habits for the rest of our summer trip.
- The traveler who brings too much baggage slows down the entire trip and merits the wrath of his or her companions. Carry one large, expandable bag that you check on each flight and a tote that can fit under an airplane seat—both of which you can carry yourself if you have to (and you probably will have to).
- You should not resent it when your traveling companion receives an invitation from a personal friend that does not include you. Never take it for granted that you will be included in everything for which your friend(s) may be invited.

I remember traveling through Europe as a college student with a very glamorous friend who kept running into American male students, who immediately asked her out to dinner. I felt pretty left out and resentful until I took hold of myself and went off alone to concerts and the theater. Each time I did, during intermission I met people from that country in the lobby. They were perplexed to see a young American girl alone, and each night a couple or a family would invite me to dinner in a wonderfully characteristic local place. Then when my friend returned to the hotel after her date with an American boy, I frankly enjoyed making her jealous by recounting my own local color experiences. They often were more interesting than hers.

• When someone invites *you* to a social event on your trip, *write the host a thank-you note* within twenty-four hours. Even if your traveling companion is also invited and writes a note, you should write one, too. If you were the guest of honor, you would send flowers or a present (with a note) to the host the next day.

• The holidays provide the perfect opportunity to renew the acquaintances you made during your foreign travels. Send each person a chatty Christmas or New Year's card, in which you mention how much you enjoyed seeing them. Give your address, and say how much you hope they will let you know when they come to the United States. If you became friends with your hotel manager or concierge, send them cards, too.

You will find that these new friends will last a lifetime if you are thoughtful enough to remember them at Christmastime. (Most people hardly ever do.)

When You're Taking a Plane

• *Dress comfortably but nicely.* Many well-heeled Americans dress like hippies when they fly today. A person clad in a beaten-up t-shirt, sawed off jeans, and monk's sandals hardly makes a great impression when he or she steps off a plane in another country. The well-dressed, neat young American, on the other hand, makes an instant, favorable impression on foreigners. "Don't disgrace your country!" my mother always used to call after her sons when they left for faraway lands, and by that she meant, "Stay well groomed while you travel, whatever you do!" She knew she did not have to give me the same advice, because I had lived abroad so many years and used to get upset at my fellow countrymen if they looked scruffy. Americans living abroad want to be proud of their compatriots.

• It also helps your image (and makes everyone who has to look at you, feel much better, too) if you *carry your personal effects in suitcases*, rather than in a series of plastic bags that look as if they just came from the supermarket. Again, some of the most affluent seem to be careless about this.

• *Check large pieces of baggage,* instead of carrying them on board. Flight attendants seem to have given up trying to make passengers adhere to the rules concerning luggage brought into the cabin, but other passengers really get upset when someone boards carrying a lot of luggage. As a result others are unable to get in or out of the aisle. When someone boards a plane and walks down that narrow aisle, looking for a seat number, with giant bags swinging from both shoulders and knocking into others, that person wins the title of "Most Hated Passenger on Board."

• *If you are seated next to a chatterer* and you not only don't like chattering, but you have work to do or a good book to read, say very politely, "I'm so sorry. I would really like to talk some more, but by the time we land I must have this work finished," or "I must return this book to the person meeting me, so I had better finish it," or some other logical excuse. When the meal is served, it is impossible to work or read your book, so that is the time to show a little kindness and converse with your undoubtedly chastened seatmate.

• *If you are a parent with a small child,* keep that child from running up and down the aisle. Not only is it very hard on the flight attendants, who must serve many meals in a short space of time and are then obliged to keep stepping over and around the child, but it is hard on the nerves of fellow passengers. In addition, it is also dangerous and against the FAA safety rules. (Many parents think their small children's running up and down the aisle, getting everyone's attention, is just too cute for words, but it is not.) A wise parent traveling with small children brings a small tote bag for each, containing favorite toys and games, to keep a child busy and happy in his seat. Snacks and a drink are also packed, because the food service may be very slow.

• *If you are traveling with a baby,* change your infant's diapers in the privacy of a lavatory and *not* in the empty seat next to you!

• *If you are sitting next to someone who is flying for the first time and frightened,* or who is an old hand at flying but still very frightened, lend a helping hand. If you just talk in a calm, reassuring voice, you can do wonders to help soothe a frightened human being. The fear of flying is very real. If you just explain what the sudden noises are, you will be a hero to your seatmate. ("That grinding noise you just heard is the sound of the landing gear being lowered.") If the person holds his or her ears and complains that they hurt, say something like, "The pressure really can hurt your ears a lot. I sympathize. Hold your nose and blow gently. Try swallowing again and again. Sipping water helps, too."

When someone is in any obvious physical distress, ask if there's something you can do, and push the flight attendant's call button.

• *When the flight attendant comes by with the drinks cart,* give her exact change for the price of your cocktail. Many people look upon the flight attendant as a convenient bank from whom they can get $20 or $50 bills changed into much needed smaller money. The attendants have a tough enough time as it is getting their regular serving chores done, without having to run up and down the aisle getting change each time someone buys a drink.

• *Help keep the lavatory presentable.* Everyone appreciates it when whoever uses the rest room last flushes the toilet, drains the water from the washbowl, stows away used paper towels, and in general leaves it looking as neat as possible. It requires everyone's cooperation to keep the rest rooms decent, particularly on long overseas flights.

• *Leave your litter in a neat pile* on your seat (newspapers, magazines, pieces of paper, candy and gum wrappers, and the like) when you leave the plane, in consideration of the cleaning crew, who may have just a few moments to do their job before the next group of passengers board.

• As you disembark, *always thank the lined-up flight attendants.* They are rarely thanked, and they usually try very hard to please the passengers. If the captain or co-captain is standing in the doorway to the cockpit, thank him for "a good flight," a "job very well done," or a "great landing, Captain." Many passengers ignore the pilot and crew, so even a few paltry words of praise mean a lot.

WOMEN AND TRAVEL

Men and Women Traveling Together on Business

• An employer ultimately assumes all of his or her secretary's or assistant's expenses on the road, even though that person may be handling all of the fiscal chores, including checking in and out of the hotel, paying the bills, tipping the bellmen, and the like.

• When men and women executives are traveling together, it is important that the woman pay her own way exactly as a male colleague would do. That includes items such as her share of the taxi to the airport and the tip for the bellmen who handle their luggage and effects. It's wrong for a woman to allow her colleagues to pay for everything (or for her male companion to try to pay for everything) as though he and she were a married or unmarried couple (even though he will be reimbursed for her share of the expenses back at the home office). They should settle their accounts on a daily basis, or one might pay for everything one day and the other person the next (which requires more elaborate accounting).

• Women should carry their own bags and packages and help carry the load of business paraphernalia they may have brought with them.

• Men should not only invite their women traveling companions to have dinner with them on the road (Dutch treat, of course), but also to join them in swimming, jogging, or using the hotel's health club. A woman executive does not have to say yes (and they may be hoping she won't say yes), but the only polite thing to do is to ask her to join them. It is particularly important if there are two men and one woman on the trip, because then it is easy for the men to make the woman feel shut out.

Once when I accompanied some young executives on a business trip (there were two other women and two men), we arrived at our destination with two hours to kill. The men said in an unnecessarily sarcastic tone, "Well, you ladies are obviously going shopping, shopping, shopping!" Then they went off to take a sauna and a nap. At dinner in the conference center later, the squash pro at the health complex came by our table and said to the men, "Well, I don't know what you did this afternoon, but these two"—and he put a hand on each of the young women's shoulders—took on the two top men players in this city, for two tough hours, and beat 'em!" I loved it. I asked the young women, "If the pro hadn't come along, would you have told these guys all about your great athletic accomplishment this afternoon?"

"Heavens, no," laughed one of them. "We would have much preferred to have them think we were shopping on the mall for two hours. It would have put them in a better mood than they will be now."

THE SEXUAL ANGLE

There should be no sexual pressures on a business trip, provided the pair from the very beginning make it plain to each other that they are making a no-nonsense, "no fooling around" trip. A traveling pair should not book a hotel suite (two bedrooms and a living room), but rather two separate bedrooms. If, however, their company's travel people book them into a multi-bedroom company-owned suite in some hotel, that is a different story. In order to protect their privacy, a locked bedroom door is all that is necessary. (The male executive may feel the need of the locked door as much as the woman does.)

If the two are occupying the corporate suite together, quite logically they will be wise not to traipse around the living room and kitchenette in their night clothes. That might be done innocently by one person but could be taken by the other as a sexual signal.

If they have their own separate rooms and meet in one of the bedrooms during the day to confer on business matters (because they have confidential material they don't wish to display in the hotel restaurant or lobby or because they need a lot of space in which to spread out papers—all over the bed, tables, and floor), they should both be dressed in their work clothes. If one of them is wearing nightclothes, the other one should say, "Look, I know you didn't have time to get dressed, so I'll be outside in the hall, waiting, until you do get dressed." (That kind of statement is enough to discourage anyone with possible intentions of adding a little romance to the work load.)

Some women are very reputation-conscious (and I am glad they are). They become very nervous about what other people are thinking when they are seen traveling with male colleagues on business, particularly when their companions are married men. A woman should erase such a worry from her thoughts, however. In the first place, her own and her colleague's behavior are all that matter, not what other people are thinking. In the second place, the woman should realize that if she and her male traveling companion had wanted to have an affair, they certainly would not have had to go to the trouble of taking a business trip to another city in order to indulge in it. It is illogical for anyone to accuse an unattached pair on a business trip in another city of being involved in making love. (Most of them are too tired anyway.)

Some women's nervousness heightens when a male companion takes one drink too many in the evening and he makes a serious or half-serious pass. (The possibility of a charge of sexual harassment begins to rear its ugly head.) The woman should keep her sense of humor at this moment but tell her colleague in no uncertain terms to lay off, that she is going to bed—by herself—and that she will have forgotten this vestige of crude behavior by the next day. If he has grabbed her in a hallway, all she has to do is threaten to scream for the hotel security if he doesn't let her go. She, of course, has had enough sense _not_ to go to his room with him after dinner (doing that with a man who has drunk too much during the evening is total stupidity), nor has she invited him into her room for any reason (including believing the old canard that, "I have some papers you really should see before tomorrow's meeting.")

If a colleague of either sex drinks too much on the road, the one who is sober should be protective of the other, get that person to his or her room and urge that person not to exit again before the next day. You really can't lock the person into his or her room—because that would be a fire hazard, for one thing—but be firm. One inebriated executive at a resort convention remarked angrily to me as I pushed him into his room, closing the door behind him, "Just who do ya think you are, my mother?" My answer was short. "Yes." That did it. He didn't emerge until the next morning, in time for breakfast but looking abashed. I whispered in his ear, "Forget it," and by the second cup of coffee, he had.

A Woman Traveling Alone

Whether a woman is on business or vacation, she should not feel intimidated about going alone into the bar in her hotel or out for an early dinner in any established restaurant in the city.

- *If you are traveling alone and want a drink in your hotel's bar,* just for a change of pace from your hotel room, bring your briefcase or some files with you, take a seat at a table, pretend to go through a couple of business papers, order your drink, and then relax. Your little performance at the beginning of your bar appearance has established you as a bona fide businesswoman and demonstrated your professional seriousness to the others in the bar. You have shown you are in town on business and are not to be suspected for one minute of being a pickup.

- *If a man starts talking to you* and you like his conversation and he then offers to buy you a drink, accept with ease. If he offers to buy you another, change the contract: You buy *him* a drink. If he offers you another, tell him two are enough. If he asks you to join him for dinner, tell him you would love to—in the hotel dining room, not outside. Then charge your dinner to your room, so he won't feel he has a right to accompany you to and through your hotel room door. Keep the relationship on an easy plane, but don't go out with a man you know nothing about, nor put yourself in the vulnerable position of having him in your hotel room—not even for a second. (A great old ploy of a man who is not staying at your hotel but wants to be with you in your room is, "Do you mind if I use your bathroom?")

- A woman traveling alone may certainly go to the theater, ballet, concert, or a play unescorted, but she is vulnerable if she leaves her hotel to go to a bar or a nightclub alone. Particularly in a foreign country, this kind of independence could be dangerous.

- *If you want to find a nice restaurant where you may go safely by yourself,* ask your hotel concierge, the maître d'hôtel of the hotel dining room, or even the hotel management. Find out about taxi transportation back, or if it is very close, ask if it is safe for a woman to walk alone back to the hotel at night.

Never feel obliged, because you are alone and staying in a hotel, to stay in your room, staring at the four walls and ordering from room service. Get out and see things, do things, but move with wisdom, always following the sage advice of someone in the hotel who knows all the answers.

A word of caution: Don't let yourself be picked up by a man you don't know in this or any other country. Don't accept an invitation for the evening. Keep meeting him for lunch or tea, until you can find out something about him. If he asks you out in the evening, accept only with the proviso that another friend or another couple you know accompanies you.

SOME PRACTICAL ADVICE

Dealing with a Travel Agent

Your dealings with a travel agent will be successful *if* you communicate well with her or him—spell out exactly where you want to go, how you like to travel, what price accommodations you can afford, and what lifestyle you prefer.

o If you have trouble sleeping with the slightest noise, tell your agent, who will book you a room in the back of the hotel on a quiet street, instead of on the noisy, bustling front side of the hotel.

o If you are too tall to fit comfortably into an airplane coach seat, mention it and the agent will book you on an aisle—and in the exit row, if possible—where there's a little more leg room.

o If the agent knows you sleep in a big bed, he or she will make sure that is what awaits you in your hotel.

o If the agent knows you like picturesque, small hotels full of the local flavor, he or she will book you accordingly; if you let the agent know you prefer the flash of a big, modern, Las Vegas–type hotel, he or she will put you in one of those.

In other words, to be effective, you have to talk to your agent and let that person know what you like. These preferences will then be entered into your personal file.

If you're like me, you regard a good travel agent not just as a necessity, but as a hero. There is no trip too complicated, no change of reservations too frequent, no cancellations too onerous for this person to handle. A good travel agent always has a smile in the voice, even if he or she would like to throttle you at that particular moment. These agents must be diplomats, culture mavens, historians, experts on gourmet restaurants, geographers who are not allowed a margin for error, travel guides, shopping savants, and psychiatrists, ready to listen sympathetically to every traveler's lament or dream fantasy. They must know as much about ocean cruises as they do about the air shuttles that fly between Washington, New York, and Boston. They have to juggle schedules in the air and be knowledgeable about everything from the dates of opera performances in Rome's Baths of Caracalla to those of the British Open Golf Tournament. You should also insist that your agent be as shrewd as the most successful used-car dealer in getting you the best deal on the complicated and ever changing prices of air tickets, car rentals, and the like.

Your travel agent works on a small commission that you do not pay—it is paid by the people who fly you there or feed and house you once you're there. So the agent does not cost you a cent. Respect for the agent means that along with all the short trips you ask him or her to use time in booking for you, you also ask for service on long hotel stays and big trips—such as an ocean cruise—on which he or she can make some money. It also means that you wait until you're sure of your plans. Don't ask an agent to work on an endless series of reservations, only to cancel them time and again.

A travel agent who has taken good care of you on a complicated trip deserves a letter of thanks from you when you return home, as well as recommendations of his or her services to your friends (and one of those many small gifts you bought on your trip, too).

A Wise Move for the Overseas Traveler

The United States government provides great services free for those who travel abroad. If you are traveling to a country where you are worried about disease or where there has been military action, civil unrest, or a natural disaster, or even if you simply wish foreign visa information, dial the Citizens Emergency Center in the State Department in Washington (202/647-5225). If you are using a touch phone, the recorded operator's voice will take you through a number of questions. You may select three countries in one region per telephone call, to listen to their travel advisories. You would not call the Citizens Emergency Center for a travel advisory on Switzerland, where nothing is ever wrong and where even the trains run on time, but you would call for the latest travel advisory on the People's Republic of China.

Those using a push button phone may call anytime for the recordings, but those using a dial phone must call weekdays between 8:15 A.M. and 10 P.M. or on Saturdays from 9 A.M. to 3 P.M. (Eastern Standard Time), when the center itself is open for individual questions and problems.

The information on which the recorded travel advisories is based comes from State Department officials living in those areas. When you call, first you will hear a general summary of the travel advisory for that region, then a detailed one, including the very useful telephone numbers of United States consulates in those areas. If you wish, you may also ask that a copy of a particular travel advisory be mailed to you.

This service may also be used to find out about Americans who are in distress abroad—including their arrests, deaths, or medical emergencies. Again, the recorded operator's voice guides you, via push buttons, through to the exact office in the State Department or to the exact number to call to obtain the information you need. If you must have information on an American in trouble abroad when the Citizens Emergency Center is closed (after hours or on Sundays and holidays), call the government operator in Washington, D.C., at 202/634-3600, and ask for the Citizens Emergency Duty Officer.

* * *

It's very difficult to be a smiling, relaxed traveler these days, what with canceled or oversold flights, hot trains on which the air conditioning has broken down, jammed highways on which your car sits for hours without moving, and buses that fill up and leave without you. Just keep telling yourself what I have to keep repeating to myself day in and day out as I fly all over this great country of ours: "Relax. Worry is not going to make your schedule any easier; fretting is not going to change weather conditions. If the planes aren't flying and you can't get a seat on the train, you will have to travel tomorrow. There's nothing you can do about any of it, so breathe deeply and relax!"

If only all of us who must travel constantly could psych ourselves into a state of acceptance of whatever happens, we would be happier, healthier people. I keep telling myself, too, that even when the clerk behind the desk is being insolent, there really *isn't* anything she could do about the situation. She could be pleasanter, yes, but she is helpless. So keep your cool. You are helpless, too, when the planes aren't flying and you have to make an important speech on the other end. Look at the people remaining calm around you. They have important engagements, too. They are under pressure, too, but they're not taking it out on anyone, including themselves. *Be like them.*

I think I've almost talked myself into it! Well, almost.

6

The Art of Tipping

Questions of tipping bedevil people particularly because the custom seems to spread ever more widely and the amounts change constantly. For example, when should you tip? When should you not? How much is proper? Is it humiliating to undertip? Is it crass to overtip? When should you withhold a tip, and if you do, should you spell out exactly why you are withholding it, or should you just say nothing?

GENERAL GUIDELINES ON TIPPING

Most people feel that their moral obligation to tip ceases entirely when the service is rendered in an irritable, sloppy, or inefficient manner.

My philosophy is that you tip a great deal less when service is rendered in a negative way. Many people rely on their tips for the major part of their income, and to deprive them of every cent of what you had planned to give could be a real hardship. I always rationalize myself into giving an unpleasant person at least a small tip, because I feel (without any supporting evidence) that each time I encounter an obnoxious person, he or she has probably just lost a spouse or found out that the bank account is hopelessly overdrawn or that the children are in trouble at school—and that is why I am being treated so badly.

- *You most certainly should not give a tip when:*

o A person is *overtly* very hostile and rude.
o A cab driver deliberately takes you the long way to reach a destination, thus running up the meter far beyond what it should read.

- *If you feel the service should have been better:*

o Tip a little less than you would have normally.
o Explain in a nice, calm way why you have tipped less.

Be ready for a possible explosion, because some people can't take criticism and will always blame you, not themselves. Others will learn by your just criticism and will perform better in the future because of it.

At Restaurants

- *When you are dining in a fine restaurant, you tip:*

o 20 percent of the bill, minus wine and taxes, to the waiter (75 percent of this tip goes to the waiter and 25 percent to the captain)
o 8 percent of the cost of the wines to the sommelier (wine steward), with a minimum of $5
o $1 to the ladies' room attendant ($2 if she does something special for you like lending you a sewing kit, finding you safety pins, brushing you off, and the like)
o $10 to the maître d'hôtel, if he gave you a particularly good table or tried hard to please you
o $1 per coat to the coat check person ($2 if you have left tote bags, briefcase, dripping umbrella, and the like in addition to a coat)
o $2 to $5 to the doorman for getting you a taxi (depending on how difficult it was to get)
o $3 to the valet parker for bringing your car around

If you become mathematically confused by having to split the bill into different percentages, call the captain and tell him you "wish to split the twenty percent of the bill tip between him and the waiter, with the waiter receiving three-quarters of it." Then explain you want them to add to your total service charge a tip of 8 percent of the wine cost. Let them do the figuring. They will be only too glad to oblige, but be sure to take a copy of the credit card voucher with you to check for accuracy. Don't, however, make paying your bill a *cause célèbre*. You certainly do not want to ruin a splendid restaurant meal by taking an unduly long amount of time to check the bill and pay the tip. That can quickly ruin the lovely atmosphere of any successful dining experience.

- *When you are a host in a modest restaurant*, there are many fewer people to tip:

  o 15 percent of the total bill, including wine, to the waiter
  o $1 to the coat check person, if there is one

Valet Parking and Limousine Service

- *When you are a guest at a large private party*, usually the only person who needs tipping is the valet parker who finds your car for you. Inquire first if the host has taken care of tips, and if he or she has, then do not add another one. If the host has not, give the parker $2 in a large city, $1 in a smaller one.
- *If you are riding in a commercial limousine*,

  o In a large city, tip 20 percent of the bill.
  o In a smaller one, tip 15 percent.

The easiest way to handle it is to tell the limo service (when you contract for the driver) to put the proper percentage tip on your bill.

When You're Taking a Taxi

In a place like New York, you should pay a minimum of fifty cents tip for a ride. For a $5 ride, tip $1. For a $10 ride, tip $1.50 to $2. For a long ride, such as out to the airports from mid-Manhattan, you would pay 15 to 20 percent of the total in tips. (If the driver really helps you with your baggage, other than just lifting it into his trunk—this is in the category of a small miracle—you would tip him more, after you have recovered from the shock.)

In a place like Washington, D.C., where drivers are paid on a confusing zone system, you usually tip the shorter rides up to the next dollar. For example, if your bill is $3.60, you would give him $4, if your bill is $4.50, you would give him $5. When your bill goes a lot higher, you would tip him up to 20 percent of the total bill.

If you are caught in a horrendous traffic jam with a zone taxi driver, forget what you should pay according to zone. Pay him up to $5 more for his time and the trauma of the traffic jam. The same goes for a meter taxi driver. Even though he is paid a small amount while waiting in traffic, tip him nicely when you have been caught in traffic, because he loses money during the waiting period. (If my New York taxi driver doesn't complain loudly all the way to the airport during slow traffic, grousing and grumping all the way, I give him an extra $2 or $3 over the regular tip; if he does gripe the entire way, I wait until I'm out of the cab, then I give him $1 extra and tell him his bad humor at my expense has cost him $2.)

When You Are Staying in a Hotel or Motel

- *If it is a fancy, expensive place in a big city, give:*

  o $2 to the doorman.
  o $3 to the bellman—or, if a lot of luggage, is involved, $5 to $10. In a first-class hotel, you do not tip the person from the manager's office, who may show you the way to your room.
  o 20 percent of the room service bill (with a minimum of $2) to the room waiter each time food and drinks are brought. (Either give cash, or write it on the bill.)
  o $2 per night to the maid ($3 if two people are in the room). Leave it on your pillow, so she will know it is for her, and not just some cash you forgot.
  o $2 every time a bellman brings something to the room, other than room service—for example, a special newspaper you have requested or a basket of complimentary fruit sent by the management.
  o $5 for the bellman who does something special for you, like go to the drugstore to make a purchase or locate a strap for your broken suitcase.
  o $1 to $5 for the valet service when your cleaning and pressing is brought to you ($1 when it is one or two items, $5 when a raft of clothes has been laundered and pressed). Of course, if you are not in the room when it is delivered, there is no tip.
  o $2 for the doorman who gets your car brought from the parking area.
  o $1 to the doorman for getting you a cab.
  o $2 to $5 for a doorman who goes out in the rain for a long time to find you a cab.
  o $5 to a concierge who has made a real effort for you (such as getting good seats for you at a sold-out performance, handling your air tickets, and the like); $10 if the service was extraordinary.

If, of course, the concierge and the bellmen are not pressed into service to answer your needs, you do not tip them at all.

- *If you are in a less expensive hostelry or one in a small town, give:*

  o $1 to the doorman when you arrive or leave
  o $2 to the bellman—or, if a lot of luggage is involved, $3
  o 10 to 15 percent of the room service bill (with a minimum of $1) to the room waiter
  o $1 per night to the maid ($2 if two people are in the room)
  o 50 cents to $1 every time a bellman brings something to your room (not, however, room service)

- o $3 for the bellman who does something very special for you
- o $1 for the doorman who gets your car brought from the parking area

• *If you wish to forego most of the service* and carry your one small bag, you are perfectly at liberty to do so, but

- o If you're in a posh hotel, you should not carry even one small bag around—that is the bellman's job.
- o If you have a very large suitcase or are struggling with several items, you really should use a bellman. If you don't, it looks as though you're too cheap to tip one.
- o You are justified in carrying your own bag if you are very late leaving for your train or airplane and feel the bellman would appear too late.

• *When you are in a luxury resort hotel where the service is included,* everyone is taken care of in this kind of plan—from the maids to the waiters, from the captains to the pool attendants. However, after a weekend of being cared for, by an excellent maître d'hôtel in the dining room, you would give him—and him alone—a tip ($10 to $15 for a weekend for a family of four; $20 to $30 for a large family or group weekend).

If You're a Weekend Guest in a Home with a Domestic Staff

If you are fortunate enough to spend a long weekend or even a week as a guest of someone who is fortunate enough to have a domestic staff in the house, it's nice to demonstrate your gratitude for good service with a tip, even if you never lay eyes on some of the individuals who served you (as, for example, the cook).

• *Give the maid from $10 to $15 if she performed personal services for you,* such as

- o Unpacking your bags
- o Bringing you tea
- o Washing personal lingerie
- o Pressing some of your things at the end of the weekend

• *Give the cook (or leave for her with the mistress of the house)* $10. If you spend a whole week there, double the tip.

• If you're a really rare creature—a houseguest in a home with a *butler*—you would give him $20 for the weekend or for a houseparty.

• One friend of mine who lives in a beautiful house with a lovely garden—and has a large staff—reported that *the staff member who gets the biggest tips in her house is the gardener.* Each guest finds specially made bouquets of flowers from the garden placed in his or her bedroom each day—a kind of pampering that has all but disappeared.

• *If someone's private chauffeur drives you for more than a half hour*—such as out to the airport or from the country into the city—you might give him $5 to $10, depending on the length of the trip.

• You can always leave a lump sum with your host and have him or her distribute it equally among the staff.

Tipping in America has become more of a habit than a reward for special service. Most of the tips I have described above are not absolutely necessary, but in my opinion, life should not consist merely of attempts to fulfill the necessaries. A tip shows your appreciation for a job well done in your behalf, and it does help supplement an income, raise morale, and make a person like his job more.

When You're at the Hairdresser

This subject used to be divided into a man's barber and a woman's hairdresser, but the two have become unisex. Many men are having their hair washed and set, blow-dried, colored, permed, and given conditioning treatments as often as women—and in women's hair salons, too— even if there are still men like my husband who would not be caught dead in such a place and still go to a plain and simple man's barber.

• *At an expensive, posh place*, you would tip:

  ○ 20 percent of the total bill to your hairdresser if you're having a cut or color or a perm; 15 percent of the total bill if you are just having it washed and set or washed and blow-dried
  ○ $2 to the shampoo person
  ○ $2 minimum or 15 percent of the cost of the manicure to the manicurist

• *At a modest establishment*, you would tip:

  ○ 10 percent of the bill to the hairdresser
  ○ $1 to the shampoo person (if your hairdresser and shampoo person are one and the same, $1 more for the shampoo)
  ○ $1 to $2 to the manicurist

• *There is much confusion over whether the owner of the shop is tipped or not*. Many shop owners charge more for their services and do not take tips, as a result. Some shop owners do not take tips but do not charge more, because they mistakenly think it is not dignified.

The only way you can discover what the practice is when you approach a new hair salon is to ask when you are making your appointment. Just come right out with the question, "Does the owner, with whom I have an appointment, accept tips?" That is the only way you'll know, because everyone has his or her own way of managing the question.

When You Are in a Railroad Club Car

When you have a first class reserved seat in club car, you may be served a meal (part of the price of the ticket), which includes service. However, as you leave the train, if the porter has given you good service and helped you with your baggage, give him a $2 tip.

For overnight and lengthy train trips, you would give your porter $5 a night tip when you leave the train. (If he does extra special service for you, you might add a couple more dollars.)

Tip the Fast-Food Deliverer

Again, you are not obligated to tip the young person who brings something like a Domino's Pizza to your home, but it's nice to do it. Give $1 for one or two regular-size pizza boxes, but if you have a large quantity or a group of oversized pizzas delivered for a party, tip $5. Large quantities are difficult to handle, and a tip helps make the job easier.

HOLIDAY TIPPING

This is a vast and complicated subject, but here's a general rule of thumb: *You give a holiday tip or present, based on*

- o The kind of place (whether it's an expensive hair salon or restaurant, for example, or a modest one).
- o Your own personal resources and ability to give at holiday time.
- o Your personal relationship with the person being tipped.
- o The section of the country in which you live. (You are obliged generally to expend more in tipping in a city like New York, Chicago, or San Francisco, than you are in smaller places.)
- o How long you have used the service (how long your car has been in that garage, how many years you have been going to that masseuse, how many years your housecleaner has been in your employ).

A holiday present or gift of money is a very personal thing. I know one woman whose entire life is wrapped up in her dog and her cats. She gives lavish presents every year to her vet, her vet's receptionist, and the three people who operate the pet grooming salon she frequents.

I know another woman who spends all day working on fitness, sometimes with a trainer who comes to her home every so often. During the holidays she tips the trainer $40, the equivalent of the cost of one session. She also works out at her health club (and has the muscles to prove it). Since everyone around there is so slim and in shape, she ironically presents the staff each Christmas with boxes of chocolates or home-made cookies!

I also know a man who last Christmas gave $100 as a holiday tip to his French teacher. He explained to me, "After a year's hard work, she accomplished the impossible. I manage to speak the language passably."

Many people have well-kept lists of their Christmas gifts and tips carefully filed in their computers, so each year they simply look at what they did last year and update it.

The amount of money that Christmas costs individuals varies widely, according to their lifestyles and ability to spend. The following is a comparison of the financial outlay for the holidays of a rich New York divorcée in her sixties and a twenty-eight-year-old woman working in New York on a $30,000 salary. This is not a comparison of what they spent on presents for relatives and friends; this is what they spent on the people who work for or serve them during the year.

What an Affluent New York Divorcée Recently Gave in Holiday Tips

- *Beauty salon*

  - Hairdresser: $100 check and $225 ski sweater. (She sees him twice a week.) $325
  - Manicurist: $25 check and $50 silk scarf. (She sees her once a week.)   75
  - Shampoo person: $20 check   20
  - $20 boxes of chocolates to ten other staffers in that hair salon who do little things for her during the year   200
  - $50 check to the receptionist   50

Note: She also, of course, regularly tips these people when they do work for her during the week.

- *Health club*

  - Trainer: $100 check. (She sees him two or three times a week.)   100
  - Four other staff members, such as the locker room attendants: $25 each   100

- *Apartment staff*

o Superintendent of the building   200
o Eighteen service employees—doormen, back elevator
  men, relief men: $100 each.   1,800

- *Garage staff*

o Boss: $200; Seven men under him: $100 each   900

- *Personal Staff*

o Private Secretary (with her for fifteen years): $1000 plus a
  gold pin ($750)   1,750
o Personal maid (with her for twenty years): $1000 and new
  winter coat ($250)   1,250
o Cook (with her for ten years): $500 and new winter coat
  ($250)   750
o Driver (with her for three years): $200 and a sweater ($150)   350
o Three regular deliverymen from the grocer's: $25 each   75

- *Donations to employees' Christmas fund of three private clubs*

o $300 to each club   900

- *Tips to maître d'hôtels of her three main restaurants*

o $100 to each   300

                                            TOTAL: $9,145

What a Young New York Career Woman Recently Gave in Holiday Tips

o Contribution toward present for her shared secretary at
  the office $20.00
o Beauty salon
  Hairdresser: tin of imported cookies   10.00
  Three others at the salon: a Christmas card ($.50) with a
    chocolate santa ($5 each)   16.50
o Superintendent (who "does *everything*" for her)   35.00
o Once a week cleaning lady: $10 and $5 bottle of wine   15.00
o Deliveryman from her grocery: $5 in a $.50 Christmas card   5.50
o Her laundry deliveryman: $5 in a Christmas card   5.50
o Newspaper deliveryman: $5 in a Christmas card   5.50

                                            TOTAL: $113.00

Tipping the People Who Serve You in Your Home

Many people have baby-sitters, others cleaning ladies. A few fortunate people have full-time cooks. Whatever you have, if that employee is an integral part of your life and helps make living easier, he or she should be well remembered at Christmas. Anyone who is part of your personal household, even on a part-time basis, deserves a personal present, not just a gift of money. Here are some suggested gifts and tips for the holidays—just to get you thinking creatively for yourself.

- *If this person has been working for you only one or two years or less,* and she comes to you

Once a Week	Five Days a Week
Cleaning Lady: Blouse and $10	Sweater and $25
Baby sitter who spends several hours: Cassette tape and $10	Two cassettes and $50
Laundress: Blouse and $20	$25 food basket and $50 tip
Cook: Nightgown (or pajamas) and $50	Bathrobe and $100
Gardener: Book on gardens and $25	Book on gardens, two bottles of good wine, and $50

Note: If these staff members have been part of your family for years, double or even quadruple their cash gifts!

OTHER CATEGORIES OF STAFF IN AN AFFLUENT HOME

- *A live-in "au pair" girl* (who will be with you a year only):
- o $50 and something personal (like a pair of costume jewelry earrings)
- o A small gift to her from the children (for example, a book, pocket agenda, some of her favorite brand of makeup)

- *A live-in trained nanny for your children:*
- o $100 check
- o Perhaps something for her room (a new TV, nice lamp, new scatter rug)
- o A gift to her from your children (such as a flannel nightgown, good hand lotion, etc.)

IF YOU ARE VERY RICH AND LIVE IN A GRAND HOUSE

- *For the nanny:*
- o One month's salary equivalent (which might be as much as $2000)

○ A TV, VCR, or credit at a nearby video rental store
○ A personal gift from the children, such as a sweater

- *For a live-in housekeeper and/or cook:*

○ One month's salary equivalent (which could be from $1800 to $3000)
○ A gift from the employers*

- *For the butler:*

○ One month's salary equivalent (anything from $3000 to $5000)
○ A gift from the employers*

- *Part-time live-out secretary:*

○ $500
○ Good quality handbag

Holiday Tipping in Your Staffed Apartment House

People who live in luxury apartment houses in big cities have a major expense at holiday time in giving cash tips to every single person who works for the building. The bigger and the more luxurious the apartment house, the more generous the tenants are expected to be. In some apartment houses, tenants tip all through the year—every time the doormen gets them a taxi ($1), for example, or that the electrician, handyman, or plumber comes to fix something ($5, $10, or $20— according to the number of hours worked on the problem). In these buildings, the men are tipped modestly at Christmas—from $10 to $50, according to how long they have worked in the building.

In the older cooperative apartments, the tenants tip generously at Christmastime, because they tip only rarely for service during the year. As December approaches, the service in the building always seems to sparkle, as the doormen, elevator attendants, and service men rush to please and serve you. It's Christmas tip time!

You tip the people in your building according to:

○ How long you have lived there
○ How long each employee has been working there. (The old-timers, regardless of their jobs, are tipped more.)
○ How luxurious the building is
○ How much the employee does for you

---

*Something like a TV, VCR, or credit at a nearby video rental store

- *When you are single and have lived in a modest walkup, without any staff other than a super, you would tip him*

  o Perhaps $50 if he takes care of your mail and packages for you, helps you carry heavy things, and fixes your plumbing and stove problems
  o Only $20 if you hardly ever see him and he is not living on the premises, ready to help you

- *When you are single and have been in a luxury co-op for only a year, for example, you might give:*

  o $25 to the superintendent
  o $10 to each of the service employees (and there may be fifteen of them)

If one of the men has been there for twenty-five years, you would give him $5 more than the others; if one is new that year, you would give him $5 less than the others.

The more years you stay in that co-op, the higher you tip everyone. Your donation eases up every year, bit by bit—perhaps $2 to $5 more, and perhaps $25 more one year to someone who has really helped you during that year.

When you have a family, particularly with small children who are demanding of the doormen and back service people, you would tip the staff more each year, according to the size of your family. For example, a lawyer with a wife and three small children, living in a nice co-op on Riverside Drive in New York, tipped the super $75 and the service employees $25 each. A banker in a more lavish apartment on Fifth Avenue, who had lived there for eight years, with a wife and three small children, tipped the super $150 and the other service employees $50 to $75 each.

Apartment house personnel tipping is a very personal thing; no one tells you that you have to do this or that. You simply adjust what most people do in your building to your own financial abilities and to how much work the staff does for you. This includes such things as

  o Delivering your newspaper to your door each day
  o Getting you and your guests taxis
  o Taking your letters to the mail
  o Distributing your mail to you
  o Signing for and delivering your packages
  o Fixing your toilet when it leaks
  o Putting new batteries in your smoke detectors
  o Keeping your dog for you while you run back to the store to fetch what you forgot

I know an elderly couple who have been living in the same splendid building on Fifth Avenue for fifty years and are barely financially surviving. The staff does not expect grandiose tips from them, nor do they even want them, because this couple is gracious and good to all of them all year long.

When You Have Your Car in a Private Garage

Many people in large cities are forced to keep their cars in garages, where they pay monthly. Some people tip the men in the garage monthly.

Unless you are a monthly tipper, remember that at holiday time the men expect a tip from you for their tender loving care of your car. Some customers of a small garage distribute envelopes to the men because they know them all well. It is easier, however, to give a lump sum to the boss and have him distribute it equitably. (A new arrival would not get the same that a longtime worker would.) You can either donate a generous sum like $200 to a four-man garage, or the equivalent of one month's garage rent (which in New York goes easily as high as $500). In other parts of the country, the costs of garage space are not so high, so your Christmas tip to a hypothetical five-man garage might be $100.

Some big city garage owners post the names of their customers and the amounts they give at Christmas in a large poster on the wall. It's not an attractive thing to do, but it sure works!

Needless to say, the owner of a Rolls-Royce should give twice as bountiful a garage tip at Christmas as the owner of a Toyota, and the owner of several cars housed in the garage should look upon his cars as spoiled children being lovingly tended by the garagemen. His tip should be very generous—commensurate with the attention that is lavished on his fleet.

TIPPING AND TRAVEL OUTSIDE THE COUNTRY

When You Take a Cruise

Since there are different tipping systems for different cruises, the best way to find out how to tip on your cruise is to

- Discuss tipping procedures with an official of the cruise line while you are booking your passage.
- Ask your travel agent to find out the information before you leave on the trip.
- Ask the advice of a friend who has just returned from a similar cruise.

   o Question the ship's purser when you're on board. By the way, *never tip the ship's officers!*

Whether you have booked a luxury cabin or the least expensive kind, here is one popular system of tipping:

   • *On embarking, establish good relations by dispensing some cash tips.* For example, give $5 or $10 when you first board to your cabin steward when he or she does some small favor for you; slip $5 into the hand of your dining steward at the first meal, and tell him "how glad you are to be in his care on this trip." This generosity will mean additional pampering while you're on board, and there is nothing wrong with that!

   • *At the end of a short cruise,* tip your cabin steward and your dining room steward $3 per day minimum.

   • Keep some dollars in your pocket to give out on an impromptu basis—for example, to the pool attendant or the tea steward, if you see them only occasionally and if you do not expect to give them a tip envelope when the voyage is over.

   • It's wise to pay for and include the tip (15 to 20 percent of the total bill) for your drinks in the bar as you go along. Of course, if you prefer, you may run up a tab that you pay on the last day. (Paying as you go makes it less of a shock to settle up when you disembark for good.)

   • Give the wine steward 10 percent of the total wine bill, although some bar regulars tip 15 percent.

   • Tip the service people (like hairdressers and masseurs) as you would on land—15 to 20 percent of the total bill each time.

   • *On a long cruise, tip some people once a week.* For example, tip the

   o Chief dining room steward $20 a week
   o Assistant dining room steward $10 a week
   o Your dining room steward $25 a week
   o Your deck steward $20 a week
   o Your cabin steward $25 a week

   • Remember, if you are a couple or a family, you should tip three-fourths more per person in your family than you would tip if you were alone.

   • Remember, too, if you are a famous, rich person, you should be generous with your tips. (Your public image begins to drop perceptibly if you're known around the ship as a "skinflint.")

   • *When your cruise is over,* put all your tips—cash or checks—into separately addressed envelopes the last day at sea, and hand them personally to each person. It's very nice to put a little note inside each envelope, expressing your thanks—"You took extraordinarily good care of us . . ."; "I will miss all those wonderful meals you served me so well . . ."; "You made the entire trip such a pleasure for my wife and me."

Yes, tipping is a complicated question on a cruise. If anyone on board was nasty to you (very unlikely), you should greatly reduce the tip—but remember, it does represent a large part of the income of the employees of the ship.

There are now cruises in operation that build a hefty service charge into the cost of the cruise, and in this case there is no tipping. That may be the wave of the future.

When You Are in a Foreign Country

It would require an entire book to cover the subject of tipping abroad. The practice is varied and custom-tailored to each culture. You must be very discreet and secretive about your tipping in the Far East— if you do it at all—and yet you should be flamboyant about it in countries like Egypt.

You tip the usher at plays and movies in Paris each time you're shown to your seat, but not at the Comédic Française, because it's government theater. You leave a small tip at a French cafe for your *café filtre*, sometimes not at an Italian espresso bar. The rules on tipping taxi drivers and gas station attendants differ from country to country. In many countries the service at hotels and meals is included (*"le service est compris"*), and in Switzerland, they take the "service included" seriously. In many other countries, it is customary to leave an additional tip on the table for the waiter even with the *service compris.*

Consult a reputable guidebook before you go to any foreign country. Chat with an American who has lived in that country, or question someone on the plane on the way over who knows the country's customs well. Write it all down—what percentage you tip the taxi driver, the waiter, the coatcheck person, the bellman, the hairdresser. Make a detailed list, get your answers, and then you'll feel secure in what you're doing. Or ask your travel agent ahead of time.

* * *

Having spelled out the proprieties of tipping, I must emphasize that a tip is not the ultimate reward. How you treat those who serve you is far more important than the size of your tip.

I have seen big spenders throwing around $100 tips in the same casual way that children stuff pennies into their piggy banks. I have also seen lavish tippers treat people as though they were chattel, ordering them around in loud, arrogant tones.

When you show dignity and respect for a person's job, and when you express your thanks and a compliment, it means much more to that individual than a handful of dollars condescendingly proffered by a rude, mean person. Anyone in a service industry—anyone who waits on you and helps you function more comfortably as you move through your day—deserves nothing less than your recognition and sincere appreciation.

Remember, too, something else that is more powerful than a tip—a letter sent to management when you wish to commend the performance of an employee or group of employees. That kind of commendation is entered into their personnel files and helps them get faster promotions in the future.

7

Dressing Appropriately

This is not a fashion book, so this short chapter will contain only a few guidelines and a fashion philosophy—my own.

It is impossible to talk about the right kind of attire without mentioning that the way you look depends not only on how you dress, but also on

- o Your posture and bearing—the way you move in your clothes
- o Your grooming (without good grooming, *nothing* is fashionable or right)

It is also better to invest in a few quality things than in a rash of lesser-quality wardrobe items. Clothing made of good fabric and in a good cut lasts for years. For example, if you amortize the cost of what a good man's or woman's suit costs, over a period of three to four years' wear, you have bought a real bargain!

PROPRIETY AND APPROPRIATENESS

Of course, you can ruin your entire fashionable image if you break the laws of propriety. If you are a woman attending a concert after the office at which everyone else in the audience is dressed in business and daytime attire while you are in a sexy black dress with a sheer black chiffon top, you are inappropriately dressed. Music-lovers don't care that you paid $2500 to buy a leading American designer's dress that you first spotted in a fashion magazine. In their eyes, you are inappropriately dressed for the occasion because people will be staring at you, to the detriment of concentration on the music. If you are ever in a quandary as to whether a certain invitation or a certain activity requires you to dress modestly, stop wondering. Dress modestly and you will always be right!

At Church or Temple

We may be living in a very relaxed, informal time, but that still does not excuse anyone who goes to services in a house of worship dressed inappropriately.

Summertime is the season that sees the worst offenses. You see a landscape of men in underwear shirts, even bare chests, and women parading on the street in short shorts with bare midriffs. Fortunately, we don't often see the worst cases of these in church or temple, but inappropriate informality is still all too common.

Men and women should really not attend religious services in shorts (except in places like Bermuda, where shorts are a summer uniform for the men, but are properly worn with high knee socks and brightly polished leather shoes). It draws attention to you and is not respectful in the house of God. A woman in a skimpy tennis dress or shorts can throw on a coverup for church. A man can throw on a pair of slacks over his shorts for the services. This advice is for those who believe in God and go to worship Him. It is little enough to ask that you dress respectfully for Him.

THE RIGHT THING TO WEAR—WOMEN

• *Remember that fashion has to fit your lifestyle, age, figure, and job.* If something is new and bizarre, don't chance it. Leave it for the models and young people in the creative service businesses. Wait until three months after some strange new fashion trend bursts across the scene. It either will fizzle out like a spent firecracker or it will be tempered into a style that will look good on you.

- *If you have a figure problem*, ask your friends which outfits look best on you. In this way you will learn the kind of styles and cuts that should guide your choices in the future.
- *Always check yourself out in a three-way mirror in the store and always sit down on a chair in front of that mirror* before you buy any dress or pants. A frank appraisal is a very good exercise before handing over your credit card.
- *Know when and where to wear pants*.

  o It's okay to wear pants for sports and physical work.
  o Don't wear them on formal occasions, such as to a wedding. (I don't think they ever look right in church, as a matter of fact, but that's a personal opinion.)
  o Don't wear pants if you have big thighs and a wide rear end and care about how you look in public.

- *Your hemlines should reach to the best point on your leg*

  o As fashion dictates that season
  o As the shape of your legs dictates
  o As your age dictates
  o As your seniority in your office and your job allows

In other words, if you're young and have great legs, wear your skirts short, but *only if that is the fashion that season*. If you're over forty, you're wise not to raise your hems far above the knees, regardless of how proud you are of your legs and even if ten-inch-long skirts are the current hot fashion. By the time you're forty, decorum should become a qualifying factor in your appearance.

What You Wear to a Cocktail Party

  o A dressy suit—sometimes called a cocktail suit or theater suit—for example, a black wool or crepe suit with rhinestone buttons or a satin or velvet suit.
  o A woman with a great figure is appropriately dressed for a cocktail party in a dressy pants suit.
  o A short dressy dress of crepe, silk, brocade, chiffon, even cotton in hot weather, either covered up or décolleté, is worn with dressy sandals or pumps. A small "cocktail bag" of silk, velvet, brocade, satin, or peau de soie is carried with this costume.
  o Accessories might be

    A satin bow or ornament in the hair
    Long sparkly earrings and bracelet
    Jeweled button earrings and a necklace or very simple, unadorned jewelry
    Never wear all these accessories at the same time.

What You Wear to a Black Tie Affair

o Long, short, or three-quarter-length evening gown; evening sandals or pumps; and an evening bag of silk, satin, peau de soie,
   velvet, or brocade material
o Jewelry—same as for cocktail party, only slightly more of it
o A fur, if you have one

What You Wear to a White Tie Affair

o A full-skirted grand ballgown
o Lots of jewelry
o Fur wrap
o Long white gloves

What you don't have, you can borrow—or rent—but the possibility
of having to prepare for a white tie occasion is very marginal.

What You Wear to Someone's Private Club

o Daytime dress or suit for lunch
o Cocktail attire for dinner

If there are going to be sports activities, ask your hosts what to
wear, because some clubs won't permit you in the dining room for lunch
in your playing clothes, and some clubs require whites for the tennis
courts. The only way you can be sure of being appropriately attired is to
ask questions of your host.

Women at Their Offices

• *It's wise not to wear pants in the more conservative areas of the
corporate world.* Pants, *but on a great figure only,* are for creative
businesses such as television, film, advertising, fashion, and retailing.
Shorts, even long shorts, are really not appropriate anywhere in business.

• *You should wear nothing glittery in jewelry or fabrics.* Those are
for evening only.

• *Wear quiet jewelry only.* The means no clanking earrings, noisy
bracelets, or dangling necklaces that jingle. Also, it is best to limit
yourself to a minimum of jewelry.

• *A minimum of makeup is also wise.* That means no false eye-
lashes, heavy mascara, or visible eyeshadow. (No bizarre nail polish,
either, like purple, or nails decorated with flowers!)

- *Never wear revealing, sexy, slinky dresses at the office.* You might get a free dinner and then some out of it, but you might also lose your job.
- *Don't dress like "Miss Prim" at the office.* You should

  o Never try to look like a man—or Little Orphan Annie, either.
  o Never be boring, with a little mannish suit, string tie, and man's shirt. If you have these in your wardrobe, throw out the string tie or necktie, buy some bright-colored or interestingly patterned blouses, perhaps a great scarf, or put a smashing clip on your lapel.

- *Dress in fashion.* When you shop, take someone whose taste you trust with you. You want to look with-it, not mousey-drab, and you want to look *right for you*, not slavishly follow the dictates of the fashion magazines.

THE RIGHT THING TO WEAR—MEN

To begin with, let me note that I am being *very* personal here in my likes and dislikes.
- *If you work for a conservative firm*, dress as the other men do— conservatively. Save your avant-garde Italian styles for your weekends.
- *If you have a weight problem*, dark-colored, single-breasted suits are best for you.
- *Wear a lightweight suit in hot summer weather.* A winter-weight fabric makes others hot looking at it, not to mention what the wearer must be feeling.
- *Brown suits are only for the fashion-secure*, so if you are not a fashion-plate, stay away from them.
- *Three-piece suits are the most conservative look of all.* They wax and wane in popularity. Sometimes you see a lot of them; other times it seems they're going out of style.
- *If you're worried about what to wear on an informal weekend gathering*, you can't go wrong with a dark blue blazer and gray wool slacks. Check with your host to see if you are supposed to wear a tie; if you are a very junior executive, forget about wearing a foulard at the neck. That's only for a senior executive or for Cary Grant's film replacement.
- *A polo shirt or sweater* looks great with slacks for a casual-dress event. A t-shirt does not.
- Remember, you can buy a $1200 suit, but it won't help you at all sartorially if you are a tonsorial disaster.

• *Never pair the top of a business suit with a pair of casual slacks*. It doesn't work. Only a blazer or a sports jacket does the job for a casual look.

• *White athletic socks* are fine when worn with loafers, sneakers, or running shoes and shorts for leisure or vacation wear. Avoid them at all other times.

Men's Fashion Disasters

• *Watch your socks when you sit down*. If there's a section of hairy leg showing between the top of your socks and the bottom of your trousers, you know it's time for action. Quick, to the store for some over-the-calf-length socks (and you may need garters)!

• *Holes in your socks* are another downer. Combine the hole-y socks with scuffed-up shoes, and you're in real trouble.

• *Short-sleeved business shirts worn without a jacket in the office* look terrible in most people's opinion, even if they don't have the courage to admit it. When it's hot and you're jacketless, you can always roll up the sleeves of your long-sleeved shirt.

• White dress socks are

    o Fine with an all-white summer suit
    o Simply terrible with black or brown street shoes and a suit
    o Even *worse* when worn with black street shoes and shorts at a resort

• Another real downer is *a shirt that's too small*, with pillows of fat bursting out between the buttons.

• *Watch those loud plaids*. Fred Astaire wore them beautifully; so do horses in their blankets.

Your Ties

If people are always teasing you about your ties, let someone pick out your next ones for you.

    o A tall man needs an extra-long tie; a heavy-set man needs a wide one.
    o Wear your most conservative ties when your suits have a strong pattern or color; wear your bright or interestingly patterned ones with your most conservative dark suits.
    o Pick up a color from your shirt for your tie, or vice-versa, so there is instant color coordination.

Your Jewelry

Less is more. A wristwatch, a gold signet ring, and a wedding ring are enough. More than one gold bracelet begins to be too conspicuous, and lots of gold chains lying in a jungle of chest hair, with the shirt proudly open at the neck to display it, is something most of us can live without viewing—permanently.

What You Wear to a Black Tie Affair

The classic black dinner suit (tuxedo) is always best. For resort wear, a man in a white dinner jacket with black evening trousers looks wonderful, but an all-black tuxedo looks trimmer, slimmer, patently more handsome. It is *always right.*

- *A white or colored (or patterned silk foulard) handkerchief* is often tucked into a dinner jacket's upper pocket to add a touch of panache.

- *Never never wear a brocaded, satin, or patterned dinner jacket.* (I also recently saw a sequin-trimmed jacket and mistook its wearer for a member of the band, not a guest.)

Winter Black Tie Variation

A jacket of a very dark jewel color or black velvet with black trousers (sometimes worn with velvet embroidered slippers in addition) would be worn only to a dinner party in someone's home, not in a public place.

- *The shirt:*

  o White, off-white, or very pale pastel
  o Pleated, never ruffled
  o Worn with a black tie of grosgrain, satin, or velvet (sometimes red or brocaded, for the holidays)

Some people like evening shirts with wing collars and small black bow ties. I am definitely not of that group, although I think such shirts look great on waiters.

- *The trousers* have black satin stripes down the sides. You may choose trousers with self-belted waists or trousers held up by suspenders (braces) that are buttoned or clipped onto the waistband.

- *An evening vest* (of black silk, velvet, or satin) or *a cummerbund* (usually matching the bow tie) is optional.

- *The shoes and socks:* Black patent dress pumps or dress oxfords are best. Black patent loafers are often worn, too, but are not as nice. Thin, long black silk hosiery is appropriate.

• *Jewelry:* Wear small cufflinks and studs of gold or pearl, and with small stones, if desired.

• *A gray or black velvet-collared Chesterfield coat, gray gloves, and a gray fedora* are stylish, if you really want to finish off your outfit with flair.

FOR A SUMMER BLACK TIE EVENT

For summer or resort wear, men often break out in plaids, stripes, or bright-colored dinner jackets, worn with black trousers; sometimes the trousers are very colorful, so a black jacket is then worn with them. A dress white shirt and a black tie complete the costume, although in summer there are often colorful matching cummerbunds and bow ties to brighten up a black tuxedo. Summer is the time for creativity, color, and pattern to take hold.

What You Wear to a White Tie Affair

Until 1960, white ties were often in evidence for grand soirées. Even if the chances are slight that you will ever have to wear this kind of formal wear—unless you get married in white tie and tails—it's fun to know what it's all about.

o Tailcoat of black wool and silk
o White piqué tie with a stiff wing collar
o Starched white shirtfront
o White waistcoat
o Black patent pumps or dress oxfords with black silk hose
o Pearl, diamond, or onyx studs and cufflinks
o White kid gloves
o Black silk top hat (optional)

A Final Word of Advice

Men should heed the same advice women are given: "Take someone with you whose taste you *know* is good before investing in a major purchase."

* * *

In summary, one might describe well-dressed people as those who dress properly for their job and their social life; who buy clothes according to fashion, but also according to their figure and age; who have good powers of observation so that they can learn good taste from others who have it; who know how to look at themselves mercilessly in a mirror before making a major purchase; and who would never ruin a terrific-looking outfit by a lapse in good posture or grooming.

You may find all this difficult at first, but with practice it becomes instinctive, and then you'll hear yourself described as someone who really knows how to dress.

8

Common
Courtesies

It is reassuring to realize that the basis of contemporary manners is not a group of rules concocted by unknown people yesterday. They are rooted in long-established principles of decent behavior toward others (even though their outer forms may have changed with the times).

We can see this well exemplified in a little book that George Washington copied and edited (as a school exercise) when he was only fifteen. It is titled *Rules of Civility & Decent Behavior in Company and Conversation*. I was privileged to be asked to write the introduction to the new edition.* George Washington's exhortations on behalf of common courtesies are still relevant. He writes in his own style, as shown here, making spelling, punctuation, and grammatical errors. However, his advice is plain, simple common sense—and timely. For example, he

- Warns us not to be party crashers. ("Go not thither, where you know not, whether you Shall be Welcome or not.")
- Tells us not to be critical. ("Reprehend not the imperfections of others for that belongs to parents Masters and Superiours.")

*On sale to benefit Mount Vernon, from Mount Vernon Ladies' Association, Mount Vernon, VA 22121. Send $5.95 plus $1.50 for postage and handling.

o Teaches us deference, something young executives would do well to heed in regard to senior management. ("When you meet with one of Greater Quality than yourself, Stop, and retire expecially if it be at a Door or Any Straight place to give way for him to Pass.")

o Promotes kindness. ("Shew not yourself glad at the Misfortune of another though he were your enemy.")

o Calls for discreet behavior in public. ("Do not laugh too loud or too much at any Publick Spectacle.")

o Advocates the proper form of address in writing business letters and in making introductions. ("In writing or Speaking, give to every Person his due Title According to his Degree & the Custom of the Place.")

o Warns against bad company. ("Associate yourself with Men of good Quality if you Esteem your own Reputation; for 'tis better to be alone than in bad Company.")

o And cautions against becoming a bore. ("Be not Tedious in Discourse or in reading unless you find the Company pleased therewith.")

George Washington's boyish *Rules of Civility* brought him to the attention of the powerful English land-owner Lord Fairfax of Virginia, who made him a surveyor and included him along with the British nobility in the estate's important social activities. It was here that Washington learned polished manners and social dexterity, assets that helped him gain the leadership of the army and eventually of his country. His rules prove that good manners, morals, ethics, and honest values are one and the same. Today's writers on this subject can only reinforce his wisdom in modern terms. If Washington were alive today, he might be addressing some of these subjects.

COURTESIES APPROPRIATE TO WHERE YOU ARE

Here are some thoughts about common courtesies we should all be practicing today to make life a little kinder and gentler all around.

On the Street as Pedestrian or Driver

• *Jaywalking and crossing against the traffic light* are illegal and dangerous and could result in a person's death. They are also rude actions. A defiance of the law by an arrogant pedestrian requires drivers to slam on the brakes, makes tempers short, and at times causes the driver to desire another meeting with that lawbreaker—this time to run him down, not save his life!

Washington would have written, with several errors in spelling and capitalization of words: "A person wishing to cross the street should wait patiently at the corner or cross-walk for the green light, and look carefully both ways before proceeding—even when the light turns green."

• *On the other hand, a driver who swings relentlessly into a crowd of pedestrians while making a turn can incite the emotions of a lynch mob in the hearts of those pedestrians.* A driver should calm down when trying to turn, will patience into him- or herself, and wait until after the pedestrians have crossed with the green light. This requires incredible self-control when thoughtless, exasperated drivers of the cars behind, who are also trying to make the turn, are blasting away on their horns to show how they feel about the slowness of the proceedings.

• *Be a considerate car parker.* A sloppy car parker makes life difficult for everyone. When you park, give yourself enough room to be able to get out of the spot, but don't park in such a way as to prohibit parking for two other cars who could otherwise fit into the space.

• *Except in cases of emergency, forget you have a horn.* An ear-shattering blast of your automobile horn just because you are irritated about something ruins the peace of hundreds of people around you, not just the person who made you angry. When you are in a traffic jam of cars unable to move, blaring away on your horn, you are doing everyone a great disservice.

• *Drive with your lights at low beam at night when cars are coming at you from the other direction.* It is really rude—and dangerous—to permit your brights to blind the drivers proceeding from the other direction.

• *If you are a slow driver (and there's nothing wrong with that), stay in the right-hand lane.* Otherwise, you can cause havoc with drivers who want to go faster and must therefore do a lot of lane-switching.

On Public Transportation

• *Say a cheery hello to the driver when you board the bus, and say thank-you when you leave.* The driver certainly deserves your recognition—and gratitude, too—because he or she has, after all, had your life in his or her hands for a short while.

• *As you board, and see someone running hard to catch this bus, notify the driver and ask him or her to wait.* (This same philosophy should motivate you to hold open the door of an elevator when you see someone running to make it before the door closes.)

• *Male or female, you should get up and give your seat to any older person who looks frail, to anyone who is blind or disabled or carrying crutches, or to a very pregnant woman.* Until the mid-1960s, this kind of rule did not have to be included in a book on manners. It was something everyone took for granted. Not any more!

• *Silence is golden on a bus, train, or subway,* which means that your well-behaved children do not play their own radios, and that they pipe down rather than become loud and boisterous.

At Movies and in the Theater

• *Silence is golden during a performance.* Don't crack gum, rattle candy wrappers, or whisper.

• *Arrive on time, so that when taking your seats you are not disrupting the view and the ambience on stage.*

• *Stay until the end of the performance.* It's very disconcerting for a performer to see and hear people getting up and leaving the theater, whatever the reason. If you have to leave early, you can always stand at the back of the theater for the last act or the last part of the program, so that your departure will not be distracting.

• *When you enter a filled row to take your seat, proceed facing the people in your row, not the stage.* In this way the people you are disturbing can look at your face, not at your rear end, as you apologize for crawling over them.

• *Pick up your candy wrappers, empty boxes of popcorn, and soda cans after the performance, and deposit them in the trash receptacle in the lobby.* Everyone will love you for it—just as they despise the person who leaves all the aforementioned litter squishing around on the floor.

In the Supermarket

• *Restrain your child from grabbing merchandise off the shelves as you push your cart down narrow aisles.* Don't allow the child to throw items down on the floor somewhere or to open packages and eat from them without your paying for that at the checkout counter.

• *When something has been knocked off into the aisle, whether it was an act of God, or a selfish human being who did it, pick it up and put it back.* This will make it easier for other shoppers to go about their business without having to run a giant slalom race with their carts.

• *Maneuver your shopping cart with grace and concern for others.* Park the cart considerately, so that other shoppers can pass you easily with their carts as you stand looking at shelf offerings.

• *When you're in the checkout line with a cart full of many purchases and the person behind you has only two or three items, wave him or her ahead of you.* It's a "do unto others as you would have others do unto you" act of kindness.

• *When you are finished unloading the groceries into your car, bring your shopping cart from the parking area to the cart storage area in the store.* Customers who leave carts out in the parking lot, instead of returning them, make it difficult for others to park their cars. The store employees then have to interrupt their regular jobs to cope with the mess.

At the Beach or Camping

The wilderness—whether it's a beach, a forest campsite, a mountain trail, or a lakeside panorama—*is precious and should be carefully protected by all of us*, so that our descendants will also have it to enjoy one day. We should also be respectful of the people around us, who have come for vacation, just some hours of peace, to fish, or to have a chance to meditate, dream, and watch for birds. Courtesies to the wilderness are courtesies to human beings at the same time. For example:

• *Every proof of your having been in any area should disappear by the time you leave it.* Every piece of litter should be disposed of in plastic bags that you take away with you and deposit in a proper receptacle (perhaps in your own garbage can at home). Not even a paper tissue should be visible.

• *Hold down the sound if there are other people within earshot, and that includes your favorite radio program or cassette tapes.*

• *If you made a fire, follow the safety rules for extinguishing it.* Don't just cover the coals or embers with sand. Throw water on them and thoroughly douse them first. (Have you ever walked over what you thought was sand but proved to be just a light covering of still-hot coals?)

• *If you're swimming in the ocean with a mattress or surfboard, or if you're wind-surfing or in any kind of a boat, watch where you're going and what you're doing.* It is not only rude but hazardous, while merrily riding the waves on your mattress, to run into a person who's peacefully swimming nearby. You could cause a serious accident that way.

It's important to teach your children that young daredevils who do outrageous things on something like a surfboard or any kind of boat, endangering the public around them, are immature show-offs and not worthy of being worshipped and adored.

At a Pool

• *The first rule concerning a friend's swimming pool is not to be forward in asking to use it. Wait until the friend invites you.* People with pools complain that their friendships with others are tested to extreme limits by "friends" who expect to be able to use the pool all the time, who want to bring along their noisy children and houseguests, and then even friends of friends. There are times when the owners of a pool want no one but themselves using it, and it is their right to demand some peace and quiet for themselves.

• *If you are fortunate enough to be invited, don't take the pool invitation as one to use the house, too.* Pool owners complain that the people they have invited "for a swim" often wander through their house at will, using their telephones, their kitchen, and bathrooms (even though there is a bathroom at the pool house). One friend told me she really resents people washing their towels in her washing machine without even asking her!

• *Remember, never use a friend's pool without knowing exactly the hours for which it is convenient for your host to have you,* or without your hosts' having given permission for everyone you bring with you (including your children). One pool owner told me that if one more person brings along a noisy, pesky uninvited dog, he is going to call the police.

• *Always shower before entering the pool.* Many pool owners die a thousand deaths as they see their friends lacquer themselves with sun oil, mix it well with sweat from hours spent sun-bathing, and then enter their pools. If there is no pool shower, use a garden hose.

• *Don't use your host's towels.* Always offer to bring your own. Some people will tell you not to bother; others will think you're the nicest guest they have ever had.

• *Be sensitive to whether the people lying around the pool want to talk, read, or go to sleep.* Play it by ear. Keep your ebullient personality to yourself if the prostrate bodies around you seem to be intent on remaining quiet or if they have their heads buried in books.

• *At the end of the season, give your pool host a gift, as well as writing a grateful letter of thanks.* It might be a useful gift that you noticed would be nice for the pool—for example, a new ice bucket to replace the old one, some lanterns to illuminate the area at night, some guest hand towels of paper, soap holders for the dressing room bathroom(s), a shower caddy for soap and shampoo to hang on a wall of the stall shower, and the like.

• *Keep your children in your view at all times—not only to keep them quiet, but also to keep them safe.* Teach them the importance of never crying "Wolf!" when they are in danger—a major lesson to learn in life.

In Golf or Tennis Games

• *Never pretend to be a better player than you are.* You can make enemies for life if you have boasted about your prowess, and then suitable partners and opponents have been lined up, but then you drag down the entire game by not being half as proficient as you said you were. It is far better to be modest and play at your own level, or to be modest but good and have your partner and opponents discover how good you are.

• *Take every game appointment you make seriously.* Don't be a no-show or cancel out at the last minute. If you must cancel a foursome, for example, find someone to substitute for you so that you don't ruin the fun of the other three.

• *Know every rule of the game before venturing out to play it.* No one should have to teach you the ins and outs of the sport while you're playing it. Get a book. Take a lesson. Talk to people, but don't go out to play without knowing the rules, how the game is scored, and how to hold and use the equipment.

• *Bring the proper equipment and clothing.* A person who arrives ill-equipped or improperly attired and then causes a great delay in the game in order to rectify the situation is a real killjoy. A person who never contributes a new can of tennis or golf balls, but always relies on the others to bring them, is regarded in the same manner as the person who never picks up the check for a meal.

• *Rigorously adhere to the rules of playing through on the golf course, of waiting to cross someone else's tennis court in order to reach your own, or of waiting to chase a ball on another's court while their ball is in play.*

• *Never give excuses for being off your game.* No one cares if you have a blister on your heel or are suffering from a hangover. They just want you to play your best.

• *Watch your language while you're playing.* Four-letter words simply don't belong in amateur sports. People within earshot immediately form a very bad opinion of you. (Bad language doesn't belong in professional sports either, but at least in that category the players are fighting for their livelihoods, not just playing a sport for the fun of it.)

• *The player who accuses or blames a partner for their combined poor scores is about as popular as someone with the bubonic plague.* A person of good character always bucks up his or her partner when that person is playing badly, and always blames him- or herself when the pair loses. After all, if you played well but your partner played badly, everyone present knows it. The nice (and sporting) thing to do is to accept the blame as part of the team. In other words, *always smile when you lose.*

• *Be very mindful of the course or court on which you are playing. Always leave it in perfect condition.* If you have cut up the green, replace the divot, smooth it, fix it. If someone has made some big dents on the court surface, smooth it over with your foot. Put the net back to the right height if it has sagged. Think of the people who will be following you to play.

• *When you take leave of the other player or players, always shake hands; thank them and leave with a smile on your face.* Some people are such poor sports that they can't bring themselves even to smile and say good-bye when they are angry at themselves (or their partners), but fortunately that is not *you*!

COURTESIES TO OBSERVE WITH THOSE YOU ENCOUNTER DURING YOUR DAY

Your Manners with the Expert Professionals Who Serve You

When you engage a professional for his or her services, naturally you want the best service for the money you will spend. But don't forget, that professional is a fellow human being, too, who looks for and appreciates signs of respect from clients. You can be sure that the client who establishes a friendly, courteous relationship will get the best service.

- o *Respect the professional* (whether your lawyer, doctor, or banker) *for that person's education and experience.*
- o *When a professional has performed a service exceptionally well for you, let that person know it.* You show you are a person of class when, even though you may have paid for the services rendered, you also express appreciation for the fine effort made for you. (This holds true whether an interior designer has made your house look wonderful, your investment counselor has made money for you, or your dentist did a great job capping your teeth.)
- o *Keep your appointments punctually.* Time is money for a professional. That also means that random chit-chat is inappropriate during an appointment with someone like a lawyer or surgeon.
- o *Don't take for granted anyone you consider to be a personal friend.* And most certainly do not try to get free advice in social situations (such as asking a lawyer a personal legal question in the middle of a golf game or cornering a doctor at a cocktail party to ask him about a health problem). Make an appointment—and pay for that advice.

Your Manners with Waiters

- o Give him (or her) your attention when he comes to tell you the specialties and take your order. Don't expect that to be done properly if everyone is joking, talking, and paying no attention to the person trying to do his job.
- o If you keep changing your mind, don't lose your temper over subsequent errors. (It's not the waiter's fault.)
- o Call him "Waiter" (or "Waitress"); don't snap your fingers at him to get his attention.
- o When something goes wrong with the order, do not voice criticisms at the waiter that everyone can hear. There are other

factors—the kitchen help, for example—that could be responsible for what went wrong. When something is incorrect, inform the waiter in a quiet voice that cannot be heard by others.

o When things go well, praise him and thank him—and tell the owner or manager, "Your waiter did a good job for us tonight."

Your Manners with Tradespeople and Salespeople

Tradespeople wish to be—and deserve to be—treated with respect and friendliness. When they are, they serve you more efficiently—and like their jobs a lot better, too.

o Don't just bark a command at a salesperson. First say hello and smile, then state what you want. Some people are so intent on having their own request satisfied that they fail to hear the clerk's nice "Good morning." Even if the clerk says nothing to you, toss a warm hello in his or her direction. It will make that person feel good, as well as eager to please you with the service.

o If you know the person's name, use it. When you remember the name of someone who serves you, it shows you respect that person.

o Communicate what you want in a clear and thorough manner. Don't expect the hair colorist in the beauty salon to be a psychic and know without being told that you wanted a golden blond instead of an ash blond tint today. Don't expect the salesclerk to know that you only buy support hose, not the regular kind. Don't expect the barber to automatically know the exact cut you want. Too often we think that people see the whole picture when we throw them just a detail. Explain everything carefully and slowly, so that those who serve you will do well by you.

o Keep any patronizing tone out of your voice. That person on the other side of the counter or the plumber working under your kitchen sink feels (and is) no less important than you.

o Make conversation with whomever is serving you whenever you are waiting for something. A stony silence throws a barrier between you. A friendly chat about anything from the weather to how the Cubs are doing this season will put you on comfortable, equal ground.

o Thank the other person for every service rendered, however small, and don't forget your smile (whether it's a smile of approval or of camaraderie is irrelevant).

o When someone has been particularly helpful to you, write a letter to that person's superior. It will be kept in his or her personnel file and could result in a promotion.

Your Manners with Strangers Encountered Along the Way

Whether you go to school, have a job, or are running a household, almost every day of your life you encounter people whose names you do not know and may never learn, people who just happen to be in the same place at the same time as you.

Your method of interacting with these people is very telling about your basic character. You can ignore every stranger you see. Or you can do just a little something nice every once in a while to bring a little happiness into someone else's life. For example:

- If you give a person a warm smile for no reason, it might give a lift to the spirits of someone who is depressed.
- If someone is having difficulty getting through a revolving door and you slow it down so that he or she will be able to get through, you just might be giving that person the one nice moment in his or her day.
- If on the bus you see someone older, looking very tired and frail, and you get up to give that person your seat, the other person may not thank you properly, but he or she will be grateful to you.
- If the person ahead of you is about to drop packages or is laden with suitcases and bundles and you step up to flag the taxi for him or her, then open the taxi door and help that person inside, you will make that person far happier than you can realize.
- When you emerge from a taxi and see someone running to hail it and you leave the door open and tell the driver to wait, you are going to be loved by that running figure for having done such a kindness, even though you may not be around by the time he or she reaches the taxi.
- When you see someone running down the hallway to catch your elevator and you hold it, you will be awarded a mental Scout badge for a good deed.
- When you are emerging from the crowded subway stairway and apologize sincerely to the woman you inadvertently bumped in your haste, she will go to her office feeling a great deal better than before.
- When you see a short person trying to reach something on the top of the supermarket shelf and you say, "Here, let me get it," you demonstrate stature of character as well as of body.
- When you suggest that someone with only two items get ahead of you in the supermarket checkout line, you ease the stress of that person's day.

It doesn't matter if it's only a momentary friendly gesture. When you say a warm thank-you to everyone who holds a door for you or "I'm sorry" to anyone you have incommoded in the slightest, and when you spring to help anyone who needs assistance, anywhere, regardless of the person's sex, age, or appearance, *you epitomize a person of good character and beautiful manners*, and I and everyone else are going to want to be around you all the time!

* * *

What a lovely world it would be if all of us would make a little effort to be thoughtful and considerate of those around us at all times, whether we know them or not. That modicum of consideration puts smiles on other people's faces (or at least, keeps the scowls away) and adds joy to our days.

Table Manners That Take You Anywhere

9

The Right Thing to Do at Every Kind of Meal

When you stop to reflect, you can see the logic in the importance to others of your own table manners. Whenever people sitting at your table or even near you glance in your direction, they can't help but notice how you are handling yourself during the course of a meal. If your table manners are graceful, their perception of you will be very favorable.

You—no one else—will teach your children. It is you who sets the example to your children for table manners. They copy you, mimic you, and you should help, guide, and remind them of the right way to get through a meal. Like everything else in life, practice makes perfect.

I will always remember a friend of mine who despaired of her teenage son's table manners. Like his coterie of friends in high school—all jocks—he ate, as his mother described it, "exactly like a gorilla." She set an 11-inch by 14-inch mirror on an easelback in front of his place setting on the family table for a period of two weeks, and she privately warned the rest of the family not to make any comment, no matter how weird they thought it was to have a mirror sitting on the dining room table. Her son could not help but notice how unattractive it was when he ate certain foods with his fingers that were meant to be eaten with a fork—such as his salad and beans. He caught his reflection, whether he wanted to or not, when he took huge mouthfuls that distorted his face while he chewed. His mother caught him frowning when he saw himself in the mirror talking with his mouth full. No matter how hard he may have tried to escape his self-image, it was there, right in front of his plate. As a result of the temporary presence of that hated mirror, he learned to eat gracefully. (I might add that the promise of a nice reward from his parents also contributed to his changed eating habits.)

TABLE MANNER BASICS

Since a person's behavior at table really signals a certain sensitivity to other people, it's very important that parents spend enough time at table with each child, right up through the teen years, to make sure that he or she is well grounded in the basic precepts of good table behavior. The environment today is not conducive to teaching manners, with everyone rushing all the time in the pursuit of his or her own agenda. After a tough day of work or school, it's so easy for each member of the family to heat up a frozen food choice in the microwave or pick up a pizza or "some Chinese" to consume in front of the television—or perhaps to the accompaniment of music tapes or a movie on the VCR. Many of us seem to spend more time in front of screens, eating à la McDonald's, than we do at a table, eating with table implements.

There's nothing wrong with doing things the easy way in the 1990s. It's just that by the time our children are in high school, they should at least know how to sit at the table and eat their way nicely through a served meal. (That kind of *savoir faire* will help their careers later in the workplace.) By the end of college an adult should be completely at ease at table.

Body Language at Table

If you are a parent, here are some pointers you might wish to communicate to your children:

• *Maintain good posture at table*. Observe to your child, "How nice you look at the table when your body sits straight in the chair, with your feet together on the floor." This doesn't mean he or she has to sit ramrod-stiff like a West Point plebe at the table, but it does mean that a person doesn't sit collapsed like a rag doll.

• *You have options on what to do with your hands when not actually eating*. You may prefer simply to rest them on the table (with the bottom of your wrists balanced on the table's edge), or you may prefer to leave your hands under the table in your lap. (Quiet hands look a lot better to others at the table than hands playing with food on the plate or with strands of hair!)

• *It's certainly all right to rest an elbow or two on the table between courses*, because that's a gesture that comes naturally to people engaged in animated conversation. While you are eating, though, it's best to keep elbows off the table.

• Sometimes (maybe often) it's boring just to sit there waiting for people to finish their plates and their endless conversations, but *keep those fingers from drumming nervously on the table* or from playing with pieces of flatware or with the glasses. You may not hear the rat-a-tat-tat sounds, but it can annoy your neighbors.

• *When cutting something, keep your elbows as close to your body as possible*, so your neighbor won't have your elbow in his or her ribs. (If possible, a *leftie* in the family should have a regular seat on the left end of the table—to make it as comfortable as possible for him and for everyone else.)

General Rules on Conduct at Table

• Food is passed or served at a family meal by a parent at the head of the table, most often in a counterclockwise movement around the table, starting with the person on the mother's or father's right—the honor guest. Take what you wish from the bowl or platter when it reaches you, then pass it on to the person to your right.

• *"Please" and "Thank you" are basic* to good manners at table. Rather than reach across the table to grab something you'd like, ask the person nearest to the item "Please" to pass it to you, and when you receive it, say a pleasant, "Thank you." You may be proud of your long reach in basketball, but if you use it at the dinner table to fetch something way across the table, you might knock something over.

• *When serving yourself, take modest portions of food*—even of the things you love most, like French fries, taco chips, and hot fudge sauce to ooze over your ice cream.

• *Adding sauces and spices can be ill-mannered.*

When you are in a fine restaurant or in someone's home, it is very rude to ask for a bottled sauce to pour all over your meat. It is an insult to the chef and to the quality of cooking. (Teach your children the difference in the nuances of dining at a hamburger chain or at a fine restaurant!) It is also wise not to pour salt and pepper all over the food put before you before you have even tasted it. Have trust in your host's or the restaurant chef's culinary talents.

• *Cut your meat one piece at a time.*

When you were a child, someone probably cut up your entire piece of meat for you into small bites. As an adult, you're not supposed to do that for yourself. Cut one small piece, then eat it before cutting another.

• *The only way to eat is quietly.* It's important to chew only small bites of food—and to swallow them with the mouth closed. It's peaceful and quiet that way for everyone else around you.

• *Don't eat too fast.* Swallow each mouthful before shoveling in the next. How can anyone understand the fascinating things you have to say at the table if your mouth is full of food and words at the same time?

• *Wipe your fingers and mouth often with your napkin.* That's what it's for. You look much nicer without greasy fingers or a crumb or a dribble of something around your mouth!

• *If you want a second helping* in your own home, ask for it. If you are a guest in someone else's home, don't ask, because if there *is* more, it will be offered to you. If there is no more of what you have just requested, everyone becomes embarrassed, most of all you.

• *Yes, you may mop up that delicious last bit of sauce* remaining on your plate, provided you spear a small piece of roll or bread on your fork, squish it around in the sauce, and then put it in your mouth— taking care not to let it drip all over you as you do that. Don't take a piece of bread in your fingers and do the mopping up, because that can be very messy. Using the bread on the fork is much neater.

• *If you are served a certain food in someone's home that you really dislike*—like beets or liver, for example—rather than making a formal protest, just leave it on your plate. Push it around a little bit with your fork, and your abstinence from that food will probably go unnoticed. If they remark outright, "Jennifer, you haven't touched your fish," you might say "I'm just not hungry, thank you," instead of "I hate fish!"

Dilemmas at Mealtime

CATCHING FOOD IN YOUR TEETH

Never use a toothpick at table, even if you feel you have a gravel pit in your mouth. Try drinking some water to help the situation, and if you feel your teeth are really decorated with food, excuse yourself for a second to go to the restaurant restroom or to a bathroom in your host's home. There you can vigorously rinse your mouth—or even use your toothpick.

WHEN A BUG APPEARS

If a little bug crawls out of your salad, pick it up quickly with your napkin, without saying a word, and dispatch it (dead) under the table. Don't point it out with great glee (or revulsion) to everyone else sitting with you, because you might ruin the rest of the entire dinner for most of the people sitting at your table.

COPING WITH GARLIC OR ONION BREATH

You may feel your presence at home, in the office, or at a party will be less than well received, given the amount of garlic you have just consumed at a particular meal. Any one of the following actions might help you deal with the problem, to everyone else's relief:

- Chew and swallow some fresh parsley.
- Rub a piece of lemon over your tongue and the insides of your mouth.
- Chew a few coffee beans.
- Take some antacid.

MEALTIME DECORUM

Saying Grace

When you are a guest in someone's home, and grace will be said before the meal (which does not happen at dinner parties), follow your host's lead. He or she will either remain standing for the blessing of the food, in which case you do, too, or the host will sit and announce that grace will be said. Don't eat or drink anything before grace has been said. Remain silent with your head bowed until the end, then put your napkin in your lap, and the meal will begin.

When Do You Start Eating?

The last person to be served should be the father or mother at a family dinner or the host or hostess at a dinner party. Everyone else at the table should wait to eat until the last person is served or has served himself. An exception to this rule is when the food on the table is hot. Then it is the responsibility of the host to urge his or her guests to begin eating at once, as soon as they are served: "Please do start. Your soup will become cold, and it tastes so much better hot!"

If there is no hostess, then the woman guest of honor on the host's right should be the first one to begin eating at the table. Everyone else will follow her, so it's her responsibility to start. If the food in front of her is cold, she should wait until everyone at her table has been served and then begin. Her male host should not start before she does. I have attended many dinners where the hostess or the female guest of honor has been engaged in animated chatter for what seems an eternity without picking up a knife and fork, leaving the rest of the guests at the table longing to begin to eat but feeling they must not "jump the gun."

Serving Yourself from a Platter

All food bowls and platters should be passed to you from the left. If you are being served something like mashed potatoes, it is easy: You simply take a glob of it with the serving spoon, put it on your plate, and put the spoon back in the bowl. (If you make the handle of a serving spoon or fork messy, wipe it with your napking before replacing it on the platter.) Serving yourself from a platter of meat slices or a small bird with a surrounding garniture is more complicated. Take the serving fork in your left hand and the spoon in your right, and scoop up the bird or slices of meat in order to transfer them to your plate. Help yourself to a bit of everything else on that platter that may appeal to you—some small potatoes, for example, or a stuffed mushroom, or a broiled tomato filled with peas, or whatever. Try not to eat something that is on the platter for decoration only. I remember the look of horror on my host's face the night I cut into a Styrofoam beehive in the center of the dessert platter. It was covered with chocolate designs, and I thought it was part of the dessert. I managed to wrest a piece free from the beehive, but it upset the entire arrangement on the rest of the platter. Our pained host whispered to me, "If I were you, I wouldn't eat that; even the chocolate sauce doesn't make Styrofoam taste good."

The main thing to remember about serving yourself from a platter is that you should leave the serving utensils lying neatly side by side in a manner that makes it easy for the next person to serve himself.

Taking Modest Portions

As a guest, serve yourself modest portions of whatever is passed or whatever is on the buffet. You should always be thinking of how many others must be served and how much food there is. If the food supply is plentiful, you can always go back for more, which makes any host proud.

When a platter abounding in tiny lamb chops is passed to you, take two. If the lamb chops are medium-size, take one. It is far better for you to serve yourself another the second time around than to watch your host's face freeze in horror because there is only enough for one lamb chop per person, and you have taken two.

When a platter with numerous small thin slices of a roast meat is passed, take two slices. If the slices are large and rather thick, take one slice. You can always take more when the platter is repassed.

Even if there is a gigantic bowl of your favorite pasta on the serving table, serve yourself a moderate portion. You can "pig out" the next time you go back—when you know everyone has food on their plates. You certainly don't want someone watching you go through the buffet line for the first time looking like a prize-winning glutton!

Tasting Other People's Food

When you are with friends in a restaurant famous for its cuisine, it is perfectly proper to exchange small samplings of the different dishes brought to the table. What is *not* proper is for a person to refrain from ordering a course, but then to sample from everyone else's plates like a hungry dog.

If your friends wish to sample one another's food, ask for two or three clean plates and transfer samples onto those plates with clean forks and spoons. Don't exchange food samples after everyone has begun eating; apportion any tasting samples *before* people have begun eating (a question of hygiene, not manners).

Two very good friends or relatives can certainly take a very quick bite of something really delicious from the other person's plate, once permission has been given, but the person sampling should use a clean utensil and do it inconspicuously.

When You're on a Diet

If you're on a diet, you should stick to it, and good for you, but if you're someone's dinner guest, it's better not to make a grandstand play of it. If you have a medical problem that makes eating normal dinner party fare almost impossible, talk it over with your host prior to the event. Offer to eat your own meal at home beforehand and to join the group right after dinner, or to be present during cocktails and then to leave as the meal is about to be served. Or you can pretend to eat and just push the food around on your plate. The one option you don't have is to force your host to prepare a special meal for you.

If you're on a weight-loss diet, say nothing about it during dinner (since there is no more boring topic of conversation nor more hostile subject to someone who is about to dive into a large piece of double fudge cake). Serve yourself well the foods that you may eat, and skip the rest. If you're brought a fattening dessert you should not touch, take your fork and push it around a bit on the plate. Your host will probably be unaware you are faking it. A vegetarian can often serve himself a variety of non-meat dishes (and sometimes non-dairy products) such as salad, rice, vegetables, and fruit, without anyone even realizing his vegetarian preferences.

If You Spill at Table

The entire question of spilling at the table is an anxious one, both for the spiller and for the host in his or her home. The spiller would just as soon have the earth open up into a great hole into which he or she could disappear so as not have to face the embarrassment. The host, in the meantime, usually tries to keep his or her cool and not show emotion—but inevitably wonders with despair just how ruined the table surface or the linens are as a result of the spill. It is a trying time for everyone.

• When you happen to spill (or a waiter spills for you) a bit of hot liquid such as tea, coffee, or soup into your teacup saucer, blot it with your napkin, so that you won't continue to spot all around you every time you pick up your dripping cup.

• *If you make just a very minor stain at your place*, like some drops of gravy or sauce, dab at it unobtrusively and clean it as well as possible with three or four pats of your napkin, taking care to return the napkin to your lap folded in such a way so as not to transfer the stain from the napkin to your clothes.

• *For a significant spill*, what happens next depends on the circumstances. In a restaurant, your host should call over the waiter to cope with the cleanup of your mess. If there is a waiter or caterer serving the meal to you in someone's home, that person will attend to the cleanup of your spill. If the spill occurs in your own home, you simply go to the kitchen and fetch whatever you need to clean it up. Perhaps a water-dampened cloth is all you need. Perhaps it is a minor stain that you can simply cover with another clean napkin. I always pour club soda on a major stain. (My definition of a major stain is something like raspberry sauce or a large blob of Beef Burgundy stew.) Blot any stain with a clean napkin or towel, making sure first to clean off the table surface beneath the table linens to protect the surface from the club soda seeping down to it.

• *If you spill badly in someone else's home*, it becomes more of a drama. A sincere apology to your host after you spill is important, but so is quick action. Ask your host if you may go into the kitchen to take care of the mess. Your host will either go with you to help gather the damp paper towels and whatever else is needed, or your host will urge you to remain seated, because "it's nothing at all, and I will take care of it." In the latter case, keep your seat.

If there's a major ugly stain *all around* your place setting, ask your host for a napkin to cover the offending area. Otherwise, anyone at the table who looks in your direction will be mesmerized by the spots.

Without making a large production out if it, it's nice to apologize to the other guests or to your family for having spilled—simply because you *have* upset the harmony and relaxation of the meal. (If you can laugh at yourself and make a quick joke about being a classic mess-maker, so much the better, because everyone else will then laugh, relax, and cease feeling sorry for you.) Start a new topic of conversation, if one of the other guests hasn't thoughtfully already started one. The sooner the party gets back on track, with the accident forgotten, the better for everyone.

If you were responsible for serious stains on your host's linens, offer to send the host's linens to an excellent dry cleaner the next day. The same rule applies if you or a member of your family is responsible for damaging any of your hosts' possessions (such as when your child throws up on their prized rug or your dog makes a mess on it). Arrange to have the damaged goods picked up, and then cleaned or repaired and brought back at the hosts' convenience.

I remember so well when as a nineteen-year-old student and the only American at a dinner party in a splendid Parisian home, I upset a full glass of red wine all over the tablecloth. In one grand gesture I shattered one of the hostess's twelve prized eighteenth-century goblets and permanently ruined her prized early nineteenth-century Venetian lace tablecloth. The duchess taught me a lesson that night that I will never forget. The guests in that dining room were frozen with horror over what the *jeune Américaine* had just done. The duchess, obviously dying inside, smiled at me and said cheerfully, "It's nothing, Mademoiselle, absolutely *nothing*." Then she called to her maître d'hôtel to "bring Mademoiselle another glass of wine," and while a footman mopped up the mess, she quickly introduced another sprightly topic of conversation to spare me any further agony. When I arrived at her door the next morning, to see if I could take the cloth to the leading dry cleaner in Paris and the shattered glass to a well-known restorer, the butler told me they had already checked. "Nothing can be done, but Madame la Duchesse wishes Mademoiselle Baldrige to know that it is perfectly all right, and she has already forgotten it ever happened." I will never forget that woman and what "real class" she showed us all that night. Through the years, whenever my children or their friends broke our antique porcelains and our good stemware (which has happened frequently), I have remembered "Madame la Duchesse," drawn myself up tall, and said to the perpetrator of the accident, "It's all right. Don't let it worry you. It doesn't matter at all."(I admit, sometimes that is very difficult to say!)

Using Your Flatware Properly

• *Hold the knife, fork, and spoon deftly*. Most Americans eat with the fork held in the right hand. You should grasp the fork with your thumb and forefinger, about three-quarters of the way up the handle. The thumb pushes against the back of the forefinger on top of the handle, and the other three fingers fit beneath the handle in ascending order. The middle finger buttresses the handle from beneath. *Hold your spoon the same way*. (NOTE: For left-handed people, the procedures described here should be reversed.)

• *When you cut something requiring a knife*, transfer your fork to your left hand and grasp it about two-thirds down the handle. The thumb

Like this . . .

Not like this . . .

The proper way to cut your meat, when eating either American or continental style, is shown here at left. Note the hand positions. You should never grasp either knife or fork in a sort of clenched fist, as shown on the right.

and forefinger work together, the thumb applying pressure from the bottom. The forefinger, applying pressure from the top, stays a little closer to the fork tines than the thumb does. In this way you can wield the fork to the left and to the right, still maintaining a firm grip on it and making the implement do what you want it to do.

The knife is held in the right hand with the thumb and middle finger (grasping it halfway down the handle), and with the forefinger pressing down firmly on the top of the blade at the point where it joins the handle. The joint operation of knife and fork working properly together looks like this:

In my travels around the United States, observing young people on college campuses and in the workplace, I find many of them holding their forks in their left hands, making pugnacious fists while they draw their knives inefficiently across the meat, as if drawing a bow across a cello!

THE CONTINENTAL STYLE OF EATING

Since we are the only country in the world whose inhabitants shift the fork, after cutting, from the left hand to the right, perhaps we should take a look at other cultures. (Where our American custom began—of putting the knife down before eating and shifting the fork back to the right hand—is still an enigma; many people in addition to myself have researched the subject, including at the Library of Congress, without discovering the origin of this custom.)

In the American style of eating, after cutting your meat you switch the fork to your right hand from the left, put your knife down on the plate, spear a piece of meat, and then eat it. (It's a lot of work, doing it that way, but that's the way we do it in this country.)

In the continental style of eating, you keep your fork in your left hand and convey the food to your mouth after cutting each piece. The knife stays in your right hand and may subtly help get the meat or any food onto your fork. This is a much quieter, more graceful, and more efficient way of eating!

• *In the continental style of eating, the fork is held in the left hand and the knife in the right all through the meal.* It is a logical, easy way of eating, and much quieter than the American system. (There isn't the clattering that occurs as one shifts the fork from the cutting position in the left hand to the eating position in the right, meanwhile laying down the knife on the plate each time.)

If you wish to eat in the continental style, keep your fork always in your left hand, usually with its tines down, and hold the knife always in your right hand—to cut food or to serve as a helper in pushing bits of food onto your fork. Even recalcitrant peas or corn kernels can be successfully captured with fork and knife working together.

• *Dessert is eaten more easily continental-style, too.* You will find that when you become comfortable with eating continental-style, it is easier to eat almost any dessert by using two implements, a fork and a spoon. Eat the dessert with the spoon in your right hand and use the fork as a buttress in the left—in the same manner you used a knife to support whatever was on the fork earlier in the meal.

When eating dessert continental-style

- Pie or cake à la mode is eaten with a fork and spoon—fork in the right hand, spoon in the left.
- Berries or any cut-up fruit is eaten with a fork and spoon—spoon in the right hand, fork in the left.
- Ice cream, puddings, and custards are eaten with a spoon only.

When I returned to this country eating continental-style after almost a decade abroad as a student and as a member of our Foreign Service, I

The proper way to eat pie á la mode is with a fork and spoon.

was chastised by certain relatives and friends for being "un-American." Since then so many Americans have traveled, lived abroad, and adopted the continental style of eating that it is no longer conspicuous. Parents should seriously consider adopting the continental style when teaching their children to eat, simply because it is easier, quieter, and more efficient. (The parents, of course, would first have to learn how to eat in this manner themselves, to make it seem natural for the children to copy.)

Position of Implements When Pausing or When Finished Eating

When you pause in eating your food, American-style, your knife (with its sharp blade side turned inward) is already resting on the right side of your plate. Rest your fork, tines up, next to it on its left. This is also the position of your implements when you have finished the contents of your plate, and are ready to have it removed.

For the rest position continental-style, the fork is laid on the left side of the plate, tines down, and the knife on the right, angled from the lower outside of the plate toward the top center. When the diner has finished completely, he or she places his or her fork and knife next to each other on the right side of the plate, as Americans do, although often with the fork tines down.

When you have paused in eating but have not finished, leave your fork and knife in this position. A trained waiter will know that you are signaling him *not* to remove your plate.

• *What do you do with your spoon?* A spoon is meant to be laid to rest on the undersaucer and not left sticking up in any kind of cup or compote. (The soup spoon does, however, rest in the soup plate.) If you are served a tall glass of *iced tea* with a tall spoon or stirrer, balance this implement on the undersaucer when not in use. If there is no undersaucer, then the stirrer will have to remain upright in your glass. Be sure to grasp it between your index and middle finger while you drink your iced tea so that it does not fall out of the glass!

When you leave your fork and knife on the side of the plate in this position (fork tines may be up or down), it signals the waiter that you are through eating and that your plate may be removed.

Napkin Etiquette

As soon as you sit down at the table, spread your napkin across your lap. A luncheon-sized napkin (for example, 16 inches square) should be unfolded the entire way, while a large dinner napkin (for example, 23 by 23 inches) should be unfolded only in half before placing it on your lap.

The most important thing to remember about a napkin is that it should stay on your lap until you have risen to leave the table. If you must leave the table during the meal for any reason, put your napkin on the seat of your chair, *not* on the table. When people are eating, the sight of someone's soiled napkin tossed on the table is very unappetizing!

When it comes time for everyone to leave the table, fold your napkin (not necessarily neatly) and leave it on the table.

USING YOUR NAPKIN AS A BIB

When you order a broiled lobster in a restaurant, the waiter might provide you with a bib to protect your clothing, but if not eating lobster, it looks pretty tacky to tie a large napkin bib-style around your neck—unless, of course, you are a child. If you are eating a food that tends to spot your clothing (soup, for example, or spaghetti or certain salads dripping in dressing), it's possible to protect yourself in a graceful way. Pull your chair in close and lean over the table when you eat this splashy kind of food. Take a corner of your napkin with the fingers of your left hand and hold it up to your throat, spreading the napkin loosely over your chest. Still holding the napkin against you with your left hand, eat the food with the fork in your right hand. If anything splatters, it will land on your napkin, not on your clothes—and other people will hardly notice that you are holding your napkin up to your neck.

A woman should not blot her lipstick on her napkin. It looks unattractive to others. A trip to the ladies' room *before the meal* to blot her lipstick with paper tissue is a much better idea—and much easier on the host's or the restaurant's laundry operations!

If your family uses napkin rings (an old-fashioned custom, since most families use paper napkins these days instead of cloth ones that are laundered once a week), teach your children to fold their napkins carefully and slip them into their rings before leaving the table.

Finger Bowls

The finger bowl—almost an anachronism today—is usually seen at a formally served dinner. The waiter brings you the finger bowl usually just before dessert is served (although in some houses the finger bowl is brought at the end of dessert, as a final ablution). This is a small bowl, often made of glass, and is three-quarters filled with cold water. A small flower or glass ornament is often floated in it. The waiter will place your finger bowl on a dainty doily (often made of linen or organdy and trimmed with lace) in the center of your dessert plate. From there on, it is up to you. Dip the fingers of each hand separately into the water and then dry them on your napkin—without making a large show of it. (You don't even have to rinse your fingers if they are perfectly clean.) Now lift the doily together with the finger bowl and place them at the

For a formal kind of dessert service, a waiter brings each guest a finger bowl filled with water, setting it on a little lace or organdy doily (optional), which in turn sits on the dessert plate. The dessert fork and spoon would be balanced on the plate in this case (instead of sitting at the top of the place setting throughout the meal, as is shown in most cases in this book). It's a nice little touch to float a small fresh flower blossom in each finger bowl.

upper left of your place setting (in the place where your butter plate would have been earlier).

The arrival of finger bowls at the table perplexes many people. At a formal dinner last year I saw the chairman of one of America's largest corporations become puzzled by a finger bowl. He noticed others removing their bowls from their plates, so he followed suit, but he forgot to remove the doily with it. As a result, he served himself a generous portion of vanilla ice cream with raspberry sauce right on top of the doily (which was ruined by swimming in raspberry juice all during dessert). Many years ago, our eight-year-old daughter, during dinner in the posh Williamsburg Inn in Virginia, having never before seen a finger bowl, picked it up and took a hearty drink from it, delighting in the "funny looking drinking glass." (The entire dining room wondered why the very dignified musicians playing chamber music close to our table were suddenly convulsed.) Recently I saw a young woman executive pick up the porcelain flower floating in her finger bowl and try to eat it. Fortunately, she did not succeed. (She explained to me afterward that she thought it was a candied flower—part of our dessert.)

In spite of such vicissitudes, finger bowls are very useful when supplied to your guests after eating certain messy foods: snails, for example, or lobster or steamed clams, or fresh corn on the cob. In this case, immediately following the course that would have made fingers messy, bring your guests finger bowls filled with warm water (and perhaps a thin slice of lemon floating in each bowl).

The guest should dip finger tips in the finger bowl, wipe them on his or her napkin, then place the doily and finger bowl to the upper left of the place setting. He or she now moves the fork and spoon from the plate to the left and right side of the plate, respectively. The empty plate is now ready to receive its helping of dessert.

Don't rush out to buy finger bowls. Use your own pretty dessert or cereal bowls. And, of course, if you are serving Oriental food, it is very nice to offer your guests *small hand towels that have been dipped into hot water scented with your favorite cologne.* The most important thing to remember about serving hot towels is for the host to have them picked up again immediately. The sight of guests forlornly holding used damp towels, not knowing what to do with them, hardly makes for a smooth dinner party.

HOW TO HANDLE DIFFERENT—AND SOMETIMES DIFFICULT—FOODS

Hors d'Oeuvres

KEEPING HANDS CLEAN

It is difficult to consume hors d'oeuvres while you're holding a cocktail glass in your hands and still look graceful. During the cocktail hour you are constantly meeting people and shaking hands. If you shake hands with fingers dappled with mayonnaise or cheese dip, people will not be delighted to meet you! It's common sense to keep a paper cocktail napkin handy, so that you can wipe off your fingers whenever they pick up the residue from the hors d'oeuvre you just ate. Even a cheesestick or a pretzel leaves your fingers in need of a napkin. I also advise everyone at cocktail parties to hold their drinks in their left hands, so that at least one hand is warm, dry, and ready to shake other hands.

DISPOSING OF TOOTHPICKS

At cocktail parties toothpicks don't just stow themselves away, although guests wish they would. When you take a shrimp on a toothpick and dip it into a sauce, don't put the used toothpick back on the platter, because it certainly isn't appetizing for someone else who wants a shrimp. The wise hostess who insists on using toothpicks (and many of us refuse to serve hors d'oeuvres requiring them because of the hassle they create) provides containers throughout the cocktail area, so that people can easily dispense with them. If there isn't an ashtray or a dish or a wastebasket nearby, put your own used toothpicks in your cocktail napkin and then leave them in the kitchen or in the guest bathroom wastebasket before you leave. I have seen people stow their used toothpicks in plants, flower vases, under sofa cushions, in the aquarium, in the cuffs of men's trousers, in women's handbags, and in other people's pockets when they weren't looking.

HANDLING DIFFICULT-TO-EAT HORS D'OEUVRES

• *When an hors d'oeuvre is hot*, test it carefully and inconspicuously with your tongue before placing the entire thing in your mouth. Many inveterate cocktail party attendees have badly burned and scarred the inside of their mouth after failing to observe this precaution.

• *When you select a puff-pastry hors d'oeuvre*, it might splash on you when you first bite into it. Wait until it cools, then try to swallow it whole. If you try to cut it in half with your teeth, you run the risk of having the soft hot contents give you—and maybe someone standing near you—an unwelcome shower.

• *When you take a raw vegetable from a platter of crudités and then dip it* into a sauce, hold your cocktail napkin beneath the vegetable until it reaches your mouth. Of course, the healthiest and the safest way, from the point of view of your cholesterol and dry cleaning bills respectively, is to eat crudités without the dip.

• *If the canapé you have put into your mouth tastes terrible*, transfer it from your mouth into a cocktail napkin, and then search for a wastebasket. Turn your back to the guests while you take the hors d'oeuvre out of your mouth.

Breads and Pastries

A ROLL AND ITS CRUMBS

When you find a basket of rolls, bread, and breadsticks adjacent to your place setting at the table, pass it first to the person sitting next to you, then help yourself, and pass it to the person on your other side, who will then pass it on.

A roll should be pulled apart with the fingers into two or more parts; it should not be cut with a knife. Don't "butter ahead"; rather, butter each piece and then eat it.

If you have a butter plate, keep your roll there. If you have no butter plate, keep the roll at the left side of whatever plate is in front of you.

Don't worry about sending a flight of crumbs in all directions as you break up the roll. Pick up as many crumbs as you can with your fingers, and put them on your plate. You can do it so naturally, as you talk, that no one will even realize you're doing it.

If someone is serving your table, the waiter will come by your place setting before the dessert course and remove the crumbs from all around the table—pushing them with a clean napkin onto a small plate or brushing them with a silver brush into a silver or metal container (a "crumber").

HANDLING POPULAR BREADS AND PASTRIES

• *A muffin or a piece of toast* should be cut in half, each half buttered separately and then eaten, perhaps spread with some jam.

• *A hot popover* should be opened, then buttered and eaten in small pieces immediately, because once it deflates and cools, it loses its charm.

• *A sticky bun or a Danish* should be cut in half with a knife—or in quarters, if it is very large—and then optionally buttered. (The term "buttered" means using butter, whipped butter, or margarine.)

• *English muffins* are already halved and toasted when they are served to you. Sometimes they are prebuttered. If you wish to put honey on the halves, take a large spoonful from the honey server, put it on your plate, and then spread it on the muffin half with your knife. This is true with jams and jellies, too. Spoon the desired quantity from the jar onto your plate, and then spread it onto your bread or roll with a knife (not a spoon).

• *A baguette of French bread* (a long thin loaf) is sometimes hard to tear apart with your fingers because the crust is so hard. A considerate host precuts it with a sharp knife into sections in the kitchen before it is brought to the table. Sometimes the baguette is preheated, sometimes even lightly prebuttered.

• *Tiny hot biscuits* are barely slit open, with a small amount of butter dropped inside. (If you take more than four of them, others around you may consider you an over-eater.)

The Relish Tray

Sometimes you will find a relish tray—containing such things as small slices of celery and carrots, radishes, olives, and pickles—on the table when you sit down. If it is directly in front of you, pick it up, pass it first to the person on your left or right, then help yourself, and then pass it to the person on your other side, who will then continue it on its way around the table. If you have a butter plate, put your choices on it. If not, put your choices on the side of whatever plate is in front of you. Items from the relish tray are picked up with the fingers, put on the plate, and then eaten one by one. (In other words, don't put food directly into your mouth from the relish tray.)

• If cottage cheese is part of the relish tray, and if you have a butter plate, spoon the desired amount onto that plate. Use your outside fork, and, when finished, balance that fork on the butter plate until you need it again for the main meal.

• When eating olives, chew the olive, and then transfer the pit from your mouth onto your fork (your tongue will do this job for you) and then down onto your butter plate (or if there is no butter plate, then the one in front of you). If you absolutely cannot handle such a delicate operation, take the pit quickly from your mouth with your thumb and forefinger, and put it down onto the plate as inconspicuously as possible. (Do not, as my brothers sometimes did when they were little and my parents were not present, spit the olive pit across the table at your adversary.)

Appetizers

Soup

Soup is a very audible food. In the Japanese culture, slurping soup is normal and natural; in ours it is not. Sip your soup quietly, and if you are blowing on a spoonful to cool it down before swallowing it, do that quietly, too.

When you are served soup in a soup plate, spoon it away from you.

When you are dealing with soup *in a cup*, with bits of food floating in it (such as croutons, shredded carrot, or egg-yolk), eat the soup until all of the food has been consumed. Then you are free to pick up the cooled-down soup and sip it directly from the cup. (Never, however, pick up your soup *plate* to drink from directly.)

You may pick up your cup of consommé and sip it, instead of spooning it, provided it is not scalding hot.

CAVIAR

There's great romance attached to the supreme status symbol food called caviar (also served at the cocktail hour). It is one of the most expensive luxuries in the world. To be served a great caviar as the first course at a dinner party is to be outrageously pampered.

The famous Petrossian caviar importing company explains that the best caviar imported into this country today comes from the Caspian Sea area of the Soviet Union. The very fine Iranian caviar, because of the political unrest in recent years, is no longer available in sure quantities.

It takes an incredibly long time for the female sturgeon to yield the prized tiny eggs, hence the exorbitant price of the following caviar varieties:

- o Beluga: The eggs are light to dark gray in color. The female takes twenty years to yield eggs.
- o Osetra: The eggs are light brown to golden. The female takes thirteen to fourteen years to yield eggs.
- o Sevruga: The eggs are light to dark gray. The female takes four years to yield eggs (hence this is the most reasonable of all).

The most luxurious food of all—caviar—is best served chilled over ice in a small bowl. Put a couple of spoonfuls onto your plate, then squirt some lemon juice on it. With your butterknife, spread the caviar on small pieces of toast or dark bread.

Caviar should be kept in a cold part of the refrigerator (never in the freezer). Once opened, it should be consumed within twenty-four hours. (For many of us caviar lovers, it is quite impossible to imagine that there would be any left over.)

• *The classic way to serve caviar* is in a beautiful crystal bowl on a bed of cracked ice, to keep its temperature properly cold. When caviar is passed to you at the table, or when you approach it at a buffet table, put a heaping teaspoon on your plate. You will also find small squares of brown bread or toast, which you may butter or not. Spread the caviar on a small toast, and if you wish, add a touch of lemon juice. Some people also add minced hard-boiled egg yolk, minced onions, even sour cream. Let's face it, by the time you pile all of that on top of the caviar, you won't even be able to taste it. Sirio Maccioni, owner of the famous New York restaurant Le Cirque, never brings all those caviar accompaniments to the table unless the diner specifically asks for them. The real caviar lover spreads it on plain toast, period.

If you are serving your guests caviar, give them glasses of cold champagne or chilled small glasses (shot glasses or liqueur glasses, for example) of ice cold vodka.

There are many lesser caviars on the market, too, including red caviar, black caviar paste, and the salty American types.

SNAILS

When a metal plate containing piping hot snails is put down in front of you as an appetizer course, you are in for a very special treat. You are also probably going to get garlic-butter sauce all over your fingers, as well as have garlic-flavored breath for at least the rest of the evening. Anyone planning a love tryst after dinner should either refrain from eating snails at dinner, or be certain that the other person orders them, too.

In some restaurants you will be provided with a metal pincer-like "snail-gripper," with which you hold the snail steady while you extract its insides with a tiny fork or nut pick. If no gripper is provided, hold each hot shell in your napkin in one hand (so as not to burn your fingers) while you extract the body with the other hand.

When the shells have cooled down and are empty, it is proper to pick them up one by one and suck the delicious juice from inside. Or, if that is too adventurous for you, turn the shell upside down on the metal plate, and then sop up the sauce with small pieces of bread you have speared on your fork.

SHRIMP OR CRABMEAT COCKTAIL

Shrimp and crabmeat cocktail are eaten with the smallest fork at your place setting (usually found on the outside left, but sometimes placed on the outside right). If there is a piece of lemon on your plate, spear it with your fork and then squeeze it carefully over the seafood. If a small container of sauce is provided with this appetizer, you may also spoon some over the shrimp or crabmeat, or you may take a forkful of the seafood and then dip it into the sauce before eating it.

If you are confronted with gigantic shrimp in a compote, you will have difficulty swallowing them whole. They may be tough, too, which means that your fork can't cut them into smaller pieces in the compote. Don't despair. Spear a jumbo shrimp with your little fork, put it down on the saucer, and then take your knife and cut it into two or three pieces. If you are feeling adventurous, you may also take a large shrimp on your fork and bite it off in small pieces.

STEAMED CLAMS

Hopefully, your thoughtful host has provided you with a couple of large napkins and perhaps even a bib to protect your clothing during a feast of steamed clams. (Steamed clams are the appetizer mainstay of a clambake, a lobster dinner, or a "shore dinner.") You should also be provided with your own empty bowl (or have easy access to a large communal bowl nearby) in which to toss your emptied shells. In addition, you should be provied with a tiny pot of melted butter and a consommé cup containing hot clam broth (made from the water in which the clams are steamed).

Your steamed clams should be open at least halfway. (If a clam stubbornly refuses to open, throw it away—it probably is bad.) Open your clam shell fully, hold it between your thumb and forefinger of your left hand, and then, with the fingers of your right hand, pull out the slippery clam body by its narrow neck. Slip the skin off the neck sheath with your fingers, discard it, and then dip the whole clam body either in the melted butter or in the cup of clam broth; then swallow it and delight in its deliciousness. It's very messy, but fun to eat. After consuming a whole plateful of steamed clams, you should be ready to rinse the fingers of both hands in water. (Guests should be provided with finger bowls of warm water for this part of the ritual.)

Real clam lovers always consume their cup of broth before leaving this part of the meal. Bits of sand from the ocean usually collect in the bottom of the cup, but an aficionado somehow manages to drink the broth without consuming a grain of sand.

RAW OYSTERS AND CLAMS ON THE HALF SHELL

Raw oysters or clam nestled into a bed of ice on the plate are an expensive culinary treat. Hold the shell steady with the fingers of your left hand, and with your right hand, use the small oyster fork to lift the oyster or clam whole from its shell. (If any part of it sticks to the shell, wield the fork to break it loose.) Then dip it into the small container of sauce in the middle of the plate. Some prefer just to squirt lemon juice on their oysters or clams, since they maintain a piquant sauce destroys the real flavor of the seafood.

You may pick up the empty shell and drain its juices into your mouth. It makes a slurpy sound and is not very pretty to witness, but in this case a purist does not care about appearances.

If you wish, drop some small oyster crackers into the container of sauce, and then fish them out and eat with your oyster fork.

MUSSELS

Smoked or pickled mussels are sometimes served on toothpicks as hors d'oeuvres. Most often they are served as an appetizer in a garlicky broth in a soup plate—a dish called *Moules Marinières*. You may either extract the mussel from its open shell with a small oyster fork or nut pick, or you may pick up the shell, put the edge between your lips, and suck out the mussel and its juice in the shell. (Discard the empty shells on another plate.) While eating the mussels, spoon up the broth, too, because it is delicious.

This is another time to hold a napkin spread across your chest while eating with the other hand, and you will certainly need a finger bowl and a clean napkin after finishing your *Moules*!

Meat

Always use a knife and fork to cut your meat, unless it is served in small, tender pieces, such as in a stew.

Cut and eat a piece at a time—don't cut ahead.

If you are served a steak or chop with a great deal of fat around it, it is perfectly proper to cut off all the fat before you eat the meat.

CHOPS (LAMB, VEAL, AND PORK)

When others are present, you should cut off pieces of the meat with your knife and fork, rather than pick up the chop and eat directly from it. (Of course, what you do at home alone is your own business!) At a meal with friends, you can always ask the host, when you have cut the meat as close to the bone as you can, if he or she would mind if you finished off the last succulent bit of chop by holding it in your fingers. The host should urge all the guests to do the same (it is a compliment to the chops). Hold the chop with one hand only, and be sure to clean off your fingers and your mouth with your napkin as you go along. (Hopefully, you won't attempt this if the chop is covered in sauce.)

CHICKEN

The same principle applies for picking up a piece of chicken, turkey, or any other kind of fowl. Of course, if you are at a picnic, a barbecue, or any informal function out of doors, it's proper to eat chicken while holding it in your hands. Indoors, seated at a table, you should cut it with your knife and fork, down to the bone, then ask your host if you may finish it off by holding it in your fingers. (It looks better not to, of course, and hopefully you won't try this at a White House state dinner, at lunch with your boss, or at your mother-in-law's the first time you meet her!)

SMALL BIRDS

When you are served a small bird such as quail, eat it with a knife and fork for as long as you can (which won't be for very long). Then pick up the little bird in one hand and eat off it until there is no more tender, flavorful meat left. Your host and everyone else at the table will be doing the same.

BARBECUED SPARERIBS

I personally feel that spareribs, which *must* be eaten with the fingers, are so messy to eat that they do not belong at a party indoors. If you serve them in your house, be sure to provide your guests with extra napkins and finger bowls of warm water.

Fish

If you are served a fillet, eat it with a fish fork and knife (fish knives are rarely seen these days, except in good restaurants, so you may use any kind of knife given you).

In a restaurant, if you are served a fish that is not filleted, and if you are not adept at filleting yourself, ask the waiter to do it. He will either do it expertly himself right at the table, or, if he is not feeling self-confident, will take it out to the kitchen and have the chef do it. To do it yourself, insert the tip of your knife under the backbone, slide the knife under the entire skeleton, and then gently lift the skeleton with the knife. Put it on the side of your plate. If any tiny bones have been dislodged by this action and you find them later in a mouthful of fish, push them forward with your tongue onto your fork, then transfer them with the fork down onto your plate.

If you are served a fish with its head, and you're like me and would never eat the head, cut it off first before you fillet the fish. You can always ask the waiter for a small plate upon which to put the skeleton and the head—to be removed from the table, so that you can enjoy your fish without its eyes staring at you. (A real fisherman would be appalled at this faint-heartedness.)

• To squeeze lemon juice on your fish before eating it, spear the piece of lemon that should be on your plate with your fork, and squeeze with the lemon still impaled on the fork tines. Cover the squeezing action with your fingers, so as to deflect any juice from squirting on your neighbor. Some restaurants solve the juice-squirting problem by covering a half lemon with a layer of gauze, so that one may squeeze it worry-free.

Lobster

Lobster is a rich, succulent delicacy, and the travails of getting the meat extracted from its shell is part of the enjoyment. No matter where you are, don't be afraid to don a bib before you attack a lobster. (Better a bib than a dry cleaning bill.)

Some people prefer to dip their pieces of lobster into a small container of melted butter before eating them, others dip them into a small container of mayonnaise. Still others prefer to put only lemon juice on their lobster meat.

If your lobster has not been thoroughly precracked for you in the kitchen (which is cheating, in my opinion), you will probably find a nutcracker and a tiny oyster fork or nut pick at your place. The nutcracker is used to crack the shell and the tiny fork to extract lobster meat from small, difficult-to-reach places. (Use a regular fork to eat the meat that comes from the larger part of the lobster.)

With your left hand, hold the lobster steady on the plate, and with your right, twist off the big claws and place them on the side of the plate. Then, still steadying the lobster, lift up the tail meat with your

To eat lobster, you twist off a part of the lobster's body, hold the part in one hand, and use a nutcracker to break the shell with the other. Don't worry if it requires two or three tries.

fork, and cut it into small enough pieces so as to be able to dip and eat them. Then break off the small claws with your fingers and suck out—from the open end, of course—the sweet meat and its juice.

Now crack open the big claws on the side of your plate. Use your fork to extract the meat, cut it into small pieces, and dip them in the sauce of your choice.

Now it's time for the good meat in the stomach cavity—the green material (called the "tamale") and the coral (or "roe"), which is found in the female and is a great delicacy. Spear this meat with a fork, cut into smaller portions, and dip it as desired. (Some people don't like the taste of this stomach cavity meat.)

Your host or restaurant should provide large bowls or platters into which the guests can throw the lobster shells as the contents are consumed. Some kind of finger bowl is also a necessity after finishing this course.

Pasta

The easiest way to eat noodles or stringy pasta is with a fork in your right hand and a large (dessert-size) spoon in your left. Pile a proper amount of pasta on your fork (not too much), and support it by pushing the spoon against it to keep it intact. Then bring the fork to your mouth. Some people use a piece of bread held in their left hand as a "pusher," to act like a spoon in keeping noodles on the fork.

Keep your napkin spread in front of you as you eat, and lean close into the table to prevent pasta spills.

If you are a purist about eating spaghetti, linguini, or any other long, thin noodles, you will not use a spoon as a support. You will go it

If you're not a "purist" about eating spaghetti, use a large (cream soup size) spoon to help you twist the strands of spaghetti around the fork. (A purist does it with deft twirls of the fork—and no other help!)

alone with the fork. The secret is in twining just a small number of strands around your fork (four or five). Keep turning your fork slowly around until all the strands are rolled compactly around it and you're ready to put it into your mouth.

When you first try this, you probably will have trails of spaghetti falling down from the fork, and you will lose as many strands as you manage to get wound around the fork. It's also common for the most professional of spaghetti eaters to err occasionally and to be obliged to slurp errant strands of spaghetti or angel hair up into their mouths. As with anything, however, practice makes almost perfect, and you will feel a great sense of achievement once you master the fork-only method of eating spaghetti.

If you find the sauce and the grated cheese sitting on top of your pasta, it is good form to mix it all up, like a chef's salad, before eating it. It is also good form to mop up the last bit of pasta sauce with a piece of bread speared on your fork.

What is *not* good form is to cut your spaghetti into small, manageable pieces with your fork—unless you are a child!

Vegetables That Are Difficult to Eat

The four vegetables most difficult to eat are:

- o Peas (because they keep escaping from the fork)
- o Artichokes (because they are complicated)
- o Corn on the cob (because eating it results in grease all over your face and kernels stuck in your teeth)
- o Asparagus

PEAS

If you are eating continental-style, it is fairly easy to shove peas onto your fork, held in the left hand, while your knife in the right hand serves as a flying buttress. If you are eating American style, it helps to use a small piece of bread or roll to shove the recalcitrant peas onto your fork. (Of course, you still have to face the problem of getting the peas from the plate into your mouth. That requires a delicate balancing act on the fork.)

ARTICHOKES

Served usually as an appetizer, the artichoke is consumed leaf by leaf. When you pull off a leaf, dip the rounded, soft, meaty end of it into the melted butter, vinaigrette, mayonnaise, or whatever has been pro-

When you confront an artichoke, grasp it with one hand near the base to steady it, and with your right hand pull off the leaves one by one. Dip each leaf into the melted butter or mayonnaise container and then eat it. Pile used leaves neatly in a ring around the artichoke on the plate.

vided in the small container at your place. Eat the leaf up to the part of it that is hard and inedible, and then discard it neatly in a pile of "used leaves" you arrange around the artichokes on your plate.

When you have eaten your way down to the central, gray, fuzzy part (the "choke"), spear it with your fork (or steady it with your fingers), hold it steady, and then cut off the gray feathery part around and under it. You should now have a "bald" round-on-top gray heart devoid of any little leaves. Cut it out from its bed of larger leaves, and dip it. (Cut it into smaller pieces on your plate before eating it, if it is a large heart.) The artichoke heart is tender and flavorful—the best part of this formidable vegetable.

Corn on the Cob

Once again, fresh corn on the cob is great for family dinners and for parties held outdoors. For dinner in your home, however, it is far easier on your guests if you cut off the kernels from the cob in the kitchen and serve the corn buttered and seasoned in a bowl.

If you are eating corn at a picnic, hopefully your host has already preseasoned and prebuttered the cobs. If not, and you have to butter the cob yourself, butter and season a few rows at a time and eat them, instead of having to hold an entire cob full of grease, which will then drip all over you.

Asparagus

Fresh asparagus may be eaten in one of two ways, depending upon how long it is cooked and how much of it is buried in sauce: either with the fingers or with a knife and fork.

If the stalks are firm and the vegetable has been steamed for only a short time, hopefully the sauce only has been put on the asparagus tips. This is the moment for you to pick it up with your fingers, stalk by stalk, eating it down to the tough, inedible part, and then placing the "used" asparagus stalks back on the plate in a neat pile.

If the asparagus is overcooked and the stalk is entirely flexible, and if sauce has been poured all over, you can't use your fingers. Cut the vegetable into small manageable portions with your knife and fork as you eat it.

Salad

Salad is a versatile food. It may be served as:

o A first course (such as chicken salad in half an avocado, or hearts of palm with lettuce and dressing)
o A side dish (such as a mixed green salad served with the main entrée)
o A separate course, between the entrée and dessert, provided it is accompanied by an assortment of cheeses and crackers

Nutritionists say that salad should not be torn into small, manageable pieces until just before it is served, because otherwise some of the vitamin content escapes. However, the host should remember to have the leaves torn into small pieces instead of forcing his guests to cope with large leaves on their salad plates.

Cut unwieldy pieces of lettuce with a fork; if they can't be cut with a fork only, use your knife, too.

If salad is served as a vegetable on your entrée plate, use your entrée fork to eat it. If it is served on a separate side plate, you may—or may not—have been provided with a special salad fork in your place setting. (If there is none, use your entrée fork.)

If you are being served a separate course of salad and cheese, between the entrée and dessert, a separate plate will be put down before you. You should have as your utensils both a salad fork and a luncheon knife. Take small portions of one or two cheeses from the cheese tray, and two or three crackers. This is no time to exaggerate what you serve yourself (everyone is watching you at the table).

Be very careful if your salad is overdressed, because it will splash on your clothes. If lettuce leaves fall off your overburdened salad plate, just pick them up and put them back on the plate. (It happens to me all the time.) If the fallen lettuce leaves behind it a big stain of dressing, dab at it with your napkin, and then forget about it.

Fresh Fruit Served at the End of a Meal

In many countries, a bowl of fresh fruit is passed to guests, either as dessert or as a prologue to dessert. The following are some tips on eating fresh fruit when you are a guest:

• *Apples.* If you eat only peeled apples, then peel your apple with the fruit knife provided you. The easiest way to handle this is first to quarter the apple. Then use the knife to peel and remove the core from each quarter. Europeans often cut the entire apple into tiny pieces with their fork and knife as they go along, but if you wish to pick up an apple quarter and eat it in your fingers, that's all right, too.

• *Bananas.* If you are at the beach or on a picnic, you simply remove the peel and eat the banana whole. If you've chosen a banana to eat at someone's dinner table, remove the skin, leave it on the side of your plate, and then cut the banana into small pieces with your fruit knife and fork. Then eat the pieces with your fork.

• *Grapes.* Usually you will find a pair of grape scissors passed with the bowl of grapes. Cut a nice cluster of grapes from the main branch, and put it on your plate. If there are no scissors, tear it off carefully with your fingers. Deposit the grape seeds into your fingers, and then transfer them to the plate as unobtrusively as possible. (Actually, it is much better if your host serves seedless grapes.)

If someone should ask you how to peel a grape, my answer is that you don't.

• *Peaches and pears.* Some people eat peaches, skin and all; some prefer to peel them. Peal first, if you must, then core the pear or remove the stone from the peach and then quarter it. It is best to eat these fruits small piece by small piece, since they are full of juice and are more difficult to eat by hand than an apple.

Sliced peaches, of course, are served with milk or cream (and optionally sugar), and pears are often poached whole in a syrup sauce. It's only when you approach the whole, fresh fruit that some manual dexterity is required to eat them properly.

• *Grapefruit.* Your host (or the restaurant) should have removed almost all the seeds before it is presented to you. Hopefully, he or she will have already precut each little section, too, so that all you have to do is slide out each section with a spoon. If the grapefruit sections have not been precut, use a small knife or the serrated-edged grapefruit spoon to do the job.

It is proper when you have finished eating the grapefruit to pick it up and squeeze its juice onto your spoon, and then drink it.

• *Oranges and tangerines.* Use your fruit knife first to remove the peel. (If the peel is thick and loose, you can pull it off with your fingers.) Then pull it apart into small, manageable sections before eating it. If your piece of fruit is covered with a network of white pulpy skin, remove that as well with your fingers. Spit any seeds into the palm of your hand, and then transfer to the plate.

• *Plums, cherries, apricots, kumquats*. A small piece of fruit with a stone in its center is put whole in the mouth with the fingers. The fruit is chewed off the stone in the mouth; the pit is then pushed onto a fork or spoon with tongue action and then brought down onto the plate.

• *Kiwis*. The kiwi is peeled and then sliced like a tomato, and the thin slices are used in fruit cups and as decoration for salads and desserts.

• *Melons, papayas, and pomegranates*. These fruits are served ice-cold and are halved or quartered, depending on their original size. A fruit like papaya, with seeds in its center, is served to you with the seeds already removed. Scoop out the fruit from its shell with a spoon.

• *Fresh pineapple*. After the ends and the outer spiny skin of the pineapple have been removed with a sharp knife, the pineapple is sliced into thin round pieces. When served on a plate (either as is, or with some liqueur like *Kirschwasser* poured over it), it is eaten with a dessert fork and spoon.

• *Watermelon*. This is too informal and messy to include on a dinner party menu (unless it is cut up, with its seeds removed, as part of a fruit cup). The problem with serving a piece of watermelon at the table is the quantity of seeds, which requires a constant spitting of seeds into the palm of the hand and then down onto the plate. This fruit is greatly enjoyed when served at an informal outdoor party—at which seed-spitting is tolerated in everyone, not just the children.

• *Stewed fruit*. If you are eating something like stewed prunes, eat around the pit by cutting away the fruit from the center. If the prune pit ends up in your mouth, remove it by fork (or spoon, if you are using a dessert spoon without a knife).

Informal Food

• *Triple-decker sandwiches*. If you have a big mouth and are eating alone, you might as well put one end of the entire sandwich in your mouth and start to eat. If anyone else is present, cut each half of this giant sandwich into yet another half. If a quarter of the sandwich is absolutely too wide for your mouth, cut it up as you go along into smaller, manageable bites.

• *Heroes*. A hero is a sharing food, a group activity. The secret to the polite consumption of a foot-long or longer hero is to cut off an appropriate-size piece for yourself, based on the number of people who will be sharing it with you, how much you like it, and how large it is. It is better to err on the side of a small portion and to return for more than to cut off too big a piece and cause a mutiny in the ranks because you took an overly generous amount. If you are the host of a gathering, precut the pieces in equal amounts. Then no one can complain about anyone else.

• *Hamburgers and hot dogs*. These are easy-to-eat finger foods. The problems that arise stem from an oversupply of sauce topping, not to mention sliced onions. Eat small portions of your hamburger or hot dog, because otherwise, your cheeks will be bulging with food (unattractive). Use napkins to hold the object, so that any sauce oozing out will hit the napkin and not your hands and clothing. If you're really worried about your clothes, stand holding the burger or dog well out from your body and lean over to eat it. (In this case, however, watch out for the shoes of everyone standing near you!)

A smart burger or dog consumer always holds it in a napkin in one hand, and has a napkin or two at the ready in the other hand.

• *Pizza*. Pizza is an informal food, not served at dinner parties, so eat it as it is meant to be eaten—each pie-shaped wedge held in your hand. As you hold it, turn up the outside edges toward the center, to prohibit the filling from sliding off and out. Lots of napkins should be on hand.

• *Tortillas*. Tortillas are also meant to be eaten while held in your hand. The flat tortilla is lightly filled with a mixture such as frijoles (kidney beans); then it is rolled up and eaten like a sandwich, from end to end.

• *French fries, shoestring potatoes, and potato chips*. These are all meant to be eaten with the fingers. If the fries are greasy or covered with catsup, you logically eat them with your fork—unless you are at an outside sporting event, in which case you use your fingers anyway. (Several napkins will also be required to repair the damage to your fingers—and possibly your clothes!)

Potato chips are in the category of "noisy foods." Be careful, when eating them at a party, to take small bites and keep your mouth as closed as possible.

• *Popcorn*. Another noisy food. The easiest and healthiest kind to eat is salt- and butter-free popcorn. When a woman takes a handful of popcorn from the bowl and puts it in her mouth, swallowing as many kernels as she can, there goes her lipstick—all over her face. (Therefore a woman who is going to indulge in popcorn would be smart to blot her lipstick first!)

I think we should all mind our manners and be concerned about the environment in our movie theaters, as that relates to popcorn! Moviegoers who do not spill their popcorn all over the floor, but instead carefully put their empty boxes in the trash cans after the film, are real heroes in today's society.

No one looks very attractive with cheeks completely stuffed with popcorn; it's also easy to choke on.

I learned another lesson about eating popcorn in my college days. I was introduced to a Supreme Court justice in his home in Washington by his daughter, a friend of mine. I had been consuming popcorn enthusiastically before being introduced, and I gave him a hearty handshake with my well-buttered, salty hand. He grimaced as if in pain, drew a large white handkerchief from his pocket, and proceeded to clean off his hand with a flourish. "Sir," I asked in an awed voice, "was I responsible for that?"

"Oh, no," he answered sarcastically, "it was Peter Pan."

*   *   *

Many parents have no idea that their children have less than passable table manners. When families do break bread together, both generations often are whizzing by each other at breakfast, or at dinnertime are consuming their meal, using their fingers, at a fast food place. I watched as my college-age son pushed his hamburger aside one day, clutched a fresh batch of french fries with his fingers, and then dipped them into a pond of catsup before plopping them into his mouth. His fingers and mouth dripping in grease and tomato sauce, he asked, "Mom, what would the manners experts say about my style of eating these fries?"

"Pretty gross, Malcolm," I replied.

He laughed and responded, "Have you ever watched yourself eating a pizza? Pretty gross, too, Mom." And that about sums up the state of America's table manners today! I guess we have to work a lot harder when we are using our knives and forks to compensate for those times when we aren't.

PART II

ANSWERS TO QUESTIONS ABOUT MANNERS THAT NO ONE HAD TO ASK BEFORE

10

New Manners for the New Society

If the writers on manners down through the centuries could be summoned from the next world back to this one to join in a seminar on recent changes in our mores, they would not only be unable to believe the dialogue that would ensue, but they would probably not even want to try to cope with it. They would never be able to accept that in today's society so much has changed so fast in so short a time, because throughout history, before these times, manners traditionally changed and adapted very slowly—and carefully.

Since the early 1960s, it's as if some Superman-like character has been hurling us through time. The Youth Rebellion of the sixties and seventies, the impact of drugs, the proliferation of sexually transmitted diseases, the increase in divorce and single-parent families, the restless mobility of modern Americans, and our increasingly time-pressured lives have all splintered many traditional family formations and altered our lifestyles.

In order to conduct our lives with confidence and grace in the 1990s, we must be clear-eyed about the changes that have taken place—and alert to those to come—and arm ourselves with knowledge about how to handle them in today's terms. This section in this book will help you do so.

DATING IN THE NEW DECADE

A real date is two people getting together at a specified time on a certain day (with advance notice and advance planning) for the purpose of doing something special. It's a date when someone asks you "to come over to my house for chili next Wednesday night," or announces, "I've two good seats for the ball game Friday night. How about it?" It's a date when you're invited "to go to the new mall opening, and then we can get something to eat." It's a date when someone of the opposite sex asks, "How about going ice-skating with me next Saturday evening, and we can get burgers there?" It's a date when someone invites you to a testimonial business dinner in a hotel ballroom, and it's a date when you're asked for a "walk in the woods to look at the autumn foliage, and maybe have some hot chocolate afterward."

A date may be just a pleasant coming together, or a payoff for a favor done, or it may be a delicate step in a courtship and mating dance.

- *Going out on a date is an opportunity to shine.*

The wonderful thing about this era in which we live is that women no longer have to sit at home passively and wait for the telephone to ring. A woman can properly pick up the telephone and ask a man out as easily as he can call to ask her out. It's an easy adjustment for the young, but a lot more difficult for women who are beyond college age. Asking a man out on a date may be a painful exercise for a woman, but she should take heart in the fact that asking a woman out on a date is just as painful for many a man! Maybe you're one of the vast world of shy people and you feel you don't stand out in group. Maybe you're a little overweight or underweight, maybe you're not a great beauty or a handsome hunk of man. Maybe you feel uncomfortable at big parties in competition with others who appear to you to be better looking, more successful, and popular. A person of the opposite sex who has caught your eye in the group may not be particularly attracted to you at that moment, so your strategy should be to get that person alone at some future time, away from the party crowd, so that he or she can get to know you—and in the process, get to like you.

Going out as a couple or in a foursome with a person who attracts you is the easiest way to show yourself at your best (with the exception, of course, of entertaining with zest in your own home, which provides your greatest showcase of all). Going out on a date allows the two of you to get to know each other in a relaxed, quiet milieu—which a party is not. The great thing about being with someone on a date is that it provides a chance to show your generous supply of intelligence, charm, and personality. You can demonstrate the kind of creative fun you know how to generate. You can display your strong points (and everyone has some of those).

But first there's this problem to resolve: How can you get someone to go out on a date with you when he or she may have no inclination to do so?

Asking the Person for the Date

Some people are so shy, they would rather live permanently in a cave than submit to the agony of asking someone out and then suffer being rejected. Here is some advice:

• *It's smart to steel yourself for a rejection to your invitation,* because the first person you ask may very well be busy, may be in a relationship with someone else, or may be working so hard that he or she literally does not have time to go out on a date. Or that person simply may not want to go out with you. That is not a serious kind of rejection. It happens to everyone, not just to you. Your goal in life should be to find the person who *does* want to and who will go out with you. That person is out there, but only you can find him or her. If you keep scanning the entire sea with your eyes, you will appreciate all the fish swimming by, and you won't have set your sights and hopes on just one of them.

• *Get organized, but be creative, too.* Make plans—fascinating plans—so that the person you want to have accompany you will really be excited at the prospect of what you have devised. Make it sound so exciting that it will be impossible to resist. Maybe you can get tickets for something that is extremely difficult to get tickets for; maybe you have an invitation to a glamorous occasion—anything from the grand opening of a restaurant to a special performance of the Bolshoi Ballet. Maybe you know a "wonderful fortune teller we can go to," and with "dinner in my favorite Thai restaurant afterward." Maybe you live in a small town that will never see the Bolshoi or a Thai restaurant—there are still different things to do and organize in your community. You simply have to be alert, as though you have eyes in the back of your head and antennae in both ears, so that you know about the new, exciting things to do or places to go in your town before everyone else does.

• *Ask the person for a date in a letter, carefully wording your invitation to sound enticing, which is often difficult to do in a telephone call.* If you were to call, asking for a date, you might sound awkward, and it would be very easy for the other person to quickly turn you down. He or she might be in a hurry and might not even try to listen to you.

Try sending a handsome piece of handwritten stationery through the mails, describing the wonderful evening or weekend activity you have arranged and asking the targeted person to join you. Your amusing letter might very well persuade that person to accept, whereas that same person might have turned you down flat at a party or on the telephone.

For example, try a note like this, which is breezy yet warm and holds out the promise of an entertaining evening.

Dear Jerry,

Someone told me that you are a contemporary classical music fan. Well, so am I—and I have two tickets to an extraordinary concert at Avery Fisher Hall on May 23rd at eight o'clock. The American Composers Orchestra will play a program of all-new works.

Along with having a modern musical ear, I am also a passable cook, so I'd like to invite you for some pre-concert chicken curry at my apartment at six o'clock.

Give me a call at my office, 000-0000, and I hope you can make it!

• *Once you have that date arranged, it's up to you to be yourself— natural and considerate*—so that the other person will be very glad to have accepted your invitation. As the nineties progress, there will be more and more reciprocation between the sexes; especially if both work, they will reciprocate in the areas of money, time, and effort expended in organizing a real date.

What Constitutes a Good Date

Sure, it's great fun to do things on the spur of the moment, but if you ask people what they feel is paramount in enjoying a date, most will say "being with someone who is organized, who is a good conversationalist, who makes me think I'm special, and who *puts me* at ease."

I recently overheard a conversation in a restaurant, when I was on a book promotion tour. I was having dinner alone and could not help overhearing the conversation at the next table between an attractive man and woman in their early thirties:

"Howard, we're just not on the same wavelength."

"Why?"

"Because I do all the talking."

"But you talk so well."

"I get tired of doing all the talking. You make no effort at all. I might as well be sitting here talking to a stone wall."

"But that's the way I am. You know that."

"You could make an effort. You could try to hold up your end, offer something, say something that might interest me for a change. I spend a lot of time preparing for an evening like this. I take a lot of care with how I look, and then you—"

"You make me sound"—the irritation was rising in his voice to match hers—"as though I bore you when I take you out."

"Howard, I have to tell you, you do. This lobster—my very favorite food—doesn't merit spending an evening like this."

"I'll get the check."

No more words were spoken, and it was probably the end of their relationship. Howard obviously should have made at least a feeble attempt at being stimulating, instead of sitting there expecting to be entertained the entire time. The young woman had obviously had it and decided, in the middle of her lobster—although I noticed she had wisely finished the best part of it before issuing her ultimatum—that she couldn't go through more evenings like this.

How I sympathized with her! I had spent so many evenings like hers during the many years I was single. It simply isn't worth going to all that trouble for someone who is *blah*, who doesn't contribute and expects you to dazzle him or her nonstop while giving you nothing in return. (There are just as many women who are blah, too; blahness is not gender-specific!) Women used to think they had to accept whatever behavior a man adopted on a date. Thank goodness this is no longer true. Today, a woman—or a man—should expect a date

- To give advance notice when making the date—at least three days before, so that there is time to prepare (to make a hair appointment, get a suit cleaned or whatever). Anyone who calls up two hours beforehand to ask for a date is hardly paying a compliment to the other person.
- To consider the other person's interests when making the plans (for example, doesn't force a baseball-only fan to a ballet or vice-versa).
- Not to try to change the plans at the last minute.
- To have original, creative ideas about things to do and places to go.
- To be on time.
- To dress appropriately, so as not to embarrass the other person. (It is normal for a person to want to be proud of the way his or her date looks and is dressed.)
- Not to make a scene in public.
- To be sensitive to the other person's financial situation when the other person is paying.
- To be philosophical when things go wrong, without knocking the other person's ideas or planning expertise—in fact, to try to find something nice to say about the place, the food, the game, the show, or the other people at the party. (With a positive attitude, you can *always* find something good, even if you consider the situation pretty disastrous!)
- Not to keep complaining (a real killjoy action) if he or she doesn't feel well or is tired.
- To thank the other person at the end of the date, whether it's to show gratitude for the money spent or praise for the planning

done or just to show pleasure for the pleasant companionship during the evening.

o To write a thank-you note after a special evening. ("You made me feel so good with that toast" . . . "I love the flowers you brought me" . . . "You were nice to fill up my car with a tank of gas when I wasn't looking" . . . "I hope some day in our lives we'll see another movie as great as that one" . . . "What a treat to have pasta like that" . . . "I really appreciated the way you took care of that guy in the stands who squirted mustard all over my dress!"

• *The best way to make a good impression on a first date is to keep your sense of humor.* People who are trying too hard to be charming can become very uptight when things go wrong. And things do go wrong. One of my goddaughters recounted the disasters on a recent date that she had initiated: The restaurant did not honor the table reservation she had made; the theater tickets weren't waiting for them at the ticket window of the theater; her date's coat got stolen from the coatroom in a nightclub where they had stopped to have a nightcap. When I insinuated that she probably would never see that young man again, she grinned and said, "I see him all the time. We just laughed all night long. I kept asking. 'Now what will go wrong next?' And something always did. He finally said that I was the kind of girl who would laugh if I lost my winning lottery ticket receipt."

Who Pays for What on a Date and When and How

The question of who pays for what on a date is as complicated and potentially embarrassing as the confusion among the parents of the bride and groom over who will pay for what in the wedding when the groom's family is assisting the bride's with the financial responsibility.

Traditionally, on a date the man was supposed to pay for everything, but like many traditions, the custom has changed and molded itself into the new society to allow for common sense. Today, with women's equality and with women earning their own money, the cost of a date is often split. What doesn't change is that when someone asks another on a first date, the one who asks should pay for that date. If a woman asks a man for the first date, she should pay for everything from the garage parking charge to the coat check. From then on, the two can compromise and split the costs according to their whims and resources. A rich man will always pay for his date; a rich woman who asks out a man who is not rich will always pay for him, too—but if she is smart, she will protect his ego and pay for the date without anyone else but him knowing it.

The important thing here is that both parties should understand who is going to pay for what on the date *before* it ever takes place. There should never be any unpleasant surprises or embarrassing moments of

"May I borrow some money?" Nothing ruins a great dinner in a restaurant faster than bickering over who gets the bill, whether someone is trying to push the bill off on someone else or trying to grab the check to pay when the other person is already trying to pay it.

People who have to watch their wallets should be honest and up-front when making the date. For example:

• A young man in school might say to his date, "I can get two tickets to the game Friday night. I'd really like to have you go with me, but things are a little tight. Can you pay for your own ticket?"

• A woman who has been taken out on a date three times by a man might say, "It's certainly time for some reciprocity! Why don't I make my famous lasagna dinner for you Saturday night, and take you to the movies?"

• A young male executive on a starting salary might say to a female colleague, "I'd like to have dinner with you Friday night. I can either buy you a pizza dinner at Joe's, or we can have a fancy dinner at Le Manoir and go Dutch. Which would you like to do?" Chances are, she would prefer to go to a nice place and pay her own way.

Since men are sensitive about women paying for them in public, a woman should be equally sensitive about it. She can slip money to her date in an inconspicuous gesture under the table. She can give him money beforehand. She can discreetly slip her credit card instead of her date's to the waiter when he brings the check.

Women in their late sixties and onward, schooled in the old tradition of a man always paying, have difficulty with the perceived embarrassment of paying for a male escort's meals and tickets. They would be better off making an arrangement beforehand with the restaurant to send them a bill for the lunch or dinner to which they have invited a male companion. They can purchase tickets to plays and concerts beforehand. It's a question of getting organized in advance.

Some rich older women, of course, solve their escort-in-the-evening problem by having a young gigolo on the staff. This kind of date seems to have no trouble at all being perceived as a man who never picks up the check!

If You're Miserable on the Date

If you're having a physically nasty time on a date (he or she is drunk and abusive or making sexual innuendoes or strong-arming you), make a quick departure. You do not have to remain out of politeness and submit to that kind of behavior just because someone is paying for your dinner. Take whatever steps are available to escape from the situation, whether that means calling a cab, asking the restaurant manager to help you, summoning the police if the situation is really out of hand, or running into the street to find a public place that is open and will serve as a momentary place of refuge.

However, the chances of this kind of danger-ridden evening are minimal in comparison to your chances of having a completely boring evening. You might be fed up, disappointed, restless, embarrassed to be seen with your date, or bothered by his or her smoking. Don't escape. Just get through the evening. It won't last forever. Be a good sport, because it's great training in self-discipline, and you can never tell when this kind of training will serve you well in the future!

• Except, of course, when dealing with someone who is abusive, *always thank your date at the end of the evening.* You don't have to be hypocritical and gush your gratitude. Just say something like, "Thank you for all the trouble you went to," or "The dessert at that restaurant was really delicious," if that was the best part of the meal. Maybe the only thing good about the meal was the bread. (I remember a friend who was miserable on a blind date and praised the only thing she found worthy of mention at the restaurant—"They have the best ice water at that place!" she said, thanking her date for an evening that in her eyes had been totally terrible.) You can always find *something* to praise during the evening. It's polite to mention that one affirmative thing and then to shut up about all of the negative rest of it. Your justifiable frankness could really hurt the other person, and the pleasure in voicing that justifiable criticism isn't worth hurting someone else's feelings.

When the evening is finally over, your date may well say something like, "Well, I'll call you again soon" or "We must do this again very quickly." At that point you should control your panic, take a deep breath, and say something kindly like, "No, I don't really think so." You might add, "I think you should ask out someone who's more on your wavelength. You see, I'm not. It's no fault of yours. It's nothing you've done. It's just that you and I don't share the same interests and attitudes. I'm sorry. Thank you for tonight." Then close the door. End of bad date. End of other person's expectations.

Give That Blind Date a Chance!

Should you go out on blind dates? The answer is *yes*—even if you have been out on eighteen of them in the past year and all eighteen were frightful disasters. For all you know, the twenty-first will be the one.

Following are some tips on how to summon the courage to go out on a blind date:

• Your friends are wonderful and loyal to arrange the blind date, even though you think they have no taste and have obviously no idea in the world what makes you attracted to the opposite sex. Be grateful to them for trying. It would be a lot worse if they never tried.

- Remember the statistics. An incredibly large number of people around the world are happily married to spouses they met on blind dates. There is always a small chance you could become one of those statistics.
- Remember that the blind date, if he or she is not totally hopeless, has friends. Many a person has found his or her true love through the friends of a blind date.
- You can be taken to wonderful new places by blind dates—places your other friends wouldn't or couldn't take you. When I was in India, I was driven from New Delhi to see the Taj Mahal on a blind date. I might never have seen it otherwise. I don't remember the man who drove me, but I certainly remember the Taj Mahal these twenty-eight years later!
- You might very possibly need that blind date in the future to round out your table at your next dinner party. Extra men, in particular, are hard to come by. One of your other dinner guests may find something redeemable, even lovable, in that person, even if you don't.
- Don't always trust your first negative impression. You might be making a wrong judgment too fast on your blind date. One of my best men friends went out on a blind date with a girl he dismissed as a total nerd. He was forced, kicking and complaining, into being her escort again a month later. He married her two months after that, in one of the great whirlwind courtships of all time.

THE NEW MANNERS CONCERNING
SEX AND ROMANTIC RELATIONSHIPS

When the Answer Is "Yes"

My own feeling is that sex is much better when there is romance lurking around somewhere. Otherwise, it can become as matter-of-fact as a computer print-out.

If you think your date tonight is going to "sleep over" and you welcome that thought, prepare for it. Have some treats waiting in your fridge. Have your bedroom straightened, with clean sheets on the bed, fresh flowers on your bureau, and fresh towels, an extra water glass, and a new toothbrush in the bathroom. A sparkling clean bedroom is enticing.

A ROMANTIC BUT POLITE POINT OF VIEW

If you have enjoyed sex with someone, thank that person the next day. Some people just arise, get dressed, and leave for their office or other appointments without waking the other person—and without leaving a note. Gone and forgotten. No telephone call, either. The sex act from the night before becomes a detached, cold, and meaningless memory. Often your or the other person's lack of communication the next day is not a deliberate snub; often it stems from not knowing what to do, as well as from being terrified of saying too much to make the other person think you are more serious about him or her than you actually are.

It's too bad, really. When two people have been intimate, and the sexual encounter was a pleasant experience for both, it should be considered a common courtesy the next day for one to get in touch with the other, if for no other reason than to say "thank you." Neither person should take a thank-you call as a profession of love or as an indication of desire on the caller's part to deepen the relationship. When you make a short thank-you call, it's nothing more and nothing less than a gesture of appreciation for a very enjoyable shared experience.

Don't call and leave a perfunctory message at your partner's office, as though you were commending him or her on a job performance in the conference room this morning. And no one is suggesting that you leave a message to be relayed through the secretary implying that her boss was really great in bed last night! What is advocated here is some signal of gratitude—whether that's a telephone call, a note, a bottle of wine, or a bunch of posies with a card that might say something as uncomplicated as "I had a terrific time last night."

A friend of mine, now in her early fifties and legendary for her beauty and her great success with men, once showed me the collection of little notes and cards she had received from men when she was young—notes that had accompanied flowers and gifts sent "always the day after a romantic interlude," she explained. One man had written, "Even if our paths never cross again, I will never forget you—or last night." ("He was anything but a poet," she laughed, "but he expressed himself rather well with that short sentence.") Another wrote on a florist's card, "It was the nicest, most unexpected, totally incredible evening." Still another wrote, "The main course at your dinner was excellent, but the dessert was *unforgettable!*"

You are not making a commitment or proposing matrimony with a short note or telephone call. You are merely instilling a welcomed note of romance into both your lives.

Of course, if a sexual encounter was an unpleasant experience from your point of view, there is certainly no need for a thank-you gesture on your part! If you're forever "busy" when the other person calls you, he or she should get the message that you don't want a repeat experience. It's easier if you're honest right away and say in your own words, "I think you're wasting your time calling me. We're not right as a couple, and in fairness to you, you should devote your energy to finding someone new."

When the Answer Is "No"

In any consideration of sexual manners, there obviously is no place for the unforgivable act of sex by force, so that is not included in this discussion. Manners come into play only in terms of sex as an act of free will.

Many people play games all the time, but sex should not be considered one of them. It is the better part of wisdom to tell the truth when you feel no attraction for a person who is pressuring you to engage in sex. It's also a kindness to that person to do so, rather than to fabricate a hundred excuses as to why there won't be any sex tonight ("I'd really like to, I really want to, but I'm just not feeling well tonight . . .").

There was a miserable period that began about twenty years ago when men tended to feel that paying the price of a good dinner gave them a license to sleep with their dates—an attitude that really put down the women who acquiesced and that made unpopular the ones who didn't. As one young friend of mine expressed it then, "It's kind of an unwritten law. You don't have to do anything for a hamburger—but for something like a good steak, wine, and atmosphere, you're really expected to put out." Today, in spite of the editorial thrust of certain magazines extolling sex as a regular necessity (and their warning that decreased regularity is "hazardous to your health, not to mention your complexion"), no unmarried person should feel *compelled* to sleep with anyone else.

It's unfortunate that it took a plague of sexually transmitted diseases to change the climate from one in which unmarried people felt a constant social pressure to engage in sex to one in which many unmarried people feel wary of engaging in sex at all.

Personally, I feel that even if kindness dictates considering the other person's ego when you reject his or her sexual invitation, it's equally important to be honest. In your own words, you might somehow communicate the message that:

- o You think the other person is *very* attractive (showing your sensitivity to his or her ego).
- o But you are not physically attracted to that person (showing your honesty). Explain that if there's a lack of chemistry on your part, it's no one's fault, just the luck of the draw.
- o You enjoy the other person's company very much, but if he or she demands more than just your company during the time you spend together, it's only fair to end the relationship.

Don't sell the other person short. You may find he or she treasures your friendship and enjoys being with you, too, even without the sex. Or perhaps he or she thinks that in time you will begin to feel a sexual attraction, too (which is not an impossibility).

Friendships between people of both sexes are very strong and powerful, but diplomacy, tact, and imagination are required to turn a would-be lover into a friend. Often the person you have spurned sexually will disappear from your life, hurt and confused. Then with time, that person may seek you out again, just wanting to spend time with you. When sexual tension decreases (it doesn't have to disappear *completely*), that's when friendship can strengthen and begin to fill a void. Men and women can—and should—enjoy being with each other without the necessity for sexual overtones to everything they say or do.

When a Woman Is Afraid to Be Alone at Home with a Man

If you are a woman who has invited a man to have dinner with you alone in your home and then you begin to have an uneasy feeling about it, don't go through with the evening as originally planned—alone with him. Invite another couple to join you, or have a sudden change of plans and take him out to dinner in a restaurant. You may have a good basis for your fears. You may have seen him in action and witnessed him drink too much or come on to you too fast; you may have heard another woman describe him as too rough. A majority of the rapes that occur take place behind a closed door when the woman is with a man she knows.

The man you don't really know but have invited to come alone to your house may be the most innocent kind of man there is, but if you have a strange feeling about him, trust your intuition and be careful.

If, for security reasons, you have invited another couple for dinner along with your male guest, you can always address the gathering when the couple makes a move to leave—something like, "Well, I think it's a good time for the evening to end for us all. Jim, I hope you won't mind if I call it a day, too." He might reply that he will only stay for "just another ten minutes—just a quick drink," to which you might announce that you need your sleep and have a tough, important week ahead of you. If you keep laughing and joking about it, your male guest won't take offense. The important thing is not to appear frightened.

It also helps if you have told the other couple beforehand that you would appreciate their making sure your male guest leaves when they do.

Women should not put themselves into vulnerable situations with men they do not know well, either personally or by reputation. When you don't know anything about someone to whom you find yourself attracted, have lunch with him and go to events in public with him. Then you'll get to know and trust him. Then it's time for the cozy evenings "at home" to begin.

Bringing Up the Subject of Condoms

We have all seen some pretty tasteless condom promotions, including ads and public relations gimmicks. I recently saw a dispenser that looked as if it contained transit tokens; another condom-holder was a child's cartoon character wristwatch with a secret compartment in the back. These gimmicks may manufacture a quick laugh for some people, but for most they constitute a "cheap shot" kind of humor.

In this confused world of ours, people need to be forthright, frank, and honest with each other. The fear of sexually transmitted diseases, particularly AIDS, is not something to treat in a cute or amusing way. If you're a woman, how do you know that incredibly good-looking man you've just begun to date hasn't been infected with the HIV virus that causes AIDS? If you're a man, how do you know that attractive woman you just met isn't a carrier, having become infected because of a drug injection with a dirty needle?

You no longer have to hem and haw about whether or not to say yes to sex with anyone. You don't have to worry about your manners in turning someone down. Saying no is very polite these days! And if you want to say yes, make it on *your* terms—safe sex only. Use a condom. Make him wear a proper-fitting tear-free, less than three-year-old (see the expiration date on the package) condom.

Anyone who writes about sexual mores writes from a personal philosophy that is impossible to disguise. Mine is very openly pro-chastity as the only acceptable lifestyle for the young. Such a philosophy used to elicit derisive laughter during the sixties. It is no longer an old-fashioned joke. Parents can once again impress this on their children. Whereas morality used to be the reason for sexual abstinence, today protecting your life is the new reason. Few people would disagree with the philosophy that love and sex ideally are at their best in marriage.

Some women are much too embarrassed even to ask a male sex partner if he has a condom, much less ready to supply him with one, but at a certain moment a woman should realize it is far better to suffer such a moment of embarrassment than to contract a sexually transmitted disease. No pleasure or moment of passion is worth that! If it is difficult for a woman to find the words to ask about her partner's preparedness prior to having sex with him, she had better learn to overcome such reticence. This is no time to be shy when her own life or that of a future child to be born to her might be affected—by this act of passion this very night. There are several ways for her to handle the situation including:

- o Supplying the condoms herself. ("Look, if you don't have any, you'll find some on the first shelf of the medicine closet.")
- o Asking him to go out to buy them. ("Since you say you're not

prepared, I think you'd better become prepared. There's an all-night drugstore a short distance away.")

o Announcing (the best idea of all) that, "Since you're not prepared, we'll just have to wait until you are. Let's skip sex tonight."

If a woman shows her partner that she is responsible for her own behavior, she will teach any man who really is attracted to her and wants her to be responsible about his, too.

Safe Sex and Bisexuality

The best of all worlds is the romantic attachment of two people who wait until they are married for sex. Since we aren't living in the best of all worlds, let's step down one level of reality and say that the best of what many adults can make of today's world is safe sex—the use of condoms for those who do not abstain. And let's really step down another great number of levels and say that bisexuality is the worst of all worlds. Bisexual acts are reportedly increasing in alarming numbers. My sense of sisterhood is showing when I say that it is totally reprehensible for a man who is bisexual to have an affair with or marry a woman who thinks he is straight. He is putting her life and that of her future children in danger because of the possibility of transmitting the HIV infection to her. There are no sexual manners that can relate to this kind of deceit.

A Homosexual Relationship

When two people of the same sex openly live with one another in a monogamous relationship they should be treated as a couple in every social sense of the word. In the evening and on weekends, they should be invited together to any kind of event. The men should not be recruited by their hosts as dates or as escorts for single women, except in the sense of friends helping out each other by providing transportation to and from a party.

When a gay man or lesbian loses his or her companion, the nice thing to do is to write a letter of condolence, send flowers to the funeral, or make a gift in memoriam to the deceased. The homosexual who loses a mate suffers a loss equal to a married couple's loss.

If you are not certain of someone's sexual preference, do not ask that person what it is. Respect his or her privacy. And remember that the most hurtful thing of all is to gossip about your homosexual friends or acquaintances. It only adds fuel to the fire of abuse that they already suffer at the hands of many people, and contributes to discriminatory behavior that goes against the very ideals of democracy and freedom that the United States symbolizes.

What to Tell the Mate of Someone Who's Playing Around

It's incredible the number of times I am asked in telephone calls on radio or TV talk shows, or in written questions (always anonymous) sent up at the conclusion of a lecture, "If you know your friend's husband or wife is committing adultery, do you let your friend know the bad news?"

I always answer, "In the first place, you have to be sure of that accusation, and that is difficult enough in itself. In the second place, let your friend find out some other way—not through you." That is the kind of accusation that you don't talk about to other people, either.

PLEASURES AND PITFALLS OF THE OFFICE ROMANCE

For many who work long hours and are dedicated to their careers, the opportunities to meet people of the opposite sex outside the office are few. In addition, working in close proximity to someone of the opposite sex is a situation that makes the job environment fertile for romantic possibilities.

I have worked in government and for corporations for forty years, and during all those years I have witnessed the following:

- o *Office romances that ended in marriage,* as everyone knew that they would. These marriages helped, rather than hindered, the careers of the couple—even if company policy decreed they could no longer work together in the same division, and even if one person, because of company policy, was forced to find a job with another company.
- o *Office romances between a married boss or senior executive and a single woman executive.* These used to result in the woman's being exploited, made miserable, and eventually fired.
- o *Long-lasting office romances* that resulted in the woman's being exploited, made miserable, and eventually fired. (Of course, in today's world, the predator can also be a female boss with a lot of power.)

- • *The office romance that could end in marriage but drags on interminably without a wedding* is injurious to the careers of both parties, because everyone in the office is speculating, gossiping, fantasizing, and spreading rumors about them every time one of them comes into sight. That cuts down on total office productivity. Suddenly the two protagonists are viewed only in terms of the status of their romance, not in terms of the work they may be producing. When this continues for months on end, the two find themselves no longer being considered for big promotions or pushed into creative new directions. A senior executive will think to himself or herself, "If those two can't make up their minds about their relationship after all this time, they won't be able to make up their minds about anything."

• *When two people do fall in love, become engaged, and marry,* it's important to their careers not to let the romance take over their work. Touching, writing each other love notes, hanging on the telephone interminably with each other, meeting by the copy machine, holding hands, gazing starry-eyed at each other in the employees' cafeteria, and entering love messages in each other's computers do not help the productivity of the company. As one executive phrased it in dressing down a pair that was being slightly nauseating in public about their romance, "Do *love* on your own time. Do *work* in this office!"

• As for the *office affair with someone who is married,* it is so stupid of the woman to permit it to happen to her that I simply have no sympathy for her. She is always the one who loses out, who gets left behind. The man keeps his job. She doesn't, and she is not what the new status of women is all about!

The work environment provides a great hunting ground for a marriage partner, but marriage, not protracted or intrusive affairs, should be the goal, and discretion is imperative in order not to derail one's career.

WHEN YOU LIVE TOGETHER AS AN UNMARRIED COUPLE

Today an unmarried couple living together no longer has to buck society as they did even ten years ago. But there are still many conservative people out there who disapprove of such relationships, even though their voices have become muted in a permissive society.

If you are unmarried and living together, even though you have not made a commitment to marriage, you have made a commitment to one another. It is a commitment that should be regarded with seriousness. Consideration of each other should be the number one characterization of your relationship. Good manners toward each other and toward each other's family, friends, and business associates are terribly important.

• As one of a couple, you should accept social invitations in the evenings and on weekends only after consulting your partner, who would probably be offended if you went to social events by yourself—without his or her knowledge. Both members of the couple should have the opportunity to accept or regret invitations. If you were to go off by yourself to your friends' parties, you would be sending them a signal (and your partner, too) that you don't consider the person with whom you share a home someone who shares equal status with you.

Sometimes it's a question of educating your friends that you are to be invited as a couple, and that you will not go out in mixed company without your partner having been invited. (Many couples, however, have an understanding that either will spend, if he or she wishes, a night out every week with just "the boys" or just "the girls," as many married couples do.)

• When the person of your choice moves into your home, make room. Give away some of the clothes that take up too much room in your house or apartment; clean out those bureau drawers. Free up half the medicine cabinet space. Don't expect another person to be happy if there is no room for his or her personal effects. Sharing means just that—splitting, dividing in two, making things equal.

• If someone moves into your home, he or she may have a completely different taste from yours. When you buy that next piece of furniture or pick out upholstery fabric, you should take into account the other person's taste.

• The household budget, cleaning, marketing, and cooking schedules should be formulated and agreed upon together, so that the work and the financial responsibilities are split fairly—according to the talents, free time, and resources or either person.

• Each should speak well—and with dignity—of the other. When you put down your partner in front of others, it casts aspersions not only on your relationship, but also on you.

• When introducing your live-in mate to people you don't know, refer to him or her as "My friend Bob Smith" (or "My friend Alice Jones"). It is not necessary to label the other person as someone who lives with you.

• Some live-togethers make fun of or mock wedding traditions by doing such things as holding a "Non-Wedding Shower" or a "First Anniversary Live-Together Party." Everyone will think it's a cheap trick to get some wedding present loot.

• If your friends ask how they should introduce you and your live-together, you might advise them, "Why don't you introduce us simply as 'Alice Armstrong and her friend Jack Mooney'?" (Introducing you as "Alice Armstrong and her date Jack Mooney" implies one thing; "Alice Armstrong and her friend Jack Mooney" implies a serious relationship.)

• When family members or close friends of either of you asks what kind of holiday or birthday presents they can give you, suggest things that you need for your household (whether it's a check, toaster, coffee maker, dinner plates, or magazine subscriptions). Any family member who may disapprove of your unmarried lifestyle should not consider their feelings a significant reason to withhold love, support, or generosity toward you.

• Be sensitive to how your mutual parents and other family members regard the relationship. You want everyone to be as accepting as possible; you want to keep the waters smooth, not storm-tossed with giant waves of anguish. I remember hearing a mother who did not approve of her daughter's living arrangement sounding off to her one day. "Look, just think of your father and me as the china closet, and you're the bull, charging around in it, doing damage. You're always on the defensive, you're sarcastic, you don't give us a chance to be nice to the two of you. Why don't you stop being the bull? Why don't you talk to us gently, tiptoe around us, and then we'll all get along just fine, and the china closet won't be rattling all the time?"

The mother had a point, but so did the daughter when she answered, "Okay, Mother, but if you and Daddy would greet us with a smile—instead of those embarrassed frowns—you would find a lot of warmth radiating back to you. You are the ones who turn us into people who are always on the defensive." (With a few more frank discussions, they worked it out and are now a close family again.)

• Welcome your partner's friends into your life, just as he or she should welcome yours. If you're slow to make snap judgments, and if you sit on your criticisms of people your partner happens to like, you'll probably end up liking them, too.

• Don't open each other's mail.

• Each person should have a certain space—perhaps a desk drawer or a section of a closed cabinet—that is his or hers alone, and into which personal papers can be filed with the knowledge that no one will pry into that area. It's a question of mutual trust.

• If one person is going to be kept late at work or on the golf course, or delayed for whatever reason, it is only considerate to forewarn the other partner. You should keep each other informed well in advance of each other's schedules and business travel requirements.

• And whatever you do—again, with my own voice ringing through—get yourself to that church or temple to get married as soon as possible. Hanging out together within the state of matrimony is much greater than without!

Making a Commitment Even Though You Decide Not to Marry

One older couple I know, who have been married and respectively widowed and divorced and both have grandchildren, made the decision to live together as permanent companions. But due to the financial and legal complications that a marriage would necessitate, they decided to forego the legal ceremony and simply have one that would express their deep commitment to one another. They gathered together all their kin and close friends, and in a ceremony at the home of the man involved pledged themselves to one another for the rest of their lives. There were flowers and music and dancing to formally mark the beginning of their lives together.

THE ROMANCE IS OVER

There's that awful moment—a serious romance is over. One lover has departed, the great passion has dissipated, and the future holds that two people who formerly thought of themselves as one are now distinctly separate individuals. The only comfort to derive from the shattering of a romance is that the breakup of a marriage is ten thousand times more difficult than a breakup between two unmarried people.

When two people involved in a romance tire of each other and feel it is useless to continue the relationship, they simply part company, usually with more than a tinge of sadness. But more often, one person walks out on the other, and that can cause an emotional upheaval that makes the impact of a volcanic eruption seem minor. And where do manners come into this situation, you might ask?

Manners come into *every* situation. Manners are simply being sensitive to and concerned about other people's welfare and feelings. From the point of view of fairness, if one person has walked out on the other, the person doing the walking has a responsibility to show as much compassion as possible.

• The person who initiates the break should quietly state to all outsiders that the breakup was a mutually agreed upon development and not boast about walking out on the other (although if he or she has a new romance, the reason for departure will be quite apparent).

• That person should not criticize the former lover in public, or even reply to nosy people who want to know why the romance is over. ("The reason we broke up? We have nothing to say about that, really," which translates to "It's really none of your business.")

• If they have shared a home, he or she should leave with all financial matters tied up neatly (such as bills paid and anything regarding real estate or other legal issues taken care of). One hears horror stories like this every day: A couple, both executives, had just embarked upon an extremely expensive redesign of the interior of their shared apartment when the woman decided to leave her housemate. She left him with all the upcoming expenses on the apartment decoration to pay by himself. When he hauled her into court to make her pay her share, there was much cheering among their mutual friends.

• The person who is leaving should put in writing a list of the wonderful qualities that made the other person so lovable. That kind of a letter can be a great source of comfort in the future to the person left behind. It helps the healing process. There is certainly a way of writing such a letter to salve the ego of the person left behind without indicating grounds for a "palimony" or breach of promise lawsuit. (You might consult your legal adviser.) It constitutes solace if the person who has left eventually goes on record with something laudatory—a letter perhaps that says how much he (or she) appreciated the attention and the love that was given to him. It means a lot to the person spurned to be told how much the laughter and the good times meant to the former lover. The person left behind needs to hear something like "You are a generous, loving person who brought sunlight into my life." You don't have to write a letter that says, "Thank you for having been the most important part of my life," which could prove legally damaging. You are just letting the other person know that the relationship *did* mean a great deal to you and that you will always have some great memories.

* * *

Today we have no choice but to step more carefully than our forefathers did. But as we enter this new decade, we should be more aware of our responsibilities, more sensitive to the feelings of others, and more compassionate toward the lifestyle choices of others.

PART III

THE RITES OF PASSAGE

Protocol and tradition begin at the moment of birth and continue all the way through your life to the end. These are the rites of passage that mark your stages of maturation. Your parents, grandparents, and great-grandparents all went through the same ceremonies, which should give even the youngest of us a sense of history, and the oldest a sense of the marks we leave in our lives.

You may chafe at some of the rituals that surround great moments in life. But you must also admit that it's nice to be the center of attention. It's nice to have people fussing over you, praying for you, wishing you well, or even sharing your grief. And it is important to be thoughtful and considerate of others going through similar rites of passage.

11

Engagements: Sharing the Joyous News

Let the world in on the happy, wonderful news that you are engaged by writing or telephoning the people you care about, by suddenly appearing (or having your fiancée appear) with a ring on the third finger of the left hand, and by having your engagement announcement published in the local newspaper.

Today the engagement process (the official "social notice" of a couple's intention to marry) is a much less important event in the stream of social rituals of a person's life than it used to be. Although in past generations a man formally asked a woman's father for her hand in marriage, many people now decide on their own to get married, without asking anyone. The young man who asks a father for the hand of his daughter in marriage is a rare and endangered species. However, it is still a wise move for the couple, once they have decided to marry, to inform both sets of parents how they plan to make it financially— particularly if parental subsidies will be involved.

The engagement period traditionally lasted from six months to a year. Today the engagement is often announced from a month to three months prior to the wedding, and in the case of people who have been living together, it simply is not announced at all.

189

TELLING THE WORLD YOUR GOOD NEWS

The first people with whom you, the engaged couple, should share the wonderful news are, of course, your parents and other members of the family. (You do not, by the way, send out engraved or printed engagement announcements cards.) If either set of parents has never met your intended, you should quickly make a visit to those parents (unless they live in another country, in which case, plan to visit them as soon as possible). For the sake of future family harmony, it is important to establish good relations immediately with your fiancé's or fiancée's parents.

• *Once you have announced to your own parents that you are engaged, it's very important to urge your parents to call the other set of parents immediately.* It doesn't matter if it's the bride-to-be's parents who call the groom-to-be's parents first—or vice-versa. What does matter is that they (divorced and remarried parents included) get in touch with each other right away to offer joint congratulations, regardless of how many telephone calls are required to track them down.

If one of the parents is disenchanted with the news, he or she should keep the disapproval hidden—at least during the first conversation with the other set of parents. In other words, if the bride's mother doesn't like the prospect of having so-and-so for a son-in-law, she should not relay this fact to his parents during the engagement announcement telephone call! It is a matter to be discussed privately with her daughter, and hopefully her daughter will be able to win her over without too much difficulty. Often a good open-ended discussion will influence people to change their opinions.

An engagement is important enough news to warrant making long distance calls to all family members, particularly those far away, who might not hear about it via the grapevine. The word should also be conveyed in writing to any family members or really close friends not reached by telephone. Anyone who feels close to either of the pair wants to hear such important news directly, because it brings such a joyful reaction to whoever hears it.

If the wedding will be a small one, both the bride's and the groom's sides would both be wise to mention this fact while conveying the happy news to family and friends. This will help avoid hurt feelings later when invitations don't appear in everyone's mailbox.

When Announcing Your Engagement Is Not Necessary

If the bride has been married before, it is not necessary to announce her next engagement. It is more tasteful to announce her wedding instead. Engagements are really for first-time brides.

The engagement process doesn't make much sense either for couples who have been living together for a number of years. Long-time live-togethers, in the opinion of many, should simply tell their friends the happiness of their plans to marry and then get married, without going through all of the engagement rituals. Usually family and friends are genuinely delighted when the couple finally makes the commitment to marry. There's no need for them suddenly to act like a starry-eyed engaged couple (which was the way young people, many of whom had never slept with each other, used to behave before they were married).

Newspaper Announcement of the Engagement

If one of the engaged couple has a high social, civic, or business position in the community, or has distinguished parents or grandparents, there is a good chance the engagement announcement will make the newspapers.

Many people, however, don't get their act together in time to have their announcement included—newspapers often require engagement and wedding information weeks in advance.

PHOTOGRAPHS

If you, the bride-to-be, satisfy the newspapers' social standing requirements and submit your portrait far enough in advance, you have a good chance of its being published. A good head shot (8 by 10 inches, black and white glossy) is what is needed. Have your photograph taken by a professional (a snapshot or an amateur's efforts just won't make it). Be sure to have the information firmly attached to the photograph (the names of both bride and groom, the wedding date, and other particulars.

For the photograph, refrain from wearing something fussy or ornate around your face; wear button or simple hoop earrings, not dangling ones. Simplicity should be the guiding factor in the neckline of your dress or blouse, your hairstyle, and your jewelry.

More and more newspapers are now publishing photographs of the engaged couple together. The man looks better in a dark suit and simple tie (no bow tie, for example, unless he always wears one).

THE ANNOUNCEMENT TEXT

The efficiency with which you handle getting the information to the local newspaper will help get your announcement into their pages. Follow the form of the regular engagement announcements in your paper. It differs in each city. For example, a hypothetical bride (or her parents) would send in to the *New York Times* an engagement announcement such as the following (you will note that the bride's parents are divorced):

ABIGAIL L. TENDERCROFT PLANS MARRIAGE
TO DR. HILARY J. WOLDEN IN FEBRUARY

The engagement of Abigail L. Tendercroft to Dr. Hilary J. Wolden, a son of Mr. and Mrs. Joseph Wolden of Poughkeepsie, New York, has been announced by Mr. Hugh Tendercroft of New York and Mrs. Peter Bordon of Beverly Hills, California, parents of the bride-to-be.

Ms. Tendercroft, an account executive at McComb Advertising Agency in New York, and her fiancé, a resident in anesthesiology at the New York Hospital-Cornell Medical Center, plan to marry in February.

The future bride, a graduate of Miss Porter's School, graduated from Vassar College. She was a member of the Junior Assembly in 1986. Her father is a real-estate developer. Her mother, Marian Boyd, is a syndicated newspaper columnist and author. Ms. Tendercroft is the granddaughter of the late Cameron H. Boyd, a U.S. senator from Michigan.

Dr. Wolden graduated from Kenyon College and the Baylor College of Medicine in Houston. His father is an executive with IBM in Poughkeepsie, and his mother is a teacher in the Pawling, New York, school system.

There are cases in which the parents are divorced and either the mother or father of the bride-to-be is detached from the family and lives far away. In this case, the parent with whom the bride lives or who is closest to her would announce the engagement in the newspapers, but the other parent must be mentioned. For example:

Mrs. Martha Wetkin of San Francisco has announced the engagement of her daughter Sarah Frances Wetkin to Jonathan Wilfrid Schoen, the son of Mr. and Mrs. Heinrich Schoen of Hartford, Connecticut. Ms. Wetkin is also the daughter of Mr. Henry Weeks of New York. . . .

WHERE ENGAGEMENT ANNOUNCEMENTS ARE SENT

The engagement announcement is always sent, of course, to the papers in the cities where the engaged couple live. If a bride's or groom-to-be's family is prominent in more than one city, the engagement announcement and photograph should be sent to the papers in the appropriate other cities also. For example, if the groom's family was very prominent and used to live in another city, and there are grandparents and other strong ties to that city, the connection should be explained in a covering memo sent along with the photograph and engagement announcement to the Society Editor of the local newspaper there.

THE ENGAGEMENT RING

Since the custom of a man giving an engagement ring to his betrothed first began, this one piece of jewelry has brought more joy (and on rare occasions, more disappointment) than any other symbol of marriage. In this age of attention to materialism, sometimes the satisfaction or disappointment is based too heavily on the degree of dazzle and the opulence of the stones. I remember a young friend of mine being teased about the small size of her diamond ring. One of her friends (obviously jealous of her engagement) said that she had better bring along a magnifying glass so that people could properly see the diamond. I whispered in my young friend's ear, "You have a terrific guy; he is so much more important than any ring!"

Here is some old-fashioned advice for the soon-to-be recipient of an engagement ring:

• *A diamond solitaire is the traditional engagement ring, set in yellow gold, white gold, or platinum.* However, you can choose any stone of your choice—ruby, sapphire, or the most expensive, emerald. If you prefer a semiprecious stone such as a green peridot, aquamarine, golden topaz, or pink tourmaline, all less expensive but exciting in color, that's fine, too. Any one of these stones or a combination of these stones also makes a beautiful engagement ring, particularly when set off by a couple of tiny diamonds in the setting.

• *If your fiancé asks you to accompany him to pick out your engagement ring, tell him yes, yes, yes!* If he is an intelligent young man, he will already have visited the jewelry store and discussed his allowable price range with a salesperson. Then when the two of you come in together, that salesperson will show you trays of rings that are in the price range your fiancé can afford. A good reason for helping him select the ring is that you can select the kind of stones you want. You may greatly prefer an emerald-cut diamond over a round one (but remember, the emerald-cut diamond is more expensive, so be prepared to choose a smaller stone). You can select your preference of design and yellow or white gold or platinum for the mounting. While you are at the store, you can have your exact ring size determined, too.

• *If he surprises you with a ring, tell him you love it—even if you don't love it.* If he picked it out, he has probably put his heart and soul into the purchase, and it would be too mean to tell him you don't like his taste. You can make yourself love that ring. Women have been doing that for centuries! However, I have known women who successfully exchanged rings at the store by telling their fiancés that the ring was too loose or tight or some such story. (They had already visited the jewelry store, found their fiancé's salesperson, explained their predicament, and selected another ring in the same price range.) When they returned to the store with their fiancés, there were no other rings of the right size exactly like the one their fiancés had purchased, so they looked around and suddenly found a ring to their liking in a totally different style. The fact that the salesperson was in collusion with them remains a secret.

• *If he (or perhaps you) are embarrassed about the small size of the stone but it's all he can afford, tell him you love it as it is*—but that you will enjoy adding stones to it someday, or exchanging it for a larger stone, when finances permit.

• *If his finances won't permit buying you a handsome ring, but your finances will, offer to contribute toward the ring.* You can even pay for most of it, if you desperately want a certain ring— provided you leave his ego intact. If he adamantly refuses to accept any money toward the ring, wear his small one with enthusiasm. (You can always buy yourself a big rock later to go on your other hand.)

• *If buying you a ring would be too great a financial strain for him when you become engaged, tell him you don't need a ring now.* I have known many young men putting themselves through law school or medical school, for example, trying to repay government loans and unable to afford an engagement ring when they marry. Their fiancées have made these men feel they were far more important than any rings.

• *If you are a woman with large fingers and big hands and your fiancé can only afford a small stone,* you may prefer to do without an engagement ring until the day comes when your husband can buy you one suitably large enough for your hands.

• *Some women prefer to forego a small engagement stone and to have instead a jeweled wedding band—in place of a plain wedding ring.*

• *If he gives you his mother's or grandmother's engagement ring, learn to love it, no matter how you feel about it.* It's not worth the risk of upsetting his entire family by refusing to wear the family ring. Years hence, you can always put it away "to save as a precious family memento for one of the children" and buy a new one for yourself. (If your future children don't want the family ring either, one of them can keep it in the vault for her children. Eventually, one of the descendants will want it!)

• *Unlike a wedding ring, the inside of an engagement ring is not engraved.*

• *Should you break your engagement, the correct thing to do is to return the ring to your fiancé,* as well as any other gifts of jewelry or family keepsakes he may have given you. (If he breaks the engagement, keep your ring!)

CELEBRATING THE ENGAGEMENT

The Engagement Party

The engagement party, usually a cocktail party hosted by one set of parents or grandparents or an uncle or aunt—or even a close friend— was often a surprise announcement of a young couple's intention to wed. It also marked the first time the young woman was seen wearing her engagement ring. This kind of reception was usually held when the engaged pair had a long time to wait—such as a year— between the announcement of their engagement and the actual wedding.

In this era of short engagements, the traditional engagement party has been supplanted for the most part by showers. (However, an engagement party can be great fun to give or attend. If you are engaged, with a long period ahead of you before the wedding ceremony, you can always hint in front of a favorite friend or relative that you would appreciate a party. Make it a surprise for your guests, so that only the engaged couple and the hosts know the real reason for the party.

I remember one engagement party I attended where none of us knew that two of our best friends had become engaged until the actual end of the evening, when we were leaving the house. Our hostess handed each of us a prettily wrapped gift. We opened our individual boxes to discover a small silver pencil inside. Then we noticed two sets of initials engraved on each. It took a few seconds to realize that these were the initials of two people in attendance at the party. Since none of us had known these two were even seeing each other, it was a secret beautifully kept—and in celebration we started the party all over again. Another engagement announcement I will never forget was a surprise cocktail party at which our host suddenly announced that he had a secret, and that the person who first discovered the nature of the secret would receive a bottle of champagne. We went scurrying all over his house, searching out clues written in poetry on scraps of paper. It was an amusing and cleverly executed puzzle, finally solved by a guest who surmised that two of our friends present were engaged.

If you can manage it, it's very nice timing to have your engagement photograph and announcement appear in your local newspaper the morning after the engagement party. Many papers will include a mention of the engagement party in the announcement.

Engagement Presents

The presentation to the bride-to-be of engagement presents by relatives and best friends is no longer a common custom. These gifts used to make sense when the engagement period lasted about a year. Some older relatives still do like to give these presents, however, as a gesture to start the bride on her marital way. The gift is usually something personal, such as a piece of jewelry, a silver compact, a handbag, a silver dressing table mirror.

The friends of the young couple seldom give engagement presents today. They are digging deep enough in their pockets as it is, paying for shower and wedding gifts.

Showers: Feting the Bride-to-Be

Showers are given by close friends in honor of the bride (but the loot collected is destined equally for the bride and groom). A female relative may host the shower (not the bride's mother or sister). It is important for a bride not to let her enthusiasm carry her away. One shower is sufficient, two should be maximum, and three becomes a travesty. People do not have enough money to be shelling out constantly for gifts. There is still the wedding gift to be given!

Co-ed showers—held in the evening at the cocktail hour, for the benefit of the bride's and groom's friends of both sexes who work—are the most popular kind of shower given today. These usually have the theme of gifts for the bar (bar glasses, wine bottle opener, bottles of wine, and the like) or gifts for the kitchen (whisks, cheese graters, carving knives, mixing bowls, and so forth). Female friends of the bride often give her a lingerie shower.

A guest does not have to spend a lot of money on a gift. It makes a lot of sense for two or more of the guests to band together to buy a more important shower present.

There are many charming customs involving the old-fashioned all-female shower, where the ribbons are saved and tied to make a ribbon rope to encircle the group of guests. (The girl with the most knots in her hand will be the next to be married.) Then there's the custom of making a bridal bouquet from the various bows on the packages. The bows are pulled through holes made in a round piece of cardboard, so that eventually the cardboard is covered with bright blossom-colored ribbons. (The bride is supposed to use this fake bouquet at the rehearsal of the wedding ceremony the afternoon or evening before the wedding.)

At a co-ed cocktail party shower, hors d'oeuvres and drinks are served; at an all-girl shower, a light lunch or tea is served in conjunction with opening the gifts.

ASKING SOMEONE TO MARRY YOU

I'm an acknowledged, nonapologetic romantic, so if you do not believe in romance, skip over this advice on how to ask someone to marry you. My first piece of advice, of course, is to be pretty sure that the other person feels the same way you do before you propose spending the rest of your lives together. My second piece of advice is, whether you are male or female, make the proposal scene a memorable one. For example, choose a first class, glamorous setting with a touch of the Hollywood of the 1930s, or devise a scenario with a touch of Jay Leno's sense of humor. Do *something* to make the occasion unusual, so the memory can be recalled as something special for years to come. Every time I see one of the old *Thin Man* movies from the 1930s, I wish I could have been Myrna Loy and had William Powell propose to me in a sophisticated New York nightclub setting. My own proposal, received more than a quarter of a century ago in Chicago, was so "unforgettable" that neither my husband nor I can remember it. (I think the dialogue went something like this: *Bob:* "Let's do it." *Letitia:* "Okay, let's.") So it is with no small amount of envy that I recount what has happened to *other* couples when they became engaged. In each case, one of the couple showed enormous imagination or wit:

• A woman in love stuck a note on top of the tennis balls in the can. When her opponent removed the lid from the can to put the three balls into play, he saw her note: "This is the 58th time we've played singles together. Don't you think it's time we played doubles instead?" Her opponent, who had been thinking along the same lines but had been too shy to do anything about it, vaulted over the net, kissed her and said "Will you *please* marry me?" (I never found out if they finished the match.)

• A middle-aged widower went to a recording studio and recorded "People," the song that was playing when he met the new love of his life. His voice was not very good, but when his lady friend listened to the tape and heard him say at the conclusion of the song, "We are two people who are meant to be together for the rest of our lives," she got the message.

• Two graduate music students spent every Saturday together, always at something musical, followed by dinner. One Saturday she was very blue because he was away. However, he had lent her his libretto to follow the opera performance, and when she came to a certain passage, halfway through the opera, she found a tiny diamond ring tied inside the binding of the book with a ribbon. At the bottom of the page, he had scribbled, "I love you. Marry me." (She did.)

• Men have surprised the women in their lives by proposing in extraordinary ways:

- o Having the proposal sky-written by plane overhead
- o Putting the proposal on a giant rented sign in Times Square in New York
- o Putting a diamond engagement ring at the bottom of her champagne glass and then bringing her the filled glass
- o Sending a mime to perform by her desk in her office, making the entire office aware that her boyfriend was too shy to propose directly
- o Proposing to her while the two of them were ballooning, or waterskiing, or ice-boating, or taking tango lessons

• One crafty young woman baked a note in her beau's birthday cake at a large party she had organized for him. She made sure he was served the piece that had the note in it, which read, "If you want to have birthdays like this forever, you had better marry me." He read her note, looked at her and smiled, and then arose from the table to toast the hostess. In his toast he announced to the group, "Janie and I are going to be married. How could I ever be apart from a woman who bakes birthday cakes like this?"

Now, I'm all for romance and, Lord knows, we need it in this cold, mechanical, technological era in which we live. But if you can't get the perfect romantic occasion together, at least get the marriage together. In other words, if you're short on imagination or wit, just summon up the courage to make one statement and ask one question. The statement is, "I love you." The question is, "Will you marry me?"

When a Woman Does the Proposing

Women have long proposed to men, in spite of the ancient canard that in order to live happily ever after, it is the man who presses the suit until his blushing love object finally acquiesces. Now, in the latter part of the twentieth century, women are unabashedly open and aboveboard about proposing. (As one young man told me recently, "Without mentioning the word 'marriage,' she made it impossible for us *not* to get married.")

Before the women's movement of the sixties, it would have been considered shocking for a woman to take the lead in marching her man to the altar, but she often did it anyway, playing a deft game of psychological warfare. She would say things such as, "You always say it's such a joy to see me. Wouldn't it make things easier for you to have that joy around all the time, without having to make elaborate plans to meet?" Or if a woman had regularly been cooking a fantastic dinner several nights a week for the love of her life, she might say, "Can you imagine your life without these great feasts prepared for you all the time? Would you like to go back to your cans of tunafish and delivered pizzas?"

While she didn't say, "Will you marry me?" she certainly was forcing the issue.

Some women still use tactics like this. Others use sex as their wedge. ("You know how great we are together, you and I. Can you imagine what life would be like without me around—available, eager, and loving?")

But today's woman really doesn't have to play those games—although she can if she wants to. If she is more honest and direct, she can put her cards right on the table: "Look, we've been seeing each other for a long time now. We're very compatible. I love you and I think you love me—at least you act like it. If we get married, our two salaries will make a neat lifestyle for us, and we could produce such beautiful children!" (There's not much romance in a marriage proposal of this nature, but, reworded to each woman's personal style, it seems to work!)

If two people have been living together a long time, it becomes harder to make the one person who has been stalling all along commit—and it usually is the man. The woman in this kind of relationship should perhaps revert to the old style of romance, intrigue, and games to influence the man into thinking that it is in both their interests to formalize their union.

It doesn't really matter who says what and who asks whom, as long as it happens—namely, that marriage license and those wedding rings!

When Your Answer Is "No"

For every proposal of marriage that is accepted, there is another that is refused. To tell someone you won't marry him or her has to be the greatest emotional rejection there is for an adult. Your kindheartedness has kept you from deflating the other person's hopes. Or is it that it's easier to be a coward and simply avoid telling the other person that there is no chance of your relationship moving to a commitment to marriage? That cowardice, however, is a big mistake, because the longer the relationship is allowed to continue, the more the rejection hurts.

It's much better for everyone if you make it quite clear early on that marriage is not possible—long before the other person gets to the stage of asking you.

But if you have let it go too far, and the other person is full of hope and excitement, turn down the idea of marriage with a sharp, clean, and swift reply. You are going to break the other person's heart—there is no more apt term for it—but do it as nicely as possible. You are going to have to find words to soothe the injured. Here are some of the things you might say:

- First, there is no way you will entertain the idea of marriage, no hope whatsoever that you will change your mind. (Make this clear, but say it gently.)

○ It is not the other person's fault, it's yours for not feeling the same emotions he (or she) does for you; you admit that you should have told him (or her) sooner.

○ You probably will never again in your whole life find anyone as sensitive, attractive, smart. (Use every complimentary adjective that could possibly apply to the other person.)

○ You will never forget him (or her), or the terrific experiences you shared together. (Explain how much you gained from your relationship, how you will always keep those memories in your heart.)

○ He (or she) deserves the finest person in the world as a spouse, and you're certain that person will soon appear in his (or her) life.

The spurned one will probably question you closely as to why you can't say yes—what's wrong, what is the missing element in your relationship, and so on. Be prepared, and be truthful if there is no spark on your part. Simply mention that you are not a match.

If there are other reasons—for example, he can't keep a job and is always broke—explain your reservation diplomatically. "You don't have the job stability I have always wanted" sounds a lot kinder than "You're a loser and you'd be on my payroll all my life."

If you feel you are simply not on the same wavelength, explain that your interests are so divergent that you would not have the foundation necessary for a marriage to work. Praise the other person's interests, and make him (or her) see that it is not those interests that are at fault. It's the fact that the two of you are too different in your enthusiasms and directions.

If you have a *serious* moral objection, you owe it to the other person to come out with it. For example, if the other person is a drug abuser, you should say that you're sorry but you could never marry a person who uses drugs, even occasionally. If he or she promises to get off drugs or alcohol, be ready to question that fine resolution. Say, "I'd have to wait several years to see if you really do get off it. You haven't conquered it during the time we've been seeing each other, and you knew how I felt about it. Please look for someone else." Your frankness may result in the other person's finally seeking the help needed to conquer his (or her) problem.

If the person you turn down thinks you did it because of his (or her) less than sensational looks, reassure that person immediately that you have enjoyed his (or her) company all this time because of other, far more important factors than looks. Maybe the other person won't believe you, but say it often. Keep reminding him (or her) of all the great personality assets that have pleased and attracted you. At the same time make the person who proposed understand that you need to be deeply in love with the man (or woman) you marry, and you are not in love with him (or her).

Think of every possible great thing about the person who has just proposed to you. After you have said no, pelt him (or her) with compliments and memories of past wonderful, shared experiences to help coat the bitter pill you have just given him (or her) to swallow. Write a letter in which you reaffirm how much the friendship you have shared has meant to you, but that you feel it is best not to see each other any more. He should be looking for someone else.

It is a difficult, even cruel time for the person who is spurned. But it is a much, much easier blow than the one a divorce delivers!

12

Weddings

The great decision has been made. The wedding date has been decided. It will be the happiest day of your life for you—the bride—as well as for the groom, your parents, and his parents. And for your friends this is a major moment, too.

The main goal for any wedding should be happiness. Regardless of the size, simplicity, or elaborateness of the ceremony, a wedding should be carefully and lovingly planned. The bride should feel it is *her* wedding, not her parents'. The groom should feel he is part of the planning, too. The weeks before the wedding should be marked by great diplomacy and tact, with everyone checking first with everyone else before making major decisions, and with account taken of the hurt feelings that might result from any exclusion.

I am a traditionalist in my attitude toward weddings. To me, the one sacred ritual that remains in this sociologically shaken world is the first wedding. The ceremony and reception are couched in such beautiful traditions that following and respecting them results in an orderly, dignified, and beautiful event. The weddings of the seventies were often chaotic, with wedding party and guests never knowing quite what to do or how to react. The old-fashioned wedding came back in 1980; I hope it will remain at least until 2001!

The pages of this book reflect the old traditions updated, but you are certainly free to follow them or change any of them as may be appropriate. The important thing is that you have a happy wedding!

CREATING A BEAUTIFUL WEDDING

There will always be publicity-seekers—usually people who have a hard time being noticed in life—who decide to get married in a helicopter or bathyscaphe or on His and Hers farm tractors. However, a truly beautiful wedding is not a media event. It is one that is carefully planned, couched in the old traditions and rituals and incorporating a harmony of design and color. A wedding consultant certainly gives the design scheme top priority, but you can handle those details yourself, too. I have attended wonderful weddings wholly handled by the bride and her mother, as well as others done by a professional interior designer or wedding consultant. Among them have been these:

• *A Victorian wedding.* At this lavish wedding the bride wore a nineteenth-century lace and silk dress handed down through her family. The bridesmaids' dresses matched the bride's in feeling, and the bridesmaids carried white paper lace Victorian bouquets. Even the white lace tablecloths (overlying garnet velvet cloths) reinforced the nineteenth-century English feeling.

• *A 1920s-look wedding.* At this one the bride wore her grandmother's flapper wedding dress. The bridesmaids wore dresses similar in cut and satin pumps that could have come from a 1925 shoe store. The bride's short dark hair was dressed in the smart bob of that period. The fabric of the circular tablecloths was printed in an Art Deco design. The music was all 1920s Charleston type, and a pair of dance instructors helped the guests learn the steps.

• *A flowered chintz wedding.* At this wedding the bride had selected a chintz fabric pattern of pink and blush peonies as the central theme. The bride's and bridesmaids' bouquets repeated the flowers in the fabric. The cushions in the church pews were slip-covered in this fabric, the bridesmaids' white dresses were sashed in this fabric, and the tablecloths at the reception were made of the same chintz. The floral centerpieces were, or course, peonies. It was all fresh, flowery, and fragrant. The only jarring moment came when two guests suffered stings from bees who were as entranced with the peonies as the guests were.

• *A country wedding.* At this charming summer wedding, held on a farm, everything was done in white mixed with pale yellow and blue gingham. The bride wore a white voile dress printed in a white-on-white gingham pattern, and a large straw picture hat with pale yellow and blue streamers down the back. The bridesmaids, carrying baskets of yellow and blue flowers, wore long yellow or blue checked dresses with two-toned satin streamers around their waist to match those on the bride's hat. The same gingham fabric was used for the tablecloths at the reception. A straw picture hat filled with blue and yellow flowers formed the centerpiece on each table. The white napkins were tied in yellow or blue checked ribbons, and each guest carried home a piece of wedding cake wrapped in a little bandana made of the checked gingham used throughout the wedding.

• *An operatic wedding.* When two people involved in the opera world were married, their twenty attendants were dressed in borrowed costumes from *Lohengrin,* and the attendants sang opera selections throughout the wedding ceremony, as did the bride and groom at designated moments. The music played at the reception was all operatic recordings, and parts of opera sets had been borrowed to decorate the plain parish hall in which the wedding reception was held. The reception was a low-budget affair—we ate cheese and drank wine—but I have never heard such beautiful voices raised in song. The entire wedding was unforgettable.

• *A silver wedding.* One extremely sentimental wedding contained a surprise element for the guests. The bride's dress and her flowers were all in white, but with a silver satin bow on each puffed sleeve. The bridesmaids wore silver taffeta and carried silver-painted roses. After the wedding ceremony was completed, the bride and groom sat down on either side of the altar. The bride's parents suddenly rose from their pews and came to the foot of the altar, where the minister awaited them, and renewed their marriage vows in an extremely touching ceremony tied into their daughter's own vows. That was the surprise—it was their Silver Wedding Anniversary! The bride's mother wore a pale gray silk dress. There were a lot of tears in that church when the wedding procession of the young bride and groom followed by her parents went down the long church aisle.

• *A skiing wedding.* This unique wedding was held up in the Swiss Alps, with the wedding party and some good skiing friends flying from Chicago to Gstaad for a long weekend. The wedding party took their skis up in the lift one morning to one of the highest slopes, where the minister had arranged a simple altar in the snow. It was a brilliant day, with the sun blazing against an azure sky. As one of the participants said, "You felt you were really in God's cathedral." The bride wore a white snowsuit, white ski boots, and a short veil; she held a bouquet of white roses during the ceremony. After the service, the entire wedding party (the parents of the bride and groom included!) took off on a long downhill run, calling out their joy. A reception lunch awaited them down in the village of Gstaad.

• *A beach wedding.* Many people who live by the sea stage perfectly beautiful informal ceremonies on the beach, with the bride wearing a white cotton Laura Ashley or Mexican wedding dress for the service. This is often followed by an informal reception—for example, a clam-bake.

• *A wedding on the water.* Some couples charter a small cruise boat, complete with a band, for their wedding and reception, sailing around a river, lake, or other body of water as they celebrate the happy union. Some couples book themselves on a ten-day cruise and are married by the ship's captain. As one bride described it, "We got married, had our reception with all the passengers on the cruise present, and we had time to write all our thank-you notes before we disembarked. It was the perfect one-stop operation. Our parents were along, but as pre-agreed, we hardly saw them after the wedding ceremony!"

It does not matter what theme or color scheme you choose at your wedding. It doesn't matter whether you serve your reception guests roast beef or snails, pasta or stuffed grape leaves. What does matter is that you plan the event in a cohesive fashion, in good taste, and that you "produce" something that none of your guests will ever forget. During this period of your lives you will be the recipients of a great deal of love. A well-planned wedding gives back a lot of that love to the participants.

Most important, your wedding should be something that pleases *you,* the bride and the groom.

YOUR WEDDING INVITATIONS

Next to a White House invitation, a wedding invitation is the most important one in the social scale. In its language and content it has remained pretty much the same down through the years. From the sixties to the eighties, many young couples gave vent to their anti-establishment feelings by sending out wedding invitations that were far different from the traditional ones used by their parents, grandparents, and great-grandparents. During that era, wedding guests received curious-looking communications in the mail—everything from rough-textured rice papers to exotic parchments. Often handwritten or printed in nontraditional inks, such as red and ochre, the text was sometimes so esoteric (ancient Japanese poetry and the sayings of Buddha, for example) that many who received these invitations had no idea they were being invited to a wedding!

Fortunately for the bridal business, conventional invitations are once again the favored kind. Anyone who receives one of these knows that he or she has been invited to a wedding and, further, knows where to be and when.

Who Receives Your Invitations?

Your wedding invitation will be much coveted, so prepare the list of recipients with great care. Hurt feelings can easily result if you overlook some people in a group while inviting many of the others.

It helps sometimes to organize your list into "Absolute Necessity" names and "Would Like to Invite if Possible" names. For example, your "Absolute Necessity" column would include:

- o Both immediate families
- o Your attendants
- o The spouses, fiancé(e)s, or special escorts of the attendants
- o Both sets of godparents, if they are close to you
- o Your clergyman or clergywoman

On your "Would Like to Invite if Possible" list, you might include:

- o Distant relatives and family friends
- o The parents or perhaps the sibling closest to you of your attendants
- o Your bosses
- o Your best friends and your fiancé(e)'s best friends
- o Close workplace associates
- o A particularly close former teacher
- o Lead figures in your extracurricular activities (for example: golf or tennis partner; certain members of your choir, music group, or art class; certain members of your garden club or softball team; fellow volunteers in your nonprofit work)
- o Close business associates of both sets of parents
- o People such as your doctor and lawyer and their spouses

The bride's and groom's families should be allowed to extend an equal number of invitations, but often it does not work out that way. Sometimes the groom's family lives far away, and not many of his family and their friends will be able to travel to the wedding. At other times, either the groom's or bride's family will be very prominent in town and will have more "necessity" invitations to extend. The balance should be worked out between the two families—with peace and harmony in mind—before the invitations are ordered.

Although traditionally the bride's family paid all the related expenses, today such matters are worked out between the two sets of parents or between the couple on an ad hoc basis—particularly where either the bride's or the groom's family sends by far the greater number of invitations.

Invitations are expensive—they can add up to $10 apiece by the time they are engraved on good stock, hand-addressed by a calligrapher, and mailed with their postage. (Add to this the cost of wining and dining each guest.) However, rather than looking on it as a matter of "How much is this person worth to me?" look upon sending a wedding invitation to a family member or good friend as a sign of affection and respect, with a desire to make that person feel good about participating in your joy.

The Various Ways of Inviting Guests to the Wedding

EXTENDING FORMAL INVITATIONS

The most expensive and traditional way is by *engraved invitations,* which are so handsome and luxurious that they are often kept by the recipients as prized mementoes of the wedding. Many brides feel that their wedding is the one time in their lives when everything must be first class, starting with their invitations.

APPROPRIATE INFORMAL WAYS OF EXTENDING WEDDING INVITATIONS

• In the case of a small, intimate wedding, you may appropriately send *notes written by hand with black ink on fine-quality white or cream-colored notepaper.* Sometimes the bride writes these herself to her and the groom's contemporaries, but her mother often writes most of them, including to family members. An example is the following note from the bride's mother to a family friend:

> George and I would love to have you both present at the wedding of our daughter, Marianne, and Jonathan Mayberry, on Saturday, May fifteenth, at Saint Cecilia's Church on Harney Street at four o'clock. A champagne reception follows at the Wayfarer's Inn on Montgomery Street.
>
> Our whole family hopes you will be with us on the fifteenth to share in this joyful occasion.

Many parents of brides who issue informal invitations for their daughters' small weddings also send out formal engraved announcements to a large group of friends after the wedding, including the small group who actually attended the wedding.

• *To cut costs, you may print instead of engrave the formal wedding text on good-quality single sheets of stationery.* Traditionally, you would choose either cream or white stock, but today you may also use color in this kind of informal printed invitation—for example, pale blue letter sheets bordered in dark blue, with black printing. It is perfectly appropriate to send out thermographed invitations (a raised printing process that emulates engraving), but I personally find invitations more honest and attractive when they are either engraved, printed, or handwritten, not replicated in a process that tries to look like engraving.

• If you do not have enough time to order invitations made, *send them by Mailgram.* Recipients will logically deduce when they read the date of the wedding that you did not have time even to write a note of invitation. You may use a formal text in your Mailgram (the same wording that you would have put on a formal invitation).

Some parents of the bride have even *faxed* their wedding invitations to their guests' offices or homes, but that is hardly within the spirit of what a wedding should be!

• A wedding invitation is extended *by telephone* only as a last resort, such as when the couple decides to marry within a couple of days of the telephone call.

The Formal Traditional Wedding Invitation

STOCK, INK, AND LETTERING STYLE

This invitation is engraved via a copper plate in black (or sometimes dark gray) ink. A print or script lettering style is used on an ecru (cream-colored) or white stock. The paper is often a heavy 40-pound weight,

ENGRAVED STYLES

Dr. and Mrs. Thomas Allen Greene

TCO-1
BELGRAVE SCRIPT

Mr. and Mrs. Richard Arthur Hyman

TCO-2
HAMILTON

Mr. and Mrs. Richard Murray Barton

TCO-3
LIGHT SCRIPT

Mr. and Mrs. Percival Harold Clayton

TCO-4
MAYFAIR

Mr. and Mrs. John Low Venable

TCO-6
LONDON SCRIPT

Mr. and Mrs. Hugh Robert Scott

TCO-7
PARSIFAL

Mr. and Mrs. Anthony Ross Hagen

TCO-8
SAINT JAMES

Dr. and Mrs. Jay Barclay Woods

TCO-11
TALLEYRAND

Reverend and Mrs. William Carlsen

TCO-14
WINDSOR

MR. AND MRS. SPENCER WOODS MILLER

TCO-16
LEHMAN ROMAN

Mr. and Mrs. Robert William Sloane

TCO-17
SPAULDING CLASSIC

Mr. and Mrs. Daniel Montgomery, Jr.

TCO-18
SHADED ANTIQUE ROMAN

and is either plain or embellished with a blind-embossed, paneled border. The stationer will show you a sample card of engraved styles of lettering from which to choose. Tiffany and Company, for example, offer the engraved alphabet shown, all of which are appropriate and attractive.

You know something is engraved if

- You rub your finger over it and feel the raised lettering.
- You find a stationer's name in raised, blind-embossed small letters underneath the envelope flap.
- You see an indentation in the paper on the reverse side.

POINTS TO REMEMBER ABOUT SENDING FORMAL WEDDING INVITATIONS

- Order them three months before the wedding, or even earlier.
- Make sure you order all the parts you will need (such as a reply card, reception card, and map card to show people how to find the church or reception).
- Be sure to include all of the necessary information in the text. Check the proof for errors *before* it is engraved, even if that entails an additional cost.
- You may certainly have the family crest blind-embossed at the top of the invitation. However, many Americans consider the use of a coat of arms on wedding invitations quite pretentious, all the more so because many people today have had fake family crests designed.
- Tissues are no longer relevant, since the new inks used in printing dry fast and do not smudge.

COMPOSITION OF A TRADITIONAL, FORMAL ENGRAVED WEDDING INVITATION

- The text is engraved on the first page of a *double-fold* invitation.
- The *outside envelope* is hand-addressed in black ink and hand-stamped. The sender's return address is written in the upper left hand corner of the face of the envelope.
- The *inside envelope*—ungummed and therefore not sealed—is addressed only with the guests' handwritten titles and family name (e.g., "Mr. and Mrs. Thomas"). All of the various parts of the invitation are placed in the inside envelope.
- If the reception will be held in a place separate from where the ceremony will be held, you will need a separate *reception invitation card*. A reception card is also useful if you are going to invite a large number of people to the ceremony but just a few to the reception held afterward in the same place (as, for example, a small reception held after the church ceremony in the church parlors).
- If you are inviting most people to the reception but few to the

marriage ceremony, you will need a separate *"Ceremony Card"* for those who should be present at the exchange of vows.

o If you do not have "RSVP" or "The favour of a reply is requested" in the lower left of your invitation, a *reply card* and self-addressed envelope must be supplied.

o A separate *"At Home"* card, giving the couple's new address and telephone number is useful.

o A *map card* may be necessary, showing guests how to find either the church or the reception.

o Other cards, such as an *admittance card* or a *pew card,* may be advisable.

Addressing and Mailing the Invitations

• Arrange for a friend of the bride to volunteer (or pay for a professional to hand-address (never type) the envelopes in black ink (with a wide pen point).

In large cities there are professional calligraphers who will address your envelopes for a price, generally ranging from $1 to $5 per envelope (including hand-stamping, stuffing, and sealing them). You can find them by asking the people who are professional party givers (look in the Yellow Pages), or the special events coordinators of businesses like large banks that use calligraphy for important parties. Or ask your church or temple, because they probably know of good calligraphers who have done other weddings. There are also computer graphics services that will address the envelopes in calligraphy (using the new technology).

Since hand-addressing a large number of envelopes is a time-consuming process, ask your stationer to supply you at once with envelopes in stock while the invitations are being made up. This allows you time to begin addressing the outside and inside envelopes well in advance of the arrival of the invitations. It's very wise to have your envelopes addressed, stamped, and ready to stuff and mail well ahead of the date you intend to mail them.

• *Hand-stamp* the envelopes with attractive, appropriate postage stamps (for example, flowers or birds). Be sure to weigh an invitation with all its parts in advance of buying the stamps so that you affix the proper amount of postage.

• Handwrite the *return address* or have it engraved or blind-embossed in the upper left-hand corner on the front of the envelope, not on the back flap. This allows a much better chance for a misaddressed envelope to be returned to the sender. The name is not necessary on the return address, but an apartment number should be included. The address normally should be that of the bride's parents, although it is sometimes preferable to use another address, including the bride's own address rather than her mother's (as, for example, when the bride's mother is ill or lives too far away from the place of the wedding). If a grandparent or another relative or a friend is giving the wedding, that person may be the recipient of the RSVPs—or may not.

If the couple itself is issuing the invitations, the bride's own address or the couple's mutual address should be provided in the return address. It is a certainty that unless an "at home" card is included, many wedding gifts will be mailed to the return address on the invitations, so you should decide whether or not the bride's parents or the bride or someone else is to receive all the acceptances and regrets.

- When addressing the outer envelopes, either center the name and address of the invitation recipient, or write it on a slant.
- If possible, mail the invitations six weeks before the wedding.

PROTOCOL ON ADDRESSING WEDDING INVITATION ENVELOPES

- The *inside envelope* is addressed to a person with his or her or their family name and title only—"Mr. and Mrs. Grant" (not "Mr. and Mrs. Jason Grant"). If children are to be invited, their given names are included on the inside envelope. For example:

Mr. and Mrs. Anthony
Mary, Beth and James

A family member over the age of eighteen should receive his or her own invitation.

- The *outside mailing envelope* is addressed either to a couple or a single person. It is proper to use "Ms." with a woman's given and family names in addressing her, rather than "Miss" or "Mrs.," if she is single or if she is married but has kept her maiden name.
- *Addressing a married or unmarried couple:* You would address a husband and a wife who has kept her own name on one line:

Mr. Charles Edward Prentice and Ms. Amy Sturgis Kendl

If their combined names are too long to go on one line, address them as

Mr. Andrew Wigglesworth Throckmorton
and Ms. Patricia Fordyce Kendleton

The use of the "and" joining their names means they are married.

In addressing an invitation to a couple who live together but are not married, you would put their names on separate lines, and place on the top line the name that comes first in the alphabet:

Ms. Caroline Breckinridge Murray
Mr. David Adam Thornton
1345 First Street Northwest, etc.

STUFFING THE CONTENTS INTO THEIR ENVELOPES

The "old-fashioned" way of stuffing invitations into their envelopes (still occasionally used today) was to fold the double-fold invitation in half, include the other pieces of the mailing, and then insert it straight up into an envelope that was just a bit larger than the folded invitation. This envelope was then inserted into a matching outer envelope that was again a bit larger—just enough to be able to slide in the inner envelope with ease.

Today the more commonly ordered invitation is a larger double-fold style, in a size from between 4½ inches by 6⅜ inches to 5½ inches by 7½ inches. Today's double-fold invitation is generally folded along the left-hand side of the invitation, rather than in the middle. This kind of invitation is inserted lying flat (instead of being folded in half) into a larger envelope, which then slides into yet a larger outer envelope.

• *This is the order of precedence within the envelope of its various parts:*

Hold the envelope so that you are facing the back of it, with the flap open. The largest part of the contents—the double-fold invitation itself—goes in first, face-up.

A double-fold wedding invitation is generally folded along the left-hand side and is inserted lying flat into an envelope, which then slides into a larger one that will be addressed and stamped.

A single card invitation of any kind is inserted in its envelope face-up in this manner.

If there is a smaller card inviting the guest to the reception, it is inserted next, on top of the larger invitation, and if there is an RSVP card, it comes next, lying face-up within the flap of its envelope (which is, of course, at this point turned face-down). A map or parking instructions or pew number card—whatever is needed—would come next.

A double-fold invitation may be folded in half and inserted in its envelope in this fashion. A smaller piece, such as a reception card or RSVP card and envelope, would be tucked inside the double-fold piece.

When you stuff an unfolded wedding invitation into its first envelope (or any invitation of two or more parts), put the smaller piece of stationery (which might be a reception card, an "at home" card, or an RSVP card with matching envelope) on top of the invitation, as shown here.

The Correct Wording on Wedding Invitations

- Names are given in full on invitations, which means no nicknames and no initials. If, however, either the bride or groom dislikes his or her middle name, it may be omitted on the invitation.
- The English spelling of "honour" and "favour" is often used in wedding invitation language, simply as a matter of tradition. If you prefer, use the American spelling and drop the "u."
- Spell out the date and the year. Spell out all words like "avenue" and "street," so that there are no abbreviations, except perhaps "Dr." or "Jr."—and you may even prefer to use "Doctor" or "Junior."
- The hour of the wedding (and reception, when necessary) is written out, following the word "at" on the invitation—for example, "at one o'clock," "at quarter after five o'clock," or "at three-quarters after four o'clock." "At eight o'clock in the evening" is used to make sure no one thinks it's an early morning service!
- Roman numerals, such as in "George Douglas Berkhardt III," are properly used on the invitation.
- When a wedding takes place in a house of worship, then the inviters use the phrase "request the honour of your presence"—a mark of respect for a church or temple. When a wedding takes place in a home, club, banquet hall, or hotel, the inviters "request the pleasure of your company." When a separate reception card is included in the invitation, the hosts also use "request the pleasure of your company."

Invitational Text

A sample wedding invitation:

Mr. and Mrs. Farnsworth Lee Maguire
request the honour of your presence
at the marriage of their daughter
Elizabeth Anne
to Mr. Tracy McLaughlin
on Saturday, the eighth of May
one thousand, nine hundred and ninety-six
at four o'clock
Saint Cecilia's Cathedral
426 Mission Street
San Antonio

A separate reception invitation card and a reply card and envelope were provided with the invitation above. In the case of a formal wedding invitation, both ceremony and reception are combined in one only when both take place in the same location:

Mr. and Mrs. Robert Agee Sundworth
request the pleasure of your company
at the marriage of their daughter
Gretchen Anne
to
Doctor (or Dr.) Cameron Aimes Johnson
on Saturday, the fifth of December
one thousand, nine hundred and ninety-nine
at half after six o'clock
and at dinner
immediately following the ceremony
The Charles Hotel
Charles Square
Cambridge

R.s.v.p.   *Black Tie*
Fourteen Linnaen Avenue
Cambridge, Massachusetts 00000

The Etiquette of Names on Wedding Invitations

• *The names of those who do the inviting are always given.* In a traditional wedding invitation, the parents of the bride do the inviting. If she divorces and remarries, the parents usually do not issue the invitations—she does. If she is widowed and remarries at a young age, they properly do issue the invitations.

• *When the two different names of the parents are too long to go on one line in the invitation,* put their names on separate lines, joined by "and" (which means they are husband and wife).

• *Generally, neither the bride's title nor surname is given on the invitation. The groom's always are.* Unless the bride's last name is different from her parents', the last name is not repeated in the invitation text. (She is simply "Elizabeth Anne," not "Elizabeth Anne Maguire" on the invitation.) The groom's full name—e.g., "Mr. Tracy McLaughlin"—*does* need to be communicated, since his parents' names are not on the invitation.

• *If the bride's parents do not have the same last names,* as in the case of divorced or widowed and remarried parents, or as in the case of the mother of the bride who has kept her own name in marriage, the bride's surname *is* given on the invitation to clear up any possible confusion. The following examples illustrate this point:

If the mother of the bride has retained her maiden name in her marriage, both names go on the same line, her name following her husband's. In this case, "Ms." is more appropriate to use than "Miss," because the mother of the bride obviously is married and is not a "Miss."

Mr. George Ames Lincoln and Ms. Serena Cooper
request the honour of your presence
at the marriage of their daughter
Leslie Anne Lincoln
etc.

• *If the mother of the bride is a widow who has remarried:*

Mr. and Mrs. George Fillmore Breckport
request the honour of your presence at
the marriage of Mrs. Breckport's daughter
Sarah Anne Simpson

etc.

- *If the father of the bride is a widower who has remarried:*

> *Mr. and Mrs. Anthony Delgas Stanton*
> *request the honour of your presence at*
> *the marriage of Mr. Stanton's daughter*
> *Marianne Lee*
> *etc.*

- *When the bride's parents are divorced* but her mother has not remarried, the mother uses her given, maiden, and married names on the first line, separate from her husband's:

> *Mrs. Marian McPherson Ormsby*
> *Mr. Robert Sims Ormsby*
> *request the honour of your presence at*
> *the marriage of their daughter*
> *Samantha*
> *etc.*

The days are past when a divorced woman had to go formally by her family name and her husband's name, as in "Mrs. McPherson Ormsby." Today she is "Mrs. Marian Ormsby" in most situations.

When both parents have divorced and remarried, the mother's name always comes first, and her ex-husband's name is on the next line:

> *Mrs. Amos Templeton Schulz*
> *Mr. Edmund Holton Draper*
> *request the honour of your presence*
> *at the marriage of their daughter*
> *Louise Marie Draper*
> *etc.*

• *If the bride has lived with her father and stepmother for most of her life, and her stepmother really raised her,* the stepmother would be listed with her husband as issuers of the invitations, and the natural mother would attend the wedding only as a guest.

Mr. and Mrs. William Agyropoulos
request the honour of your presence at
the marriage of their daughter
Olympia
etc.

• *When grandparents or another relative (or even a godparent) gives the wedding,* their relationship to the bride is always made clear:

Mr. and Mrs. Stephen Miller Blaine
request the honour of your presence at
the marriage of their granddaughter
Stephany Lee Blaine
etc.

• *The question of who is paying for the wedding is not relevant to the invitations.* It is petty for one of the divorced parents to say, "Since I'm paying for everything, I don't want the other parent's name on the wedding invitations." Both parents of the bride should be the issuers of the invitations in one way or another, and the mother of the bride should have her name at the top of the invitation to the wedding ceremony regardless of what bad feelings there may be or who is picking up the bills.

There is an exception to this rule, of course, just as there is to everything. If a woman abandons her child and suddenly shows up just at the time of the wedding, she should not expect to assume her role as mother of the bride—either on the invitations or at the reception—but must defer to the bride's stepmother, who raised her. The natural mother in this case would be present at the wedding as a guest only and would not stand in the receiving line at the reception. (The same holds true for the natural mother or father of an adopted child or for the surrogate mother of the bride if she is invited to the wedding.

- *If the bride's first marriage was annulled,* she uses her maiden name on her new wedding invitations, just as before.
- Adult children of a widow or divorcée who is remarrying may issue the wedding invitation, as in this example.

Frederick H. Chatfield, Jr.

Christopher R. Chatfield

Elizabeth C. Gilmore

Alexander D. Chatfield

request

the honor of your presence

at the marriage of their mother

Lansdale

to

Thomas Gardiner

on Saturday, July the fifteenth

nineteen hundred and eighty-nine

at four o'clock

Trinity Church, Copley Square

THE USE OF TITLES IN INVITATIONS

- *Using "Esq." on an invitation.* If either or both parents of the bride are lawyers who normally use "Esq." after their names, *do not* use it on a wedding invitation.
- *When the mother of the bride has a title,* her name with title follows her husband's name on the same line:

> *Mr. Andrew Ellison Tate and Dr. Susan Peters Tate*
> *request the honour of your presence*
> *at the marriage of their daughter*
> *Linda Sue*
> *etc.*

• *When both husband and wife are doctors,* they may issue the invitations in one of two ways:

> *The Doctors Shannon*
> *request the honour of your presence*
> *at the marriage of their daughter*
> *Marilyn Edna*
> *etc.*

or:

> *Dr. Ralph Wolcott Shannon*
> *and Dr. Eve Gaines Shannon*
> *request the honour of your presence*

The above use of "Doctor" refers to medical doctors, not people who hold Ph.D.'s. However, it is appropriate for people in academia who hold Ph.D.'s to call themselves "Dr." when issuing invitations.

• *When the bride herself has a title such as "Doctor" or "Judge" or military rank, she should use it with her full name on the wedding invitation:*

> *Mr. and Mrs. Cornelius Robert Jones*
> *request the honour of your presence*
> *at the marriage of their daughter*
> *Grace Ellen Jones*
> *Major, United States Air Force*
> *to*
> *Mr. Alan Greenberg*
> *etc.*

• The appropriate honorific precedes a public dignitary's name on the invitation. In the following example, the mother of the bride is a Congresswoman who merits the title "The Honourable" before her name on any formal invitation, and who, because of her important official rank, precedes her husband on the invitation:

> *The Honourable Cynthia Wyciekiwiski*
> *and Mr. Stefen Anthony Wyciekiwiski*
> *request the honour of your presence*
> *at the marriage of their daughter*
> *Annemarie*
> *etc.*

WHEN THE COUPLE GIVE THEIR OWN WEDDING

More and more people are marrying for the first time—as well as for the second and third times—at an older age today, and therefore issue their own wedding invitations, as well as pay for the wedding themselves. Their parents may be retired and living on reduced incomes, while the couple is able to afford the cost of the wedding far better than their parents.

- The woman's name is always placed first on the invitation regardless of whether it is she or he (or the two equally) who is paying the bills for the wedding:

> *Cristina Falchi Bonvento*
> *and*
> *Peter Mark Norgren*
> *request the honour of your presence*
> *at their marriage*
> *etc.*

Neither Cristina Bonvento (whether she is a Miss, Ms., or a Mrs.) nor Peter Norgren needs a title on their own wedding invitations. An optional way of issuing these invitations is as follows:

> *The honour of your presence*
> *is requested at the marriage of*
> *Cristina Falchi Bonvento*
> *to*
> *Peter Mark Norgren*
> *etc.*

- A widow has an option on the wording of the wedding invitation she issues with her husband-to-be:

> *Mary Belle Smith*
> *and*
> *Gregory Concord Dee*
> *request the honour of your presence*
> *etc.*

Or, an older widow, used to using only her husband's name, might prefer to do this way:

Mrs. Peter Philip Smith
and
Mr. Gregory Concord Dee
request the honour of your presence
etc.

INVITATION TO A DOUBLE WEDDING

A sample invitation for two sisters would be:

Mr. and Mrs. Anthony Longo Gucci
request the honour of your presence
at the marriage of their daughters
Grace Anne
to
Mr. Donald White Burton
and
Jennifer Tod
to
Mr. George Holland Tree
on Saturday, the tenth of May
etc.

The older daughter is listed first on the invitation.

A sample invitation from two sets of parents to the double wedding of their daughters, who are cousins, would be:

Mr. and Mrs. John Wilson Kramer
request the honour of your presence
at the marriage of their daughter
Felicia
to
Mr. Hans Franz Schmidt

Mr. and Mrs. Gregory Theodore Juergen
request the honour of your presence
at the marriage of their daughter
Denise Louise
to
Mr. James O'Neil

Saturday, the twentieth of December
etc.

The Separate Reception Invitation Card

Separate reception invitation cards are often issued when the religious ceremony is held in one place and the reception in another.

An invitation to a "reception immediately following the ceremony" can indicate any of several possibilities. Catholic and Protestant morning weddings are usually followed by a "wedding breakfast," which is really a lunch. After a four or five o'clock Christian wedding, a cocktail and hors d'oeuvres reception is usually hosted, while at Jewish weddings, almost always an elaborate meal is served. After a Christian or Jewish six o'clock black tie wedding or a very formal eight o'clock service (before 1960 men used to wear white tie and tails for this), a seated dinner is usually given, with the guests attired in evening clothes.

The reception card inserted in front of the wedding ceremony invitation in the envelope may read as follows:

Reception
immediately following the ceremony
1120 Fifth Avenue

The favour of a reply is requested
1120 Fifth Avenue
Apartment 16-X
New York City 10128

- If you plan to serve your guests a meal instead of just a cocktail buffet, say so on the invitation:

Lunch Reception (or Luncheon)
immediately following the ceremony
Omaha Country Club

R.S.V.P.
139 East Farnam Street
Omaha, Nebraska 00000

- If you want to have both the ceremony and the reception (held in different places) to be on the same invitation, it is certainly all right to do so. It makes the invitation less formal. You wouldn't have to include the year, spelled out, for example. Since the invitation is for the wedding in a church and for the reception in another place, you would not use "request the honour of . . ."

Mr. and Mrs. Gregory Anthony Jenkins
request the pleasure of your company
at the marriage of their daughter
Evangeline Lee
to
Mr. Stephen Patrick Smyth
on Saturday, the first of June
at five o'clock
Saint Patrick's Church
Seaway Avenue
and to the dinner reception immediately following
The Pavilion Restaurant
1320 Jones Street
Annapolis

WHEN THE RECEPTION IS HELD MUCH LATER THAN THE CEREMONY

Sometimes there are too many weddings booked in the desired church on a certain day, and the bride can not obtain the hour she prefers for the ceremony. In this case, she accepts what is given her, everyone comes to the wedding ceremony at the hour stipulated, goes home (or wherever they may be staying) afterward, and then returns to another place for the reception at the specified hour. The invitations for the religious service and for the later reception may be mailed together.

In the case of a daytime service and an evening dinner reception, guests would be dressed in daytime apparel and return for the reception in evening clothes. (The wedding party would remain dressed in their special attire for both ceremony and reception.) The card for a later reception following a wedding held at "twelve noon" in a church might read as follows:

Reception Dinner
at eight o'clock
The Mansion
Dallas

R.S.V.P.

Black Tie

WHEN THE FATHER OF THE BRIDE HOSTS THE RECEPTION WITH HIS WIFE, THE BRIDE'S STEPMOTHER

When a man remarries and his daughter has a wedding, his present wife, the bride's stepmother, often feels left out. If he is paying for the entire reception, he and his present wife should list their names as hosts of the reception party, and she would act as the proper hostess of the party. However, she should not stand in the receiving line with the bride—the bride's mother should do that.

Mr. and Mrs. Jonathan Arnold Miller
request the pleasure of your company
at the marriage reception
of his daughter, Sally Anne
immediately following the ceremony
The Standard Club
Chicago

Reply card enclosed

TO WHOM ARE THE REPLIES SENT WHEN THE BRIDE'S PARENTS ARE DIVORCED?

When the father of the bride and his present wife give the reception, it is silly to demand that the guests reply separately to the bride's mother for the wedding ceremony, and then to the bride's father and present wife for the reception. One reply card is enough, and it should be for the reception.

The reply card for this reception invitation should go either to the mother of the bride's home or to the bride's father's home—whichever the divorced parents decide is the most efficient way to handle it. This is a time for the mother of the bride and the father of the bride's present wife to bury any animosities (at least for the moment), and to cooperate on the arrangements for the better functioning of the wedding and a happier bride.

If the bride's stepmother and father will be receiving the RSVPs, it is incumbent on the stepmother to make sure the bride's mother knows of every acceptance or regret as it arrives in the mail. If it is decided that the bride's mother will receive all the replies, then it is incumbent on her to inform the bride's father or his wife of the status of the acceptances. No one should feel left out or ignored. It is too important a time in the life of the bride to have infighting over who receives the replies—or handles the wedding gifts. Everything should be worked out in the most efficient manner.

The Ceremony Card

When the major invitation piece will be to the wedding reception and very few people are invited to the religious service, a "ceremony card" should be included in certain invitations. This card is to invite those who are family or are particularly close to the bride and groom to be present at the exchange of vows. (This is particularly appropriate when the bride has been married before.)

A ceremony card enclosed in an invitation simply gives the name, time of ceremony, and address of the place where it will take place:

Ceremony

Saturday, the fifteenth of April

at half after five o'clock

United Methodist Church

3400 Baylor Boulevard

Syracuse

Soliciting a Reply to an Invitation

In order to solicit a reply to your invitation, put "R.s.v.p." or "R.S.V.P." or "The favour of a reply is requested" in the lower left-hand corner, with the address beneath. Telephone numbers are not given on formal engraved invitations. However, the rule is broken in the case of a prominent bride and groom for whose wedding several hundred invitations are being extended. It is appropriate in this case to list the bride's mother's telephone, the office of one of the bride's parents, or, in the case of the couple extending the invitations themselves, one of their own office telephone numbers.

THE REPLY CARD

Many (myself certainly included) decry the apparent need for a reply card on which recipients simply check to notify their hosts of their acceptance or regret and then mail it back in its preaddressed, sometimes prestamped envelope. However, the "RSVP" card seems obligatory in today's fast-track world. If a reply card and self-addressed envelope are to be included in the invitation, you may engrave in the lower left corner of the wedding invitation: "Reply card enclosed." This removes from the invitation recipient the responsibility to write a formal acceptance or regret note.

The text of a reply card is typically simple and to the point:

M/M _____

Accept _____ *Regret* _____
for the eighth of July

Some people put "The favour of a reply is requested before the thirtieth of June" (two weeks to ten days before the wedding) on their reply cards, but I feel that is unnecessary. It is simply a testimonial to the fact that the parents of the bride think their guests are so lazy that they have to be jostled into replying before the wedding is upon them.

As for prestamping the return envelope, many of us are at odds with those who feel the return envelope must be stamped before the proposed guest will consider mailing back the reply card. A wedding invitation does not require the hosts to coddle the guests. The guests should feel so privileged to be invited to the wedding that they at least come up with a stamp for the envelope.

The Formal Acceptance or Regret

The formal acceptance or regret, handwritten and carefully centered on nice stationery, may be disappearing from the social scene, but it is still the really correct way to reply to a wedding invitation. For example:

*Mr. and Mrs. Gregory Samuel Pontius
accept with pleasure
Mr. and Mrs. William Andrew Touletas'
kind invitation
for Saturday, the sixth of May*

or

*Mr. and Mrs. Gregory Samuel Pontius
sincerely regret that
their absence from the city
prevents them from accepting
the kind invitation of
Mr. and Mrs. Gregory Samuel Pontius
for Saturday, the sixth of May*

In the case of extra-busy people, formal acceptances and regrets may be typed by a secretary, rather than handwritten.

When Portions of the Invitation Are Accepted and Portions Regretted

On occasion, one member of a couple will be able to attend, but not the other. On occasion, a guest will be able to attend the reception, but not the ceremony. On a reply card, these variances should be noted by writing a note at the bottom of the card: "Julius Rose will be able to accept the wedding and reception, but because of illness, Mrs. Rose will be unable to accept."

In a proper, formally written reply, the wording would be as follows:

Mrs. Gregory Samuel Pontius
accepts with pleasure
Mr. and Mrs. William Andrew Touletas'
kind invitation
for Saturday, the sixth of May
Absence from the city
(or illness or whatever)
prevents Mr. Pontius from accepting

"At Home" Cards

When these are sent with the wedding invitations, they simply state the address of the couple and, if they are not already living together, the date after which they will be in joint residence. For example, an "at home" card of a couple who do not live together already might read:

At home
after the fifteenth of January
335 Amory Road
Apartment Fourteen A
Des Moines, Iowa 00000

If you wish, include the telephone number, if it is known at the time. Some people will wait to send their wedding presents to the couple after they are in residence at their new home, so the "at home" address is very useful.

A Pew Card

Pew cards are a nice touch to include in an engraved invitation to a large church wedding at which a certain number of pews are reserved for special guests down front, on both sides of the church. A pew card would be included in invitations to family members, parents and spouses of the wedding party, and VIPs. The small card would read something like this:

Cathedral of Saint John the Divine
Saturday, the fourth of December
Pew number _____

Present this card to an usher

The number of each family's or guest's pew is written in by hand. These reserved pews will also be recognizable by virtue of special floral decorations or ribbons marking them. The ushers' job is to get the right people into them.

• *Admission cards* are necessary only for the wedding of a super-celebrity, such as a star of the entertainment world or a famous government official, when some kind of control at the church doors becomes necessary. Otherwise, the guests might find all their seats taken by curious fans.

Please present this card
Unitarian Church
Saturday, the twentieth of May
(Name of guest or couple written here)

Other Enclosures

• *A separate card may be included to communicate alternate plans in case of bad weather.* For example, if you are planning an outdoor wedding and worry that it may rain, you might enclose an engraved card in the formal wedding invitation that reads:

> *In case of rain*
> *the wedding will be held*
> *in Old Saint Mary's Church*
> *1300 Rosewood Avenue*

• *A separate map card* may be included if either the church or the wedding reception address is difficult to find. You might think it would not be necessary to provide separate directions to the reception if the plan is that everyone will be going from the ceremony straight to the reception. Then you'd expect those who don't know the way to follow those who do. However, sometimes people are unable to attend the wedding ceremony, for one reason or another, and go directly to the reception. This is the reason for providing the map.

• *An engraved "directions card"* is a good idea when a map is not necessary, but exits off freeways and express highways are involved. For example:

From Main Street to Easton:
Take Route 14 to the Southern Beltway. Go 1¾ miles to Exit 37. Turn right onto Jones Boulevard. Go 2½ miles to Hathaway Avenue. Turn left, and enter Grace Church parking lot immediately on the right.

WEDDING ANNOUNCEMENTS

Wedding announcements, often engraved on the same high-quality ecru stock as wedding invitations, and similar in size, are sent to people who were not invited to the wedding but with whom you want to share your good news. For example, you would send announcements to people who live far away and could not possibly come to your wedding. If you are married with only your family and a very few friends present, you would send announcements to your entire list of friends who ordinarily would have been invited to your wedding. The parents of both bride and groom would also send them to all of their friends, past and present, who were not sent invitations.

You might send an announcement to your old teachers, baby sitters, to your doctor, classmates, business associates, and the alumni magazines of any school you attended.

Second-time-around brides find the announcements particularly important as a way of communicating the great news in their lives.

• *Recipients of wedding announcements are not expected to send
a gift* (as recipients of invitations who accept are). However, many
people who feel close to the bride or groom do send gifts—even a small
token—to show their pleasure over the news.

• *In formal engraved wedding announcements,* a separate card
giving the couple's address (and telephone number, if desired) is
enclosed with the announcement. The "at home" cards are a perfect
way of showing that the bride had kept her own name after marriage, if
that is the case. For example:

At home

Martha Renwick Ashton

George Ralston Leigh

1435 Second Avenue

Atlanta, Georgia 00000

000-000-0000

Anyone receiving that announcement in the mail will know that the bride
has retained her own name.

In formal engraved announcements, an inner envelope as well as
the outer one used for mailing is customary, just as with a wedding
invitation.

• *In an informal printed announcement,* the bride and groom's
return address on the envelope removes the necessity for a separate card
giving their address.

• It is important to remember that *wedding announcements should
not be mailed until immediately after the wedding ceremony.* Many
brides ask a friend to be responsible for them and to take them to the
wedding in a tote bag—stamped, sealed, addressed, and ready to mail.
The friend then goes to the post office to mail them on the way to the
wedding reception. Friends who receive the announcements postmarked
the day of or the day after the wedding know that the bride and groom
had them in their thoughts, and that is what matters.

The Announcement Text

The announcement text for formal engraved or for printed announcements would be as follows:

Mr. and Mrs. Remigio Grant Ashton
have the honour of announcing
(or *have the honour to announce*)

the marriage of their daughter
Martha Renwick

to

Mr. George Ralston Leigh
on Wednesday, the first of June
one thousand nine hundred ninety eight
(in printed invitations, the year is given in numbers)

Saint George's Church
(naming the place is optional)
Des Moines, Iowa

If the couple are announcing their own marriage, which is often the case with divorced, widowed, or older couples, the text would read:

Mary Simpson Bartlett
Henry Thatcher Jones
have the honour to announce
their marriage
on Saturday, the tenth of January
etc.

Some people send flowery announcements with texts such as "We have the joy of announcing happy news we wish to share with you, that we have joined in matrimony," and so on. Anyone is free to do what he or she pleases, but you will not find help on sending that kind of announcement in this book!

HOW MUCH WILL IT COST AND WHO WILL PAY?

First, the Budget

In the past, after a couple decided to marry, the groom nervously went to the bride's father to seek her hand in matrimony. Later the wedding would be planned, and a budget would be set by the bride's father, who would be responsible for paying for almost everything.

Today, once both have agreed to wed, the bride's father is consulted only in terms of how much he will pay toward the wedding—certainly not in terms of the young man's asking permission to marry his daughter. Today the rules are no longer strict about the protocol of payment for the wedding. Often the bride's and groom's parents sit around a table and talk about who will (and is able to) pay for what expenses for the upcoming wedding. There is a give and take, which is common sense. There are still some brides whose parents incur tremendous debt by hosting lavish weddings—to give the appearance of being rich and successful—but the majority of weddings today are the result of shared expenses, even including costs borne by the marrying couple.

The budget is important to establish—and adhere to—at the very beginning of the planning activities, because otherwise expenses can get completely out of hand. A wedding can easily cost $50 per guest, $300 per guest, or $1000 per guest by the time all the expenses are factored into the total amount. If you have 300 guests, that can add up to a great deal of money!

In drawing up your budget, remember these expenses—some of which occur in any wedding, and some of which occur only in very lavish ones:

o *The invitations*

Cost of paper, engraving or printing (stationers)
Cost of hand-addressing the envelopes, perhaps by calligraphers
Cost of postage

o *Possible expenses involving the attendants*

Paying for their lodging (if they aren't staying with friends)
Paying for the dress and for the airfare of a much-loved brides-

maid or the rental of the usher's suit and the airfare of a much-loved groomsman (who could not afford to be in the wedding otherwise)

o *Church or temple services*

Payment to the church pastor or rabbi
Payment to the church organist, choir, and regular staff of the house of worship

o *The reception*

Rental of room or banquet hall or whatever kind of area
Preparation and service of food and liquor
Rental of equipment needed, including tabletop accessories, tables, and chairs
Optional services of party designer or coordinator
Special linens made for the tables (optional)
Construction of tents for outdoor receptions (including heaters or air-conditioners if necessary)

o *Flowers*

For the bride's bouquet
For the bridesmaids' bouquets and perhaps flower girls' baskets
Boutonnieres for the groom and the male members of the wedding party
For the church
For the receiving line area at the reception
For the tables at the reception
For decoration of the tent for an outdoor reception
For the handle of the wedding cake knife
Corsages for the mothers of the bride and groom (done rarely now, fortunately, since they can ruin the look of a dress)

o *Photography*

Bride's formal portrait made in studio
Candids of the wedding
Video recording of the wedding (optional)

o *Transportation*

Limousines to take bride and groom to and from the ceremony and the reception
Limousines for their families and the bridal party

o *Music*

In the church (organ, choir, chamber music, or other)
At the reception (trio, dance band, or other)

o *Gifts*

From the bride and groom to each other
Their individual wedding rings
For their wedding attendants

o *Groom's special expenses*

The cost of the rehearsal dinner the night before the wedding
   (usually given by the groom's parents)
The purchase of the wedding license
Clergyman's fee (often paid for by bride's parents)
Traditionally, he paid for the bride's bouquet and his ushers'
   boutonnieres, but it has been proven easier and more efficient
   to let the bride's florist also handle these flowers.
Wedding trip

Paying for It

Traditionally, the bride's family bore the brunt of almost all of the wedding expenses. Today, so many people are getting married at a later age, and so many people are divorcing and remarrying that these customs are changing. The following are today's options for paying:

o If the groom's family is rich and the bride's is not, the groom's family pays all or almost all of the expenses, even though the invitations are still sent out in the bride's parents' names.
o If the bride's family is rich and the groom's is not, the bride's family pays for everything, including the rehearsal dinner that is customarily the groom's family's responsibility.
o If the bride's and groom's families both have modest incomes, the groom's family may offer to pay as big a portion as possible of the wedding expenses to help out.
o If the bride and groom are both working and in their thirties or older, their parents may be retired and living on limited incomes. The bride and groom would pay for their own wedding in this case.
o If the young bride has been divorced and her parents are not in comfortable circumstances, she and her new groom might divide the costs between them.

The important thing to remember is that all details of who pays for what must be ironed out before the wedding is planned! If expenses are to be split between the two families or between the bride and groom themselves (as is often the case in second marriages), it should be recorded in black and white (with a copy for each) as to who is going to be responsible for what.

Another option for a couple splitting the costs of their wedding is to have one person pay all of the bills, with the other member of the couple reimbursing the "treasurer" for half the expenses.

PLANNING FOR A PERFECT WEDDING DAY

Choosing the Time for the Religious Ceremony

There are special days that are traditional wedding days, such as Saturday for Christians and Sundays for people of the Jewish faith. In some Catholic churches, it is considered in questionable taste to be married at a large wedding during Lent. In most religions it is perfectly proper to be married in a religious ceremony on weekdays, but it is difficult for guests who work to be able to attend.

Choosing the Place for the Wedding Service

As noted, people get married at home, at City Hall, on board ship, and in a judge's chambers. They get married in the bride's family's living room, in a garden, in a hotel parlor, in a public park, or in front of a famous monument. I've even been to a wedding on a grass tennis court. But most often, people marry in a house of worship.

Traditionally, the wedding is held in the bride's or the bride's family's place of worship. Today, with the tremendous mobility of Americans, brides often find themselves being married in a new city or in a house of worship where neither she nor her family is known. An early discussion with the minister, priest, or rabbi is of paramount importance, because the church or temple may already be booked for the time you'd like for your own wedding. You may have to choose another time of day or even another week for your ceremony. Sometimes there is a great deal of red tape to unravel, so allow plenty of time to accumulate records and perhaps provide copies of everything needed— from birth to baptismal certificates. You both may be required to attend an obligatory marital counseling course—sometimes an all-day session, sometimes classes taking place over a period of several weeks.

Once you have found your house of worship, establish a good pattern of communication with the clergyman. He will be able to give you the rules of his parish regarding certain areas—such as what kind of music you may or may not have and what restrictions there might be on photographers, video cameras, and special lights. He will discuss the kind of service you want to have—and what you may and may not do to alter or add to the official rites of marriage. He will arrange to show the church facilities to your wedding coordinator or florist, and coordinate with them as to when they should gain access to begin their decoration of the church. He will facilitate on your wedding day the optional laying down of the red carpet ("canopy") from the church door to the curb, and the optional installation of a white "runner." (Just before the bride makes her appearance, two ushers or church employees roll the runner down the aisle on which the bride will walk, each helping guide the huge carpet.

Options That Make for a Happy Day

When you plan your wedding, you want to make it beautiful, sentimental, and, above all, fun for everyone. And you want your families to be happy, too. There is no question but that all of this can be realized—if everyone gives a little, makes an effort not to voice dissatisfaction with arrangements, and compromises here and there to accede to the bride's and groom's wishes.

You have some options in the planning that make for a happy day:

• Take into account strong feelings of both the bride's and groom's parents, because, even though it is *not* their wedding, they may feel it is.

• Take care to invite as guests all those who love you and who would feel deeply hurt not to be included.

• When your parents buck you on your decisions, gently bring them around to your way of thinking, rather than dismiss their suggestions or criticisms out of hand as having no value whatsoever.

• Use your wedding as a great family healer. Tell those members of the family who are estranged that you expect them to be present as full-fledged members of the family circle, with everyone in communication with one another, and with family feuds put to rest.

All too often in weddings one family feels the other family does not have the proper background and educational advantages. The family who feels superior should, to use the vernacular, "sit on it" and keep those feelings in control. The bride and the groom are what matter, not the social prestige and wealth—or lack of it—on one or other side. I remember one mother of the bride who was worried sick that the rehearsal dinner, given by the parents of the groom, would be improperly hosted and embarrassing to the bride's family friends. A sister of the bride cornered her mother and told her to stop being so wrought up: "Mom, let the rehearsal dinner be reflective of the groom's family, and let the wedding be reflective of our family, and then the bride and groom can reflect on each other and forget about all of us!" (A wise philosophy!)

• Become a planning expert in the *human* aspects of your wedding, not just the straight logistics. For example:

- ○ Arrange to have Aunt Mathilda, who is fragile, picked up at the airport and given VIP treatment during the wedding celebration. Don't expect her to fend for herself.
- ○ Assign a good friend to introduce your clergyman around at the wedding reception and make him feel comfortable.
- ○ Tell a good friend sitting at each table to take home the beautiful centerpiece at that table when the reception is over.
- ○ Call both sets of parents late, on your wedding night, to tell them how much you appreciate the wedding, how much you love them, and how happy you are.

- Remember that the best way to avoid hurt feelings when you extend your invitations is to establish a firm policy and then stick to it— for example, "It's a very small wedding, only families and a small group of the bridal couple's closest friends."

- A *wedding consultant* is very helpful for those who would like to turn the entire coordination over to a professional. A wedding consultant or planner knows who the best vendors are and can get the best prices. A wedding consultant does not forget important details, and on the actual wedding day he or she is supervising everything with a practiced eye—unlike the mother of the bride, who will be busy with her guests. This person may charge a flat fee or may take a percentage of the gross cost of the wedding.

KEEP TRACK OF IMPORTANT DETAILS WITH A WEDDING PLANNER

Devise your own wedding planner to help you get organized. You might buy yourself an ordinary notebook with subdividers, and make yourself entries such as these:

Invitation List

- Include under this heading an *alphabetical list of names and addresses of all recipients of invitations,* with each title correct, and with each word written out (example: "Street" instead of "St.") exactly as the envelope is to be addressed. Give a copy of this list to:

- ○ Yourself, for yourself
- ○ Whoever is addressing the invitations
- ○ Your parents
- ○ The groom
- ○ His parents

- Include this additional information:

  o Name of printer or engraver
  o Address of printer or engraver
  o Telephone number
  o Name of your contact with the company
  o Date when invitations promised to be delivered
  o Names of addressers or calligraphers to address envelopes
  o Date when finished envelopes to be delivered to you
  o Type of stamps purchased, how many purchased
  o Date of mailing of invitations

- Set up two sets of RSVP pages—one to record names of those who accept, one to record those who regret.

The Wedding Party

Put first in this section *an alphabetized list* of members of the wedding party.

Give each attendant his or her own page, and include the following information:

Name _____

Name of spouse or date attending _____

Address and home and office telephone numbers

_____   _____

Name of spouse or date accompanying _____

Wedding costume

    (1) Size information:

      For bride's attendants:

        Dress size _____Shoe size _____

      For groom's attendants:

        Pants: Waist _____Inseam measurement _____

        Coat size _____

        Shirts: Neck _____Sleeve _____

    (2) Date and hour of fittings _____

Arrival and departure information

    Arriving how _____What day _____ Hour _____

    Departing how _____What day _____ Hour _____

Address and telephone number during wedding festivities

_____   _____

Name of parents (if to receive wedding invitation) _____

Address _____

The Wedding Ceremony

Place _____

Clergyman _____

Assistant clergyman or secretary _____

Address _____

Telephone number _____

Time and date of rehearsal _____

Time of ceremony _____

    Time for groom and best man to arrive _____

    For ushers _____

    Time for bride's mother to arrive _____

    Bride, attendants, and bride's father _____

Music:

    Soloists or group _____

        Telephone number _____

    Organist's name _____Telephone _____

Program _____
_____

Flowers:

    Where _____   Type _____

    _____   _____

    _____   _____

Fees:

    Sexton's _____Clergyman's _____

    Organist's _____Other musicians' _____

Instructions for photographer during ceremony:
_____

Reception Planner for a Large Wedding

If you have a wedding consultant, you don't need to make a reception planner. You can take a look at your consultant's planning notebook whenever you wish.

If you are doing your own, you might follow these charts, to work with in conjunction with your caterer.

PROTOCOL CHECKLIST

Staff needed to check in at door _____

No. of tables needed _____

Table cards? _____ In stock _____ To order _____

    No. needed _____ Person in charge _____

Seating charts to be made? _____ Blown up to what size? _____

    By whom? _____

Place cards: No. needed _____ In stock or to be ordered _____

    Names to be: Handwritten _____ Typed _____

    Done in calligraphy _____

    Person responsible _____

Menu cards: No. needed _____ Handwritten _____

    Typed _____ Calligraphy and offset _____

    Person responsible _____

Person in charge of seating _____ Tel. _____

Receiving Line: Where? _____ Names (in order of standing in line)

    _____

    _____

    _____

    _____

Will there be an introducer? _____ Name _____ Tel. _____

Names and tel. of "party workers" _____ _____

                                    _____ _____

                                      _____ _____

No. of copies of guest list required _____

CATERER'S CHECKLIST

Name _____ Address _____ Contact _____ Tel. No. _____

	Food to be served	Liquor, wines, nonalcoholic drinks to be served	
Cocktail Hour	_____	_____	_____
	_____	_____	_____
	_____	_____	_____
	_____	_____	_____
	_____	_____	_____
Dinner	_____	_____	_____
	_____	_____	_____
	_____	_____	_____
	_____	_____	_____
	_____	_____	_____
	_____	_____	_____
	_____	_____	_____
After Dinner (in the tent)	_____	_____	_____
	_____	_____	_____
	_____	_____	_____
	_____	_____	_____

Help hired:
   No. in kitchen _____ No. of waiters & waitresses _____
   Coat-checkers _____ Valet parkers _____
   Restroom attendants _____

Restrooms:
   Suitable for guests? _____ Need guest soaps, guest
   towels? _____ Are portable facilities necessary? _____

Extra security:
   Necessary? _____ Will caterer provide? _____
   No. needed _____ Name of outside company handling _____
   Contact _____ Tel: _____

Flowers:
   Room decor plans _____
   Table centerpieces _____ No. _____
   Style of container _____

Transportation Arrangements

Name of Car Service: _____ Contact _____ Tel.: _____

Date	Names of People to Meet	Terminal	Flt/Bus/Tr. No.	Time

Rehearsal Dinner	Pickup Points:	Riders' Names
Date:	1.	
_____	2.	
Address:	3.	
_____	4.	
Hour:		

WEDDING DAY   Date:

To the Church	Pickup Points	Car #	Riders
Address:	1.		
_____	2.		
Hour:	3.		
_____	4.		
	5.		
	6.		
To Reception			Riders
	Car 1:		
Address:	Car 2:		
_____	Car 3:		
_____	Car 4:		

WORKING WITH THE CATERER

When you hear that a caterer's meal costs $150 per person, remember that that sum represents not only his or her profit and the cost of the food and its preparation, but also the service of it and the rental of equipment involved in the serving of it. It never ceases to amaze me how one can eat the same delicious menu at two separate wedding receptions and find one caterer has charged the bride's parents $250 per person, while the other has charged the bride's parents $75 per person. The expense of doing business in a particular location, the cachet of the name of the more expensive caterer, plus perhaps an extra measure of style in service all add to the price of the food.

Remember to add service charges and tax onto the prices you are quoted by the caterer so that you will understand what your true charges will be. Generally a service charge of up to 20 percent is added to your bill (as well as sales tax). If you were *very* well pleased with the reception, arrange to have the director of operations and the captains receive an extra tip of from $20 to $50.

The caterer will provide coat checking facilities, if you request those. Some caterers even handle such details as the music, the entire floral and table design of the party, including the lighting, and the organization of valet parking.

The best way to find a great caterer is by word of mouth. When you are ready to settle on the firm, look carefully at the samples of their rented equipment, including the kind of chairs they will provide for your guests at the table, the style of their serving platters, the color and condition of their table linens, and the quality of their glassware, china, and flatware. Sample what they suggest for your menu, so that you know exactly what will be served and how it will be presented. Most caterers will prepare free tastings for you at their establishment. It's preferable not to hand them recipes of dishes you would like served, because without the caterer's having practiced those dishes several times before, the results could be unsatisfactory, if not disastrous. Have your caterer prepare the kind of food he or she knows how to serve with a flourish.

• Be sure you understand everything written down in the contract before you sign it. Know what all the costs of equipment rental will be. Read the fine print about the cancellation charges. (Sadly enough, there *are* weddings that are called off at the last minute, for one reason or another.)

• Since the cost of drinks and wines is a major part of the contract, make sure the contract stipulates that *quality brands* are to be served.

Otherwise, you might find Uncle Freddie's Homestyle Bourbon and Platinum Star Plus Scotch being served at your open bars instead of the recognizably good brands.

• Be sure there will be enough waiters or waitresses to serve your guests. New York's Glorious Foods, one of the top catering firms in the world, believes that the food cannot be served properly and at the right temperature if there are not at least one and a half to two waiters per table of eight or ten people. For a cocktail buffet for a hundred people, they feel five waiter/bartenders plus a working captain are needed to handle the crowd. The number of people serving is of paramount importance, because if guests have to fight to get a drink and if the meal service is interminably slow, the wedding reception will be considered a flop.

THE FOOD AT THE RECEPTION

Whether you hire a caterer or make other arrangements, the food you serve your guests should be

- o Delicious
- o Plentiful
- o Unusual—or at least not cliché
- o Beautifully presented

Wonderful wedding reception food is not stereotyped; there is no traditional wedding fare today. Instead, there is as much variety in the choices as there is in the bride's family's tastes. You can be as imaginative as you wish—within the limits of your budget and the capabilities of the person preparing the food. I have enjoyed an extraordinary clambake wedding reception at the beach (steamed clams and clam broth, roast corn, boiled lobsters), and a delicious roast goose with cornbread pudding at a wedding lunch in snow-blanketed mountains. I have delighted in the taste of perfectly prepared couscous at an Arab reception; I have savored vegetarian sandwiches served with pink lemonade at a reception in Ohio on a hot summer's day. It was all *wonderful*.

Planning the Menu

The menu for your reception should suit:

- o The budget of whoever is paying for it.
- o The time of day when the food is served. (A breakfast requires a very different menu from a dinner.)

- o The region of the country. (The menu might feature fresh fish at a Cape Cod wedding, Creole dishes in New Orleans, a barbecue in Texas, and a special ham dish in Georgia.)
- o The degree of formality of the wedding. (You might serve paella for a reception on an outdoor patio in Arizona, but you would not serve it at a dinner at the Waldorf in New York.)
- o The ethnic preferences, if they exist, of the couple to be married.

There are simple nonalcoholic receptions held in the parish hall of a small church after the wedding ceremony; there are celebration picnics set up on a grassy knoll after an outdoor service; there are Chinese, Indian, Italian, Greek, and Mexican banquets served in restaurants; and there are five-course dinners served in hotel and club ballrooms after services in large cathedrals or temples. All of them owe part of their success to careful planning of the menu.

BREAKFAST

If your wedding reception will be a breakfast following an early morning service, while you are greeting your guests (and before anyone sits down to eat) have your guests offered a tray with their choice of plain fruit juices, sparkling water, Mimosas (champagne in orange juice), and Bloody Marys (vodka in tomato juice). You might serve a menu like the following:

Creamed chicken crêpes
Broiled tomatoes stuffed with pâté, crushed bacon, or grilled mushrooms with herbs
Hot brioches, croissants, bran muffins, and biscuits with a choice of butter, honey, jam, and cream cheese
Hot baked fruit with optional whipped cream
Wedding cake (with which coffee is always served)

By the time the bride and groom cut the cake, it will probably be close to noon. Have champagne served to each guest who wishes it, for toasting purposes and for consumption along with the wedding cake.

An Informal Reception in the Parish Hall or Rectory

Fruit punch (with or without alcohol)
Sandwiches, including cream cheese on orange bread, smoked sturgeon in puff pastry, pesto tartlets, and sliced turkey on tiny hot biscuits with cranberry chutney
Ice cream and wedding cake

A THREE-COURSE LUNCH

Cold Potage Saint-Germain (cream of pea soup)
Chicken Breasts Véronique (with mushrooms, white wine, and seedless grapes)
Puree of spinach in avocado halves
Endive and arugula salad vinaigrette
Frozen mocha mousse and wedding cake
White wine until dessert; champagne served with dessert

A FOUR-COURSE DINNER

Stracciatella soup (chicken broth with beaten egg)
Salmon timbales (small molds of salmon mousse with hollandaise sauce)
Roast loin of pork with hot prune sauce
Green beans
Baby carrots
Banana sherbet and wedding cake
Champagne served throughout the meal

Of course, if you are among the very rich, you can have a "simple" wedding lunch of only three courses, like that of Mercedes Kellogg and Texas billionaire Sid Bass when they were married at the Plaza Hotel in New York in December 1988. Their menu cards read at the top, "Celebrating the marriage of Mercedes and Sid Bass." The menu consisted of:

Caviar de Beluga aux Blini (accompanied by vodka and a Pouilly Fumé La Doucette 1985 white wine)

* * *

Carré d'Agneau Rôti au Romarin
Gratin de Pommes de Terre Dauphinois
Flageolets (served with Château Latour 1982)

* * *

Soufflé Glacé aux Pralines
Coulis de Poires
Gâteau de Mariage (served with Krug Rosé champagne)
Café

This menu translates to lots of fresh caviar, lamb chops with potatoes au gratin and white beans, and an ice-cream praline soufflé with wedding cake.

At the opposite end of the financial scale, at a wedding lunch held the same day in another part of New York, the menu read:

Cream of tomato soup with croutons
Spinach-filled ravioli
Ice cream with chocolate sauce
Wedding cake and coffee
One red wine served throughout

No one could say which lunch was the more delicious.

"GRAZING"

During this kind of reception, some small tables with chairs are set up at random, but the majority of guests dance or stand and talk, eating off little plates with food selected from the buffet. In most cases, guests consider the ample choice of hors d'oeuvres their evening meal.

It's very important to instruct the waiters to keep the buffet table replenished and to keep picking up used glasses, plates, and silverware from around the entire party area as guests come and go. The kinds of grazing food that might be found at this kind of reception:

Small open-face rye bread sandwiches with rare roast beef, topped with a thin layer of horseradish sauce
Circles of smoked salmon with fresh dill
Crudités (fresh vegetables, mostly raw, but some of which—like broccoli and cauliflower florets—are lightly steamed, with a dip of choice
Small sandwiches (crusts removed) with any kind of filling (for example, mushroom paste; shrimp mashed with mayonnaise, shallots, capers, and seasoning; red caviar and sour cream)
Shrimp and crab claws
Poached salmon
Platter of assorted cheeses and crackers
Broiled water chestnuts wrapped in bacon on toothpicks (must be served piping hot)
Curried crabmeat tarts
Turkey bouchées (turkey salad in tiny pastry shells)
A pâté of choice
Sliced baked ham
Prosciutto and fresh figs on toothpicks
A cold pasta or rice salad
Bowlfuls of balls of different flavors of sherbet
Wedding cake
Coffee
Champagne served throughout

The Presentation Is Important

Often, all you have to do is explain to the caterer or the hotel banquet manager that you care very much how the food is presented, whether it is individually served by waiters or whether it is presented on the buffet table on platters. For example, it looks pleasing to the eye when:

- A large cold fish, its skin removed, is embellished on its side with a flowering branch (made with fresh dill and vegetable flowers).
- A container of pâté is beautified with geometric designs or even the bridal couple's monogram, made from scallions and sweet red peppers.
- A fresh green sprig of an herb lies across the face of half a hard-boiled egg.
- A bunch of marinated beans is tied like a bunch of logs with a strip of pimiento.
- A hollowed-out cucumber boat carries a cargo of salade Niçoise.
- A baked half acorn squash is filled with anything from paprika-sprinkled hot creamed chicken to *pasta al pesto.*
- A grilled skewer is made colorful with cubes of lamb or chicken alternating with slices of red pepper, yellow squash, and green zucchini.
- A mound of yellow molded rice is decorated with a garland of Chinese pea pods, mushroom halves, and cherry tomatoes.
- A large roast on a platter is framed in clusters of fresh (not overcooked) decorative vegetables and watercress.
- Poached pears swim in a creamy custard sauce, each pear topped by a sugar violet or other candied flower.
- A mound of butter pecan ice cream, sprinkled with powdered cocoa, sits on a plate covered half in caramel, half in chocolate sauce (the two sauces meeting in the middle).

The Wedding Cake

Fresh flowers are often used on today's wedding cakes. New York's famous wedding cake baker, Sylvia Weinstock, finds that most brides ask for a chocolate layer cake with chocolate filling, a chocolate hazelnut torte cake with mocha praline filling, or a yellow cake filled with apricots and Grand Marnier liqueur. Brides are getting away from the more traditional—and boring—white cake with white frosting.

It is a nice tradition, however, to have the decoration of a first

The wedding cake deserves its own skirted table, which can be wheeled into the center of the room when the bride and groom cut the cake. This multitiered carrot cake with marzipan frosting, decorated with fresh flowers, was made by Cheryl Kleinman for our daughter Clare's wedding.

bride's cake all in white. (Second- and third-time-around brides should properly have cakes decorated with touches of color.)

Be sure, when ordering your wedding cake specially made, to have good references from other satisfied clients of the cake-maker and to have seen color photographs of his or her work. It is preferable to order the exact design you liked in a photograph.

FLOWERS

Sometimes a floral designer rather than a wedding consultant is the mainstay of the wedding organization. Sometimes a floral designer is hired by the wedding consultant as part of his or her coordinating duties.

A good florist is one thing; a good floral designer is another. He or she will first survey the premises of every single place that will need flowers or greenery (including the wedding cake), then work with the bride and her parents in drawing up a proposal and budget. After that the bride's family can relax.

Some of these professionals design the entire wedding, not just the flowers. Sometimes they buy their flowers in the wholesale market; sometimes they stock and retail flowers themselves. If you choose a floral designer to do your wedding in conjunction with your own planning endeavors, be sure to find one of excellent reputation. Word of mouth is very important or, as with a caterer whose food you may have enjoyed at someone's big party or wedding, a floral designer may have done a very impressive party that you or a friend of yours attended recently.

Flowers are an important item—not only for the church, but in the bride's and her attendants' bouquets, tucked into the men's lapels, decorating the place of the religious service, centering the tables at the reception, and embellishing the tent or the room where the reception is held. They are a major factor in the wedding budget.

• It is possible to hold down the budget for the flowers at the reception by using few flowers and a lot of greenery in the centerpiece and in the flowers on the serving table. Tall plants or even trees in tubs can be rented to flank the receiving line and to disguise ugly parts of the room. I was once helping a bride by putting the place cards on the tables for her dinner reception in a hotel ballroom when I noticed the distress of the floral designer, who had just seen the bandstand put in place. "This is the ugliest bandstand I have *ever* seen," he said. He disappeared for half an hour, returned with tall flowering quince branches in glass vases, put these on the floor in front of the bandstand, and suddenly you couldn't see it any more.

• It is a nice touch, of course, if the flowers are integrated into the design scheme of the whole wedding, so that the colors repeat those of the bridesmaids' dresses, the linens used at the reception, and other color-coordinated items. I remember a reception lunch at which people sitting at the round tables noticed suddenly that the flowered table cloths repeated the design theme of the wedding. There were large white flowers printed on the fabric (the same flowers carried by the bride in her bouquet), and there were small yellow, pale blue, and peach-colored flowers in the rest of the fabric design—the same flowers and colors as in the bridesmaids' dresses and in their bouquets, and in the flowers of our table centerpieces. There were peach napkins and peach linen seats on our chairs. It was all beautifully thought out and executed.

• The bride should have as large or as small a bouquet as she wishes. She can carry a white prayer book with streamers or an armful of calla lilies. This is the time for her to have the loveliest flowers in the world—her own fantasy fulfilled.

The bride's bouquet, symbolic of all that is beautiful in a wedding, may be all white or touched with pastel colors. It should be beribboned so that its effect, sailing through the air at the end of the wedding when the bride tosses her bouquet to the next young lady to be married, looks all the more sensational. This is our daughter Clare's wedding bouquet, by floral designer Ann McIlvaine.

Bridemaids' Bouquets

The bridesmaids' bouquets, of course, are an integral part of the design of the wedding. They are usually less costly if chosen to reflect the season of the year, such as peonies in May, mums and autumn leaves in the autumn, and white, pink, or red poinsettias at Christmas. In today's shipping-by-jet world, you can have any out-of-season flowers you want from any part of the world—as long as someone can pay for it!

Boutonnieres

The men in the wedding party wear boutonnieres in their left lapels. The bridegroom's and the best man's might be based on the flowers in the bride's bouquet, such as a pink rose with a sprig of stephanotis. The boutonnieres of the ushers and the fathers of the bride and groom might be different, such as carnations, roses of a different color, or lilies of the valley.

PHOTOGRAPHY REQUIREMENTS

The Bride's Portrait

It is nice to have a formal full-length portrait made for posterity. It should be shot in a photo studio, showing the bride in all her regalia (in color or in black and white). This photograph (8 inches by 11 inches or 11 inches by 14 inches in size) might be given by the bride as a present, framed, to her husband to grace their own home, as well as to both sets of parents and grandparents for their homes. The maid of honor will want a smaller one (5 inches by 6 inches) of her best friend or her relative, in a double frame, with a photograph of the entire wedding party on the other side of the frame. The groom may well want an additional smaller one of the bride for his office.

Usually the bride's actual bouquet of flowers will not be shown in this formal photograph. Rather, she will be holding a bouquet of rather nondescript artificial flowers. It doesn't matter, but what does matter is that her hair and veil be shown in the photograph exactly as they will be on her wedding day.

This is usually the photograph the society section of the local newspaper requests for their Sunday bridal section (in an 8- by 11-inch black and white glossy form) although some newspapers request an informal photo of the bride and groom taken together on their wedding day.

The Candid Photographer

The candid photographer handles the most important part of your wedding—the official record. Whatever you do, use a professional to take your candid pictures. If a well-meaning friend or relative volunteers to assume the role of official wedding photographer, he or she might make disastrous amateur mistakes. Also, when the photographer is socializing with family and friends and enjoying the reception, important pictures are not being taken.

IN THE CHURCH

Many houses of worship will not allow flashbulbs popping during the services. Some will allow the photographer to come down the aisle only twice—once to photograph the bride and groom at the altar, and once to catch them on their way out, walking joyfully to the back of the church as man and wife. Sometimes the photographer can perch in the choir loft and capture important parts of the ceremony noiselessly and inconspicuously with a long lens. If you intend to have a video camera recording everything, be sure to get permission before it is used at your wedding ceremony.

GROUP PHOTOS

Usually the wedding party is photographed at the place where the reception is to be held, just before all the guests arrive from the church services. The members of the wedding party and the parents should be well warned ahead of time that this is a priority project and that nothing must interrupt it once everyone has arrived at the reception area.

- o The entire group should be photographed together (no glasses in hands, please).
- o The bride and groom should be photographed with each set of parents.
- o The bride should be shown with all her bridal attendants.
- o The groom should be shown with his attendants.

COVERING THE FESTIVITIES

Instruct your photographer well before the wedding. Give him or her a list of the members of the wedding party and all relatives and out-of-town guests. Assign a friend who knows everyone to help scout the important people for pictures at the wedding reception, and to stay at the photographer's side. Go over the wedding schedule with the photographer in advance, so that he or she knows what must be covered:

- o The bride getting dressed?
- o Hugging her mother before her mother or a beloved relative leaves for the church?
- o Talking to her little sister?
- o Chatting with her father in the limousine on their way to the church?
- o Any pictures of the groom and best man behind the scenes at the church before the ceremony begins?
- o Photos of the ushers in action?
- o Guests going through the receiving line?
- o The first dances on the floor?
- o Bride and groom in first dance?
- o Father dancing with bride; groom dancing with bride's mother?
- o Bride tossing bouquet?
- o Groom tossing garter?
- o Couple pelted with rice or flower petals as they leave?
- o Kissing parents and friends good-bye as luggage is loaded into their car?
- o Waving good-bye from back window of getaway car?

LOGISTICS AND PAYMENT FOR CANDIDS

Usually the photographer presents you with a book of proofs of all the photographs, and you order desired prints by number. The bride's parents are supposed to make a gift of eight to ten photographs to the groom's family, but usually the latter will want many more than that. The best way to handle it is to let the bride's parents and the groom's parents handle their own orders for everyone in their families, and then let each side pay the photographer directly for their prints. It is a gracious gesture to send each member of the wedding party an 8- by 10-inch photograph of the group—but then it is also gracious to allow each member of the wedding party or close family members to view the book of proofs and to order (and incidentally pay for) additional photographs.

A WEDDING PICTURES ALBUM

It is a very nice gesture if a family member purchases three attractive photo albums to hold the various wedding photographs and presents one to the bride and groom; one to the parents of the bride; and one to the parents of the groom. Each album should be lettered with the couple's name or initials and the date of their wedding. It becomes a treasured keepsake to be handed down to future generations.

MUSIC

If there is going to be dancing at the reception, the music will be as important as the food—maybe even more so. The music sets the ambience and motivates people to mix and dance with each other. People suddenly feel good. Romances start at weddings. Music makes the party come alive.

The choice of your music for the religious service is one thing. Your choice of music for the reception is quite another. First, you must decide if you want to have music to listen to, not dance to at your reception. (This is often the case for a morning wedding followed by breakfast or lunch.)

For your listening music, do you want a chamber music group? A pretty young harpist? A pianist singing sophisticated, low-key love songs? A jazz combo of guitarist, bass, and pianist playing Cole Porter, Steven Sondheim, and George Gershwin softly in the background?

If you have retained one of the orchestras of the great band leaders (such as Lester Lanin, Peter Duchin, Michael Carney, Vince Giordano, or one of the top local groups, you know what kind of music they are going to play. If you hire a band that plays South American music, you know what you're going to get. What matters is your own choice. I went to a June wedding where the bride and groom, who had recently taken lessons to learn how to waltz, hired a waltz orchestra, and that was a tremendous hit with the guests. The older guests got by dancing a sedate foxtrot: the younger guests managed to move happily to a hidden rock beat.

The following week I attended the outdoor wedding of my niece Megan Baldrige to Craig Murray, at my brother Mac's and sister-in-law Midge's farm in Woodbury, Connecticut. Mac was the Secretary of Commerce in the Reagan administration, but his heart was always in the ranchlands, not in the protocol caverns of our nation's capitol. There was nonstop dance music provided by Bob Mobilio and his Waterbury band, alternating with a bunch of cowboys who drove up in their old bus all the way from Coleman County, Texas. The latter group was headed by Red Steagall and his country and western band, well-known musicians on the rodeo circuit but totally unknown on the formal wedding circuit. The wedding guests danced sedately and happily to Mobilio's great beat, then lost every inhibition while stomping to the cowboy's music.

• If you want music for dancing, before hiring the group, either listen to it live or listen to its tapes. Look at the outfits the musicians plan to wear (and make them rent alternative clothing if the look is not right). Make sure the orchestra leader knows the kind of music you want played. Perhaps you could strike a deal with your daughter (or, if you are the bride, with your mother) to have a rock band play softly during the seated meal, and then let the amplifiers on the sound system be turned up several decibel points while the young really take to the floor.

• If you want a conga line at your wedding reception, have a conga line. But make sure the band you hire plays conga music.

TRANSPORTATION

If you are planning a high-budget wedding and will transport the wedding party in limousines to and from the rehearsal dinner, as well as to the church and to the reception on the wedding day, or if you are planning a small wedding and will ask friends to help out by transporting the wedding party in their private cars, make the plans well ahead. Put a transportation sheet in your wedding planner and keep it current.

Today many families hold down costs by ordering one limousine to transport the bride and her father from home to the church or temple, and then to transport the bride and groom from the ceremony to the reception. The rest of the wedding party travels by sedans provided by the limousine service or by cars driven by friends or by a combination of both.

• If you are dealing with a limousine company, send them a typed list of the names of all the people who are supposed to be in any one car at any one time, going to each location. Give them specific times. Make sure the best man has a copy of this sheet, as well as the bride's parents, because among them, they should see that everything goes smoothly. Each member of the wedding party should know the number of the car in which he or she is supposed to ride every time there is a movement of people from one place to another.

• It is very nice if, at the conclusion of the religious services, there is a bottle of champagne well chilled in an ice bucket in the back of the limo—plus two champagne glasses—for the bride and groom on their ride from the church to the reception. (The limo service will handle that, or the best man or the father of the bride can make it happen.)

WEDDING ATTENDANTS

The Bride's Attendants

You need only one attendant for your wedding, but if you are having a big wedding, several more are certainly appropriate. Since a first wedding is such an exciting event in your life—and in the lives of your friends, too—you might wish a scenario like this:

- Ten bridesmaids (we are talking about a wedding for 350 guests or more)
- Matron of honor
- Maid of honor
- Junior bridesmaid (a sister or a little cousin from age nine to thirteen)
- A ring-bearer (someone like a nephew aged three to five) or little boy pages or both
- One or two flower girls (nieces or children of good friends perhaps, ages three to five)*

An easily manageable number of bridesmaids for a normal sized wedding (up to 150) is anything up to six. Don't forget that each out-of-town attendant requires a complicated logistical support system (such as having her met when she arrives in town, and transporting, housing, feeding, and entertaining her for three or four days). When a bride has an overly large number of bridesmaids, they begin to look like a line of Rockettes from New York's Radio City Music Hall. (One wedding I attended recently included fifteen bridesmaids, and the guests, I noticed, spent all their time comparing the height, physiques, and hair styles of the bridesmaids—completely forgetting to look at the bride!)

*The use of small children is a European custom and only makes sense when the bride and groom have many small relatives.

If you have only one attendant, she may be single or married. Normally you invite a sister close in age or your best single friend to be your maid of honor, and a sister or a close married friend to be your matron of honor. (Your matron of honor, by the way, may be a widow or a divorcee today.)

In deciding on your other attendants, you might choose a sister of the groom's and among your other close friends. There is often a dilemma in trying to pick from among your old chums from childhood in your hometown versus your close friends with whom you have graduated from school in another town. Your attendants' ages should be close to your own, so if you are in your early twenties, don't feel you have to invite someone in her thirties or older to be in your wedding. If you have to leave out good friends who you know feel they should have been asked to be your attendants, talk to them about it. Tell them how much their friendship means to you. Give them important tasks to do in your wedding; make sure they're invited to the wedding parties, if possible. Brief your parents on what to say to them to make them feel they *are* part of your wedding, even if not actually attendants.

THE PREGNANT BRIDESMAID

A slightly pregnant bridesmaid brings the joy of creation to the wedding pageantry. A very pregnant bridesmaid can't find a dress to fit, in the first place; in the second place, guests will be distracted from the bride—wondering when the baby is due, whether it's a boy or a girl, if the baby is kicking inside right now, and so forth. A good friend of the bride who will be far along in her pregnancy on the wedding date should, in my opinion, take it upon herself not to accept the bridesmaid role. The bride in turn can include her friend in all of her wedding events, consider the friend a member of the wedding party even if she doesn't march down the aisle with the others, and have her stand with the bridal party of the group wedding picture. In this way, anyone looking at the picture will realize that the "pregnant one" is an honorary attendant who would have been dressed as a member of the wedding party if her blessed event had not been so imminent.

BRIDESMAIDS' DUTIES

Between them, the matron and maid of honor should organize with the other attendants the bridesmaids' party that is optionally given for the bride on the same night the bachelors' dinner is held for the groom. The lead attendants also organize the joint gift for the bride (which entails the selection of the gift, the solicitation of the money, the possible engraving of the object). They also run errands to assist the bride before her wedding and help her get dressed on the wedding day. They make sure her "going away" costume and honeymoon luggage are safely ensconced in the room at the reception place where she will dress after she and her groom leave the party. And they see to it that her white dress and veil are taken safely back to her home when she and her husband have left. In general, the bridesmaids help make the wedding a success by assisting the mother of the bride with whatever needs doing and by being gracious to all the guests, particularly the couple's relatives. The bridesmaids can do all this and still have a good time with the ushers!

The Groom's Attendants

The groom has only one honor attendant—his best man—who is often his brother or best friend, sometimes even his father. (The father acting for his son is part of tradition, but recently, in an overreaction to the women's movement, there have been examples of mothers serving as their daughters' only attendant, too.) The groom should try to match the number of bridesmaids with ushers, but if he has fewer attendants than his bride, it really does not make any difference.

THE BEST MAN

To be asked to be someone's best man is an honor that is not to be refused, if possible. The job carries responsibilities, too, for helping bring off a smoothly run wedding. The groom should pick as his best man not only a brother or a close friend, but someone who is gregarious, aware, and a good manager. He should be an expert, briefing the ushers and making sure they know what to do and when to do it. He should have eyes in the back of his head so as to be aware when anyone from the mother of the bride to the maid of honor might need assistance. If someone becomes drunk and abusive at the wedding reception, if the groom loses his suitcase, if the bride's family runs out of champagne and needs someone to make a quick trip to the liquor store, the best man should see that it's taken care of.

• The best man communicates with the ushers and makes sure they show up for the fittings on their wedding suits. The best man organizes the groom's attendants' joint present to the groom. During one of the days prior to the wedding, he helps the groom organize the optional bachelor dinner (at which the groom's gifts to his ushers and the ushers' gift to the groom are exchanged). He should also make sure the groom emerges from any mayhem that may occur at this party unscathed and in good physical shape.

• On the wedding day, the best man helps the groom get dressed. He makes sure he has the bride's wedding ring in his pocket in order to be able to give it to the groom at the proper moment in the service. If the groom, not the bride's family, is paying the clergyman's and church fees, the best man makes sure the money is in envelopes in his possession, ready for the groom to present just prior to the ceremony. He makes sure the wedding license has been brought to the church.

• He helps the mother of the bride coordinate all the limousines and family cars that may be put to use to carry people to the church, to the reception, and away from the reception.

• The best man also sees to it that the ushers have their wedding ties and boutonnieres in place, have their gloves (if gloves are to be worn), and have their seating lists in hand, and he ensures that they get to the church an hour before the ceremony. He also makes sure he and the groom reach the church twenty minutes to a half hour before the ceremony.

• The best man leads off with the first toast to the bride at the rehearsal dinner and at the reception. He not only starts the toasting, but he regulates the order of toasting that follows. He already has in his pocket a list of those who have agreed that they want to be called upon to give a toast. The groom and the family members give their toasts first. He gives everyone in the wedding party their cues. I have seen best men send scribbled messages to toasters, telling them to sit down when, as a result of having drunk too much, they rambled on boringly and aimlessly. The best man usually succeeds in his mission. I remember one night when a college roommate of the groom was giving a stupid, drunken, and endless toast. He didn't have his glasses and couldn't read the best man's note to him when it was given to him. Thereupon the best man rose and took over the microphone. Holding his own note in his hand, he read it: "This note says 'Finish and sit down—*now*.' " (The toaster did just that amid great laughter.)

• The best man helps get everyone in the wedding party into a group for the official posed photograph of the group. These photos are usually taken at the place of the reception before the other guests start arriving from the church. When the wedding party has arrived ahead of everyone else, it is usually the *only* time the entire group is available for the photograph.

• Besides organizing the toasting at the reception, the best man makes sure the ushers perform their duty dances (with the bride, mother of the bride, grandmother of the bride, little sister of the bride, and all the bridesmaids).

• He oversees the transfer of the luggage to the getaway car, makes sure the groom has the airplane tickets, and that everything goes according to plan for the departure of the couple from the wedding reception to begin their honeymoon.

THE ROLE OF THE USHERS

If there is an equal number of men and women attendants in the wedding, the ushers escort the bridesmaids back down the aisle at the conclusion of the ceremony. If there are fewer ushers than bridesmaids, the latter walk down the aisle two by two.

The ushers are usually the age of the groom and comprise his own brothers, perhaps a brother of the bride, and his best friends. Since their main duty is to seat guests for the religious ceremony (and give the bridesmaids a good time during the parties), a family member who is to be an usher should be at least a mature seventeen- or eighteen-year-old.

At a very small wedding, it is nice to include a young usher of ten or more—especially if it is the bride's or bridegroom's child by a previous marriage.

THE REHEARSAL

One or two nights before the actual ceremony in the church or temple, a rehearsal should be scheduled with the officiating clergyman. Everyone practices walking down the aisle, and the service is briefly described, so that the wedding party knows what to do, and so that the pageantry is unified and dignified. The organist or at least one member of the musical group to play during the service should be present for the rehearsal to learn the music cues, too. When the rehearsal takes place on the night before the wedding, generally it is scheduled before the wedding party attends the "rehearsal dinner."

The Rehearsal Dinner

This party, usually hosted by the groom's parents, but also optionally hosted by a relative or even a good friend of either the groom or bride, may be as formal or as informal as you wish it. Separate invitations are mailed for this party to members of the wedding party, the relatives of the bride and groom, and to close friends who are coming from out of town for the festivities. The rehearsal dinner may be anything from a black tie dinner in a hotel or restaurant to a barn dance or a picnic in the park. It can be a hamburger dinner at the ice-skating rink or a cookout on the beach. It is meant to be fun, and usually the best toasting of the bridal pair occurs on this evening.

A sample invitation for an informal rehearsal dinner and an evening of lake sailing follows:

Peter Parkinson
cordially invites you
to the Rehearsal Dinner
for Mary Beth Brown
and his godson Peter Wentworth, Jr.
Friday, June twenty-third
at five o'clock
"Gull Lodge"
23 North Lake Road
Lake Minnetonka

R.s.v.p.   *Sailing before and after dinner*
000/000-0000   *Dress: Shorts, slacks, sweaters, boat*
                   shoes

THE WEDDING DAY ARRIVES!

Getting to the Church

Just before the ceremony is to start, the bride's mother is driven in a limousine (or a friend's car, if several limos are not in the budget) from her home to the church. She may be accompanied by other immediate members of her family. Immediately following are the bridesmaids in their limo or series of cars. Then the bride and her father leave for the church in a limousine (the same one that after the ceremony will transport the bride and groom alone to the reception).

Meanwhile, Inside the Church

By now the ushers, of course, have already been at the church for an hour, seating guests, and the guests are listening to the organ music or other type of music that has been provided. The groom and best man are waiting backstage, so to speak, in the church parlors or rectory, for the signal to walk from the side into the front of the church for the start of the wedding procession from the back down the center aisle.

The main job of the ushers consists of escorting lady guests down the aisle to their seats for the ceremony—and in general overseeing the seating of all the guests for the services. They should have been thoroughly instructed about special seating arrangements. They should have been briefed on the guest list by the best man, who has been briefed by the couple's parents. They should be clear on who sits where, who's important, and who needs special attention. ("Great-Grandma Mullens is ninety-four years old and totally deaf. She'll keep shouting 'What?' at you, but don't try to answer. Just take her down and put her on the aisle in the second row, right-hand side.")

At important weddings with pew cards, a guest hands the pew card to the usher when he or she arrives. People often forget to bring their pew cards, so the usher should be able to consult his alphabetized seating list and find the proper pew number with ease. The front pews for the family and special guests are usually marked off from the others with markers of flowers and ribbon—an important decorative detail in the church.

Each usher escorts as many ladies down the aisle as is possible in the time period. The protocol works more or less like this:

- o The usher greets the guest. If there is special seating and if he does not know this person, he asks for the name and checks his list to see where the guest should be seated.
- o He offers his inside arm to the lady; a male companion or child would follow behind.
- o If several women arrive at once, he offers his arm to the more senior one or the one he knows personally. (If a whole group of women arrive at once, they have their choice of staying in the back to await an escort or of walking down by themselves. (Needless to say, young women choose the latter option.)
- o The front pews (the ushers know how many are to be saved) are kept for family members (bride's on the left, groom's on the right).
- o If there is no special seating, the usher guides guests to pews down in front on a first-come, first-served basis, but again, bride's friends on the left and groom's on the right. He might ask, "Are you a friend of the bride or of the groom?"

If there are few of the groom's friends attending the wedding (as is often the case for a groom who lives far away), the ushers should split up the guests so that there looks to be an equal number of guests on each side of the church.

Seating in the Front Pew on the Bride's Side

In the easiest of situations, the bride's mother and father occupy the front pew on the left. However, with so many deceased, divorced, and remarried parents, it is often not that simple. If the bride's parents have been divorced, regardless of what hard feelings may exist between them and their present spouses, it is very considerate of everyone to put aside their personal animosities in favor of the bride's happiness and allow tradition to be served during the ceremony. In other words, it makes the nicest of weddings if the bride's own mother and father sit side by side in the front pew, with the bride's stepfather and stepmother in the pew behind. If that is too much to ask, it is nice if both the bride's parents (or the groom's parents, if there has been a remarriage), and their present spouses occupy the front pews together. If that is impossible because of animosities, then the bride's mother and stepfather should occupy the first pew, and the bride's father and stepmother would occupy the second pew. Their various other children, siblings, and grandparents should also occupy the front pews on the bride's (or groom's) side of the church.

THE WEDDING SERVICE

Music for the Ceremony

In some churches the liturgical music is rigorously prescribed, and in many churches you must pay the organist, even if you don't use him or her. In other churches you are allowed a free hand in your musical preferences—anything from a chorus of guitars to a harp to a group of trumpets to Aunt Hortense singing "I Love You Truly." You must find out from your clergyman how to plan for the music of your service.

If you have an Aunt Hortense who wants to sing at your wedding, diplomatically lay obstacles in her path—unless she's a professional. Many a wedding ceremony has been ruined because a relative or close family friend insisted on providing the music and, in doing so, either left the guests flinching or laughing outright.

The Service Is About to Begin

THE MOTHERS ARE SEATED

About five minutes before a Christian wedding procession is about to start, an usher escorts the mother of the groom to the front right pew.

Her family and husband should follow her into the front pews, her husband sitting on her left in the pew. Then, a few minutes later, the head usher escorts the mother of the bride into the front left pew. There is an anticipatory stillness in the church. The music has now ceased, so that when it starts again to announce the procession, there will be a greater dramatic impact.

The place in the pew next to the bride's mother on the aisle has been left vacant, for the bride's father will occupy this seat after escorting his daughter to the altar. The bride's mother is the last person to be seated in the church before the doors are closed and the pageant unfolds.

THE RUNNER IS LAID

If the bride has a long train, an optional white runner (sometimes supplied by the church, but usually by the florist) is rolled down from the front of the aisle to the back, to protect her dress when she walks down to the altar. It is rolled by two ushers or a church employee on the right-hand side of the aisle, because that is the side the bride will use as she walks down on the right arm of her father. (Going out of the church, she should walk down on the left arm of her husband, so that her dress will once again sweep along the runner.)

THE WHITE SATIN RIBBONS ARE PULLED ACROSS THE AISLE POSTS

Next, another option: Two ushers, one on either side of the aisle, pick up the folded pieces of white satin streamers behind the front pews where the families are seated. Working at the same speed on either side of the aisle, they pull back the ribbons, weaving them in and out of the aisle posts in a straight line, placing the last loop of their ribbon over the last aisle post on their side of the aisle. This "seals in" the wedding guests, so to speak, and the ribbons remain in place until the end of the ceremony, and until the wedding party and the bride's and groom's families have left the church. (After the ceremony, the same ushers carefully roll up the ribbons as they remove them from the aisle posts. When they have completed this job, the wedding guests may rise, depart from the church, and head for the reception.)

The Processional Begins

Out walk the clergyman, the groom, and best man from the side of the church. They proceed to the altar and turn to face the back of the church, where the procession will begin.

The first people to come down the aisle as the processional music is played are the ushers, who march down briskly, hopefully smiling, two by two, and then take their place on the right-hand side of the altar

The bride comes up the aisle on her father's right arm, preceded by the flower girl (and ring-bearer, if there is one), the bridesmaids, the maid of honor and matron of honor, and the ushers. The bride-groom, best man, and the minister, in the meantime, have come in from the side of the altar and await the procession.

as you face it—next to the groom and the best man. Next come the bridesmaids, two by two. Then comes the ring-bearer, if there is one; the pages, if there are any; the flower girl, if there is one; the junior bridesmaid, if there is one; then the maid of honor and matron of honor. They group themselves on the left-hand side of the altar in a row—or curve or whatever formation the clergyman has decreed is the most efficient and attractive way to do it. They all remain standing. (In a Catholic ceremony, there may be kneelers for the entire wedding party to use later.)

Now comes the great moment everyone has been waiting for: the appearance of the bride on her father's right arm. Hopefully, she will be smiling broadly, looking directly at her husband-to-be, who probably will be looking back at her with a dazed and extremely happy, proud expression on his face. (He should not try to practice this in the mirror at home beforehand.) I myself was not a smiling bride, since I was crying with the emotion of the beauty of the church and what was happening down the entire length of the church—I probably looked as though I had lost my best friend. Some brides are nervous coming down the aisle and look almost angry with tension. (All brides look smiling and relaxed on the way out after the services.)

• *If the bride's father is in a wheelchair,* he may be in place at the foot of the altar when the processional begins, and she may be escorted

The wedding principals, once they have marched to the altar, usually form a semicircle, facing the minister and the altar. Their backs are now to the congregation and remain this way throughout the ceremony. The best man (in this case the groom's father) stands to the right of the groom, and the other ushers stand in order of height (tallest to shortest) to the best man's right. The maid or matron of honor stands to the left of the bride, and the other bridesmaids follow to the maid or matron of honor's left.

down the aisle by another male member of her family before joining him. Or she may walk down the aisle alone. I once saw a very touching wedding processional in which the father of the bride pushed his own wheelchair as the bride walked proudly beside him. There was not a dry eye in the congregation on that day, nor was there the day another bride went down the aisle with her father, who was blind, accompanied by his faithful Seeing Eye Dog.

The Role of the Bride's Attendants

• The *matron of honor* "outranks" *the maid of honor* in that she walks closer to the bride in the procession down the aisle. (In other words, the maid of honor walks first, then the matron of honor, and finally the bride on her father's arm.) Either the matron or maid of honor hold the bride's bouquet during the ceremony; they both straighten out the bride's train when she turns around at the altar. If one of these attendants is the bride's sister, it is she who lifts the bride's veil for the husband's kiss (if the kiss is part of the religious service). At the conclusion of the ceremony, when the wedding party starts to walk back down the aisle, the best man escorts the matron of honor, followed by the head usher escorting the maid of honor.

• A junior bridesmaid precedes the maid of honor in the procession. She also walks by herself back down the aisle in the recessional— unless there is an extra usher, in which case she has an escort, too.

• The *flower girl* (or the pair of them) wear dresses either in the same color and fabric as the bridesmaids, or they are attired in pretty white organdy or cotton dresses in the summer or velvet dresses in the winter. They often wear wreaths of flowers and carry baskets of flowers. When coming back down the aisle in the recessional, they scatter some wild flowers or rose petals in the aisle from their baskets. If in the excitement they forget to do this, it is not important!

• The *ring-bearer,* often dressed in satin or velvet shorts (or even knickers with white knee socks) and a silk shirt with a Peter Pan collar, precedes the flower girl or the junior bridesmaid. An option to having a ring-bearer is having one or two little boy *pages.* (If possible, all the children wear black patent leather or white Mary Jane shoes and white socks.) The wedding ring(s) borne by the ring-bearer on a ceremonial satin pillow are sewn firmly into it, because a little boy could certainly not be responsible otherwise for delivering them safely to the best man and matron (or maid) of honor.

If there is a junior bridesmaid behind the ring-bearer, she will usually keep him from running off in all directions and make him do his job properly. I will never forget one nine-year-old junior bridesmaid who suddenly departed from her dignified walk, darted off and caught her three-year-old brother by the arm after he had run off into a pew on the far side of the vast church. She gave him a scolding and a hard slap on the seat of his pants. Immediately he became obedient and followed her back across the church and into the procession. The bridal party, of course, had come to a halt during this drama. The entire congregation, the bride included, were laughing, but it did not at all detract from the beauty of the wedding. It added to it.

Variations on Who Acts as the Father of the Bride

The man who customarily walks the bride down the aisle on his right arm is her father. However:

• If her father is ill or deceased, the bride's teenage brother, an uncle, her grandfather, her godfather, or a close family male friend may properly do the honors. If the father is dead and the bride's mother has remarried, her stepfather acts in her father's place. (However, if the bride's relationship with her stepfather is strained, she may ask another male relative to take her down the aisle.)

• If the bride's parents were divorced when she was young and she was raised from early childhood by a loving stepfather, it may be a last act of kindness to her natural father if she consents to be given away by him—unless there is very bad feeling between them. If there is bad feeling, then she should ask her stepfather to take her down the aisle.

Giving the Bride Away

In a Catholic ceremony, once the father has taken his daughter to the foot of the altar, he gives her to her husband in a symbolic gesture of taking her left arm out of his as she reaches out her right hand to her groom. He then returns to his seat in the front pew, next to his wife.

In Protestant ceremonies, the minister asks almost at once, as the bride and her father stand together with the groom, some form of the question, "Who gives this woman in matrimony?" The father of the bride answers "I do" or "Her mother and I do" and puts the bride's right hand in the clergyman's. Then, after sometimes giving her a kiss on the forehead, for which he must lift her veil but then replace it, he steps back and rejoins his wife in the front right pew. His place at the bride's side is now taken by her husband-to-be.

Today there are variations on this part of the ceremony. The bride's mother may join the bride and her father when they reach the altar, and may reply *"We* do," with her husband, in answer to the minister's question. Then both parents go to the front pew to sit down. I have also seen a wedding where the bride was "given away" at the foot of the altar by her remarried birth mother and remarried birth father, and by her stepfather as well, who had really raised her. The "giving away" answer was a resounding "We do" by three people.

Once given away in a bridal ceremony, that's it for the bride. If she remarries later, she is not given away again.

The Wedding Ring Is Placed on the Finger

An important part of the ceremony is when the groom places a wedding ring on the bride's finger, or when both exchange wedding rings. (The bride should *not* be wearing her engagement ring.) Normally, the best man guards the ring that will go on the bride's finger in one of his pockets until it is needed, while the matron or maid of honor either wears the ring for the bride to give her groom on one of her fingers, keeps it stowed in her dress pocket, or has it tied to her sash on a small, thin ribbon.

If a ring-bearer brings the rings on a pillow up to the altar, the best man should produce a penknife from his pocket to cut the threads that have sewn the ring or rings to the pillow. The best man then puts the bride's wedding ring in his own pocket for safekeeping, and gives the wedding ring that will go on the groom's finger either to the maid or matron of honor standing nearby.

I wonder how many times, while nervously handing the little ring to the groom or to the bride, someone, either the giver or the receiver, has dropped the ring on the floor of the church. The nice thing is that it is always found again!

Recitation of the Vows

The vows, the choice of prayers, the music playing during the ceremony, and any creative ideas for special words to be spoken during the service should all be discussed well in advance with the clergyman performing the service. Some religions allow great freedom in what is said and not said; others are dogmatically strict. Different parishes have different interpretations of the wedding service, and the bride and groom must fit their own wishes into the rules of the church.

The Kiss

If and when the groom and bride are supposed to kiss near the end of the wedding service, the matron or maid of honor should lift the bride's veil. Sometimes she forgets and the groom lifts it. Sometimes he forgets and the bride lifts it. It really doesn't matter!

At a Catholic Mass, when it is time for the Kiss of Peace, the bride and groom often give each other a kiss and then go down to both front pews to kiss their parents. This is also done in some Protestant ceremonies. Sometimes bride and groom stop to kiss their parents in the front pews as the recessional begins at the conclusion of the ceremony.

The bride and groom leave the church in a joyous (and usually brisk) recessional. They are followed by the flower girl (and ring-bearers or junior bridesmaids, if any), and maid or matron of honor and best man. Then the bridesmaids and the ushers marching in pairs follow.

A nice tender kiss at the altar when the clergyman says to the groom, "You may now kiss the bride," is enjoyed by everyone present. However, the clergyman does not enjoy standing there while bride and groom, still on the altar, engage in a long, passionate kiss worthy of an X-rated movie.

The Recessional

For the recessional, at the conclusion of the services, the positions in line are reversed. The bride and groom walk first, followed by the matron of honor with the best man, the maid of honor with the head usher, the ring-bearer (who may have gone to sit with his parents by now), the junior bridesmaid and the bridesmaids—each paired off with an usher. (As noted, if there aren't enough ushers, the bridesmaids walk out two by two.) If there is no runner, the bride may go down the aisle on her husband's right arm; as mentioned earlier, if there is a runner, she would take his left arm in order to walk on the runner.

A DOUBLE WEDDING CEREMONY

When two couples marry in the same ceremony, they are usually sister brides or brother grooms, cousins, or two very close friends marrying two very close friends.

A sister bride may act as her sister's attendant, and vice-versa; a brother groom may act as his brother's best man, and vice-versa. Or each may have his or her own set of attendants. I remember one beautiful wedding of twin sisters who had the same six bridesmaids act for both their weddings.

Twin brides may dress in identical dresses, if they wish, or in different styles (but these should harmonize with one another).

The two sets of bridesmaids' dresses do not have to match, but it looks much more harmonious if they do—not necessarily in color, but in style. The two grooms and the ushers should wear identical wedding apparel.

In a double wedding of sisters, each with her own attendants, the ushers would march in first in the processional; then would come the bridesmaids, followed by the maid and matron of honor—all belonging to the older sister. Then would come the older sister bride on her father's arm, followed by the younger sister's attendants, then the maid and matron of honor; then the younger sister bride on the arm of a brother, uncle, grandfather, or cousin.

If both girls wish their father to take them down the aisle, the father takes the older one down first, walks briskly back, and then comes down slowly again with his younger daughter. (In the case of twins, one baby was born first and is therefore older.)

If the church has two side aisles, rather than a center aisle, both wedding parties may proceed slowly down the side aisles in unison.

The wedding service of the older daughter takes place first. In the case of two unrelated girls marrying two brothers, the older girl's wedding ceremony takes place first.

The mothers of two brides who are close friends would sit with their husbands together in the first row. The mothers of two grooms marrying sisters would sit in the first row together with their husbands. The mother of the older bride would walk down the aisle and be seated first—since her daughter will walk down the aisle first and will be married first.

• A double wedding calls for two sets of limousines and two wedding cakes. Friends of one bride who do not know the other one or the other's husband well do not have to give a wedding present to both couples. Only family and friends who are close to the brides or grooms of both couples should give two presents.

A difficult task is that of the best man or of the two best men, to make sure that neither couple receives short shrift in all of the toasting at the rehearsal dinner and at the wedding reception.

THE PREGNANT BRIDE

A bride who is up to four months pregnant can get away with wearing a simple, loosely fitting, long white dress that does not shout her happy, blessed state to the guests at her wedding. A bride who is markedly pregnant but nevertheless marries in a large ceremony, dressed in a long dress with a train, looks—in the opinion of many—ludicrous. It is in better taste for a bride who "shows" quite a bit to be married in a long or short white, dressy maternity dress. Restraint and good taste are important primarily in the religious services and in the way the bride is dressed.

A SMALL OR BIG WEDDING AT HOME

How nice to be able to have your wedding at home or in the house of a relative or special friend.

A home wedding is usually small, and the bride's and groom's parents are wise to keep the guest list smaller than they would ordinarily think is required, because the available space is quickly utilized by:

- o The clergyman's requirements for the ceremony
- o The need for a place for the members of the wedding party to assemble before the procession

- Chairs for older, frail guests, even if the rest of the guests are standing
- Racks for coats and umbrellas, perhaps even for boots
- A place to stash wedding presents (even though they should not be brought to the house on the wedding day)
- The need for changing rooms for the bride, groom, and attendants
- Space to set up the reception food and drink before the service (assuming the reception will be at home, too).

In the best of situations, the guests are seated on portable chairs set up auditorium-style in the living room (or the largest room in the house). If the ceremony lasts longer than ten minutes, those chairs are really needed.

The altar can be improvised in front of the fireplace or a picture window or any focal point in the living room. It is better to clear out most of the furniture before the ceremony. One lovely floral bouquet on or at the foot of the altar is all that is needed. When there is seating auditorium-style, the chairs should be placed on two sides, with an aisle in the middle. White satin ribbons can mark off the first row or two on each side for the bride's and groom's families to occupy.

The music may be supplied by a pianist (with or without a soloist singer), a trio or quartet, or an electric organ—anything dignified and appropriate for a religious service. At the sound of the processional music, if there is a large staircase, the bride's attendant descends it, followed by the bride. Her father waits for her at the bottom of the staircase, and they follow her attendant on the short walk into the living room, down the center aisle to join the groom, clergyman, and best man at the altar. The bride may wear a long white dress and veil or a street-length white dress or suit. She may wear a late afternoon dress or a dinner gown. (If the wedding is a very small one in the home, she would be dressed in white, but not necessarily in a long formal gown; at this kind of small wedding, there need not be music.)

After the ceremony, the bride and groom walk back down the aisle to appropriate recessional music, and go immediately to the area where the reception will be held. When there is a tent nearby, the receiving line is stationed in the house or near the tent entrance. (There is no need for a receiving line if the wedding and reception are very small.)

On occasion, the bride has a ceremony in the presence of just family and a handful of close friends in the house, followed by a large reception in a tent on the grounds. Her parents would invite guests to the wedding reception only—for example, "at five o'clock." Then family and a few very close friends would be invited by handwritten note to the ten-minute ceremony at a quarter to five. The first reception guests would probably not arrive until ten or fifteen minutes after five, which would give the bride and groom the chance to sit down and relax for fifteen minutes with or without their families before the receiving line would begin.

Tenting Your Yard or Garden

If you plan to hold your reception in your own house and have invited a large number of guests, you would be smart to plan on having a professional tenting company erect a tent off to the side of the house, or in the backyard or garden. Tents can be heated in winter and air-conditioned in summer. The kind with side flaps that can be raised or lowered is essential in case of inclement weather. The see-through plastic kind allows people to enjoy the grounds around them to a certain degree. (It's a nice touch to have rented lights illuminating the trees and shrubs outside the plastic tent for an evening wedding.)

Any kind of tent looks much prettier when at least the interior posts are decorated with greenery and flowers. The florist can make a harmonious decorative plan to include items such as decorated tent poles, table centerpieces, colorful tablecloths, flowers on the serving tables, flower-decorated chandeliers, and a boxwood or flowered hedge around the dance floor. (I remember a Christmas wedding reception where fresh holly ropes cordoned off the small dance floor in the tent. There was only one drawback: Anytime the women went near the ropes, we caught our dresses on the sharp-leafed holly. We loved it anyway.)

THE RECEPTION

The order of events at the reception goes like this:
- The wedding party's group photographs are taken.
- Arriving guests check coats and sign the guest book.
- Arriving guests go through the receiving line while music plays for guests and libations are passed.
- The receiving line breaks up, and the wedding party goes into the reception area to join the other guests.
- The bride and groom dance the first dance; everyone dances from then on.
- Everyone eats and drinks.
- Toasts begin and follow through the eating period.
- Bride and groom cut the cake.
- Bride and groom depart the reception to change into "going-away clothes."
- On their way out, the bride tosses her bouquet to an unmarried

bridesmaid; the groom optionally tosses her garter to an unmarried usher.
- o Bride and groom say good-bye to their parents and best friends and depart for their honeymoon in car containing their luggage.
- o Everyone else goes home.

When the Wedding and Reception Place Are Combined

If you plan to hold both your wedding and reception at home, there are no problems of scheduling. If you plan to hold both or just the reception in a hotel, restaurant, or club, you must fit into their schedule of already booked events. If you plan to hold your wedding and reception in an informal park or gardens, a museum, an historic home, or any revered and protected site that is open to the public, you must adhere to a list of rules and regulations laid down by those entrusted with the administration of the place. However, the visual riches of the gardens or the sweep of the fields in the distance, or the awesome history and the beauty of the interiors of an old house or mansion dating from the eighteenth or nineteenth century is well worth all the restrictions, including some of these:

• Your event must not conflict with any other one scheduled for that day (and some weddings are booked a year in advance). Your event must be scheduled after the public hours are over (which is often 5 P.M.)—or perhaps you may rent the facilities only on the one day of the week it is closed to the public.

• Some properties, because they are not properly heated, rent only from April through November.

• Some historic sites require that you be prepared for rain, and therefore you must tent the gardens—because the house is too fragile to hold a large number of guests coming inside from the rain.

• There is often a fairly rigid maximum number of guests you are allowed to invite for either a standing or seated event. For example, at a historic Greek Revival mansion with formal gardens and terraces where only 75 guests may be accommodated indoors (12 seated), but 450 may be accommodated in the gardens outside, tenting is required for more than 75 guests.

• There is a wide range of rental fees for these properties. For example, a corporation pays New York's Metropolitan Museum an annual Corporate Patron fee of $30,000, which includes, among other pluses, permission to use the museum premises for a party. (To host a press-related event at the Met costs $35,000.) The bride's parents pay $1,875 for five hours for the rental of the lovely house and gardens at Woodlawn Plantation at Mount Vernon, Virginia, overlooking the Potomac. Some other historic places charge $3,000 for six hours. Other smaller gardens or historic places around the country charge anywhere from $25 to $100 an hour to rent their facilities.

• Many properties and gardens request an extra fee to cover the security requirements and cleanup of the grounds.

• Some institutions allow alcoholic beverages to be served only in the house, others only in the gardens. Some prohibit the serving of alcohol at any time.

• Some institutions allow you to choose only from their select list of caterers; others oblige you to use their own restaurant facilities on the place.

• Some institutions will not allow amplified music in the gardens, but only indoors (because of neighbors complaining about noise); others will allow it only outdoors; others will not allow band music and dancing anywhere.

Guest Book

A nice custom, but not mandatory, is the signing of names in a handsome leather book purchased just for the wedding. Guests sign the book with their formal names ("Mr. and Mrs. John A. Howe, Jr."—not "Jack and Joanie Howe"). The book should be placed on a table (of a reasonable height) near where guests check their coats at the reception (or at the wedding itself, if it is held in a home). The book should ask for the guests' addresses, too—so it becomes a useful resource of updated addresses for the future. A young member of either the bride's or groom's family (twelve years or older) might be stationed by the book to invite people to sign. It's very difficult to hurry past a twelve-year-old requesting you to sign his or her book.

The Receiving Line

The fathers of the bride and groom may cut in and out of the receiving line. Even the bridesmaids may cut in and out of it after the first half hour. But the bride and groom and their mothers should certainly stand through all of it. Their friends can keep everyone supplied with glasses of champagne on the table behind them, and they can turn around occasionally and discreetly sip from their glasses—but members of the receiving line should not be seen in the act of drinking too often.

Likewise, guests going through the receiving line should not have glasses in their hands. If the line is long, a guest can always take a glass from a passing tray; then, as he or she approaches the bride's mother, the glass should be disposed of or hidden somewhere. It should not be in the guest's hand.

In a receiving line without fathers, the mother of the bride is first, then the mother of the groom, then the bride and groom and the bride's attendants.

The Order of the Receiving Line

- *If both fathers stand in line at a very large formal wedding:*
  - Bride's mother
  - Groom's father
  - Groom's mother
  - Bride's father
  - Bride
  - Groom
  - Matron of honor
  - Maid of honor
  - Junior bridesmaid (if there was one)
  - The other bridesmaids, oldest ones first

Flower girls, pages, and ring-bearers do not stand in the receiving line—they wouldn't have the patience. Nor do the ushers. (The fathers of the couple often don't, either!)

- *Usually only the father of the bride stands in the line—and he sometimes for only the first forty-five minutes.* The father of the groom, if he is not in line, goes around the reception making sure everything is going all right.

- *If the reception is held at the home of the bride's stepmother,* the latter should stand first in the receiving line *in her own house,* to help introduce the guests. The presence of the stepmother would change the lineup, since the stepmother and the mother of the bride probably would not wish to stand next to each other. In this case the order would be:

With both fathers in the receiving line, the mother of the bride is the first to receive guests; then the father of the bride; then the mother and father of the groom, the bridal couple, and the bride's attendants.

○ Bride's stepmother
○ Groom's mother
○ Bride's mother
○ Bride's father
○ Bride
○ Groom
○ Matron of honor, etc.

• *If the bride's father is newly remarried* and the reception is held in his home, his new wife does *not* stand in the receiving line, but plays the role of a guest. The bride's mother stands first in line in this case.

• *If the bride's mother is dead and her father has not remarried,* her father would stand first in line to greet the guests, with the groom's mother next to him, and the bride and groom next to her.

Going Through the Receiving Line

Generally, the conversation going through the receiving line should be short and sweet—and it is pretty pedestrian. It's important for women guests in greeting the bride and her attendants *not* to get lipstick on them. It's important for men not to kiss the bride on the mouth, for several reasons. The cheek will do. Women guests, because of their lipstick, should hug the bride, rather than kiss her on the cheek. People who are not close friends of the bride should clasp her hand warmly and not try to kiss her at all. Sample receiving line conversations:

Guest to bride's mother: "Mrs. Gaines, I'm Holly Reynolds, a college friend of Abigail's. What a lovely wedding it was—perfectly beautiful. And Abigail is so radiant!"

Bride's mother to guest: "Thank you so much, Holly. I've heard Abigail speak of you often. We're so glad you could come. I know how much it means to Abigail to have you here."

Holly to bride: "You look absolutely gorgeous, old friend! Your dress—your veil—Abigail, you're so beautiful. And George is such a handsome guy. I'm so happy for you both!"

Bride to her friend: "Thanks, Holly. It really went well, didn't it? And we're going to be so happy. I'm so glad you're here! I want you to have a good time, too, Holly. There are lots of great single guys here. I'll see to it that you meet some."

Holly to groom: "Congratulations. I'm Holly Reynolds, Abigail's friend from Vassar. We saw each other when you used to come up to Poughkeepsie to visit her. No wonder Abigail married you. And you have the most beautiful bride in the world, you lucky guy."

Groom to Holly: "She is beautiful isn't she? Yes, I am a lucky guy—and I remember you from those college weekends, too. Great to have you here, Holly."

Holly to father of the bride: "I'm Holly Reynolds, Mr. Gaines, a friend of Abigail's from college days. You have the loveliest daughter in the world, and I can see where she gets those great looks—from her parents. You must be so proud of her."

Father of the bride to Holly: "Thank you for that, Holly. Yes, her mother and I are very proud of Abigail. This is a great day for her, but it's both a sad and wonderful day for us."

Holly to father of the bride: "You're gaining a wonderful son-in-law. He's quite a guy."

Father of the bride: "I know he is. Abigail has great taste, and he's a fine young man. We're glad you could come today, Holly."

Holly to bridesmaid: "You look perfectly lovely. I'm Holly Reynolds, a college friend of Abigail's. What a beautiful wedding this has been!"

Bridesmaid to Holly: "I'm Suzanne Smith. Abigail and I went to school together, and we've been friends a long time. It's so nice you could make it to the wedding. I know Abigail is really glad you're here."

And so it goes. Pleasantries, niceties, and compliments. No dilly-dallying—the line must keep moving quickly. It makes it much more interesting to those standing in the receiving line if the guests passing through give their names and mention how they are connected to the bridal couple. Otherwise, it becomes boring listening to a chorus of "Wasn't it lovely!" "Don't you look pretty!" "Isn't this a happy occasion!"

Seating the Tables at the Reception

THE BRIDE'S TABLE

After their receiving line duties are over, the bridal party enjoys the chance to be seated and to dance, eat, and drink. Even if the reception food only consists of hot and cold hors d'oeuvres with ice cream and wedding cake, the wedding party should have a *bride's table* to give them the opportunity to sit, relax over their food and champagne, and dance when they wish. There are place cards for them at even this kind of informal reception. For the rest of the guests there should be small tables scattered around for those who wish to sit when they're not dancing or socializing. (Some of the older people will wish to sit and observe all the time, instead of dancing.)

For a formal seated lunch or dinner, there are place cards and table numbers for *all* the guests, as well as for the bridal tables.

The bride and groom would, of course, be seated side by side at their table. The groom would have the matron of honor on his other side; the bride would have the best man and next to him the maid of honor on her other side. The ushers and bridesmaids would sit in a male-female alternating pattern. If there is room, it is nice to invite the spouses and dates of the ushers and bridesmaids to join this table. If the wedding party is large, there would probably not be room at the table for spouses and dates, so they could have their own separate table nearby.

At most wedding receptions there is a Bride's Table, at which only the bride and groom and their attendants are seated. For example, the bride and groom are in the center of this rectangular one-sided table, which allows all of the reception guests to have a good view of the newly marrieds. (Frequently, when there is a Bride's Table and a Parents' Table, both are round.)

THE PARENTS' TABLE

There is also usually a *parents' table* at any type of large reception. The mother of the bride would have the father of the groom on her right; her husband (or if she is without a husband, her brother, uncle, cousin, family friend or boyfriend) would sit opposite with the mother of the groom on his right. The bride's mother might have the clergyman who performed the service on her left; the mother of the groom might have

Sometimes there is a Parents' Table at the wedding reception. The mother of the bride (facing us) is in the center, with the father of the groom on her right and the clergyman on her left. Across from her is the father of the bride, with the mother of the groom on his right and the matron of honor on his left.

the bride's grandfather on her other side, and so on—alternating family members and any distinguished guests or very close friends.

It is also appropriate to have one very long rectangular Bride's Table, at which the entire wedding party, parents included, would be seated.

Wedding Toasts

At a certain moment in the process of eating and drinking, the best man begins the toasts, which continue on and off, under his control, for as long as there are people who wish to offer their good wishes publicly. At large weddings it is important that there be a microphone for everyone's use—either a portable mike passed around from guest to guest, or a standing mike that each person uses to give his or her toast. It is also an excellent idea to have the toasts at your wedding taped— that provides a fabulous souvenir of a terribly important event in your lives to enjoy in future years.

Toasts are really an important and integral part of the rehearsal dinner and the wedding reception. Like everything else in the field of ancient rituals, there is an etiquette to be followed. For example:

• The person being toasted never drinks at the end of the toast, but simply remains seated and smiles at the person making the toast.

• When you are the one who is toasting, rise to your feet if there are ten or more people at the table. Otherwise, at a small intimate dinner, you can make your toast while seated. You can get the others' attention by saying something like, "Ladies and Gentlemen, I have a toast to make," or more informally, "I have" (in a louder tone than usual) "something to say tonight." (Don't rap too hard on the rim of a good crystal glass to get people's attention, as I have done on at least three occasions, because you will break the glass!)

• A wedding toast should be *no longer than three minutes,* so don't get carried away. You may appropriately be loving, amusing, sentimental, or teasing in your remarks. You may be serious or clever and amusing. Above all, you should be self-rehearsed and practiced. (Practice giving it to yourself in a mirror.)

• The order of toasting either at the rehearsal dinner or at the wedding reception is as follows:

  o The best man toasts the bride.
  o The groom toasts the bride.
  o The bride toasts her groom.
  o The father of the bride toasts the couple.
  o The bride toasts her groom's parents.
  o The groom toasts his bride's parents.
  o The matron or maid of honor toasts the couple.
  o The father of the groom toasts the bride.
  o The mother of the bride toasts the couple.
  o The mother of the groom toasts the couple.
  o Other relatives and close friends of the bride or groom continue toasting.

The reason for a list of the order of toasts is that it brings order out of chaos, makes the performance work smoothly, and gives courage to people who are shy—and who desperately want to make a toast but are afraid. (When the shy person knows he is on the list, he usually manages to summon his courage when the moment comes, rise to his feet, and get out the words.)

This list is in the hands of the best man. It is he who commands the toasts. Once it starts—once he has made the first toast—he signals each person in the wedding party who wants to make a toast. (He has, of course, asked the individuals beforehand if they wish to make a toast, and if the answer is yes, he explains that they should wait until he calls on them.) Then, at the completion of a toast, he looks over to the next person and nods a signal that means "You're next." That person should then rise and do his or her stuff.

A successful rehearsal dinner or wedding depends on following a list of the order of toasts because unless the family and really close friends are allowed to toast the bride and groom first, wedding guests who are not at all close to the family are likely to jump in ahead and upset the members of the wedding party.

NOTE: The toasts for the rehearsal dinner may be a bit longer than those at the wedding reception. The ones on the day of the wedding, if there are a hundred or more people, should be kept short and snappy.

The Bride's First Dance

It doesn't matter whether there's a piano or a full band at the reception. There may have been music playing during the entire reception, but people should not be dancing until the receiving line has been terminated and the first dance can be performed by the bride and groom. When the receiving line is broken and the wedding party is now free to take seats at their tables and to dance and eat, that's the moment for the bride and groom to begin the dancing. The orchestra strikes up the tune the bride and groom have asked the orchestra leader to play (perhaps a sentimental song for the couple, played to a beat to which they can comfortably dance). If they are good dancers, they should hold the floor alone for at least five minutes. If they are not, then after about one minute, the bride's father and mother should join them on the dance floor, and the bride's father can cut in on them and dance with the bride while the groom dances with the bride's mother. Then everyone gets out on the floor, and anyone can cut in on anyone else. The more informal and the more changing of partners there is, the better time everyone has.

WEDDINGS IN THE JEWISH TRADITION*

Marriage is one of the most important institutions in Jewish tradition. A strong, loving family unit continues to be of paramount importance to those of Jewish faith everywhere, so weddings are regarded as solemn occasions, worthy of careful planning. They do not take place on the Sabbath or major Jewish holidays (with the exception of Hanukkah). The ceremony often takes place in a temple or in a hotel or hall where the wedding feast will also be given.

Invitations

Invitations to Jewish weddings are often issued in the names of both sets of parents, with the bride's parents listed first. The preferred form is the following:

*My good New York friend Holly Pearl Pressman has contributed much of this information.

Mr. and Mrs. Jacob Feldman
request the honour of your presence
at the marriage of their daughter
Rebecca Anne
to
Mr. Roger Nathan Greller
son of
Mr. and Mrs. Warren John Greller
on Sunday, the sixth of June
etc.

Another form is the following:

Mr. and Mrs. Jacob Feldman
and
Mr. and Mrs. Warren John Greller
request the honour of your presence
at the marriage of their children
Rebecca Anne Feldman
and
Roger Nathan Greller
on Sunday, the sixth of June
etc.

Preparation for the Wedding Day

In preparation for the wedding day, traditionally the bride and groom fast and repent, just as they do on the Day of Atonement. After serious reflection and purification, the couple is ready to enter a new stage of life together. If the ceremony is to be held in the evening, the bride and groom may eat a light snack before the ceremony at sunset, the beginning of the next Hebrew day.

The Chuppah

Traditional Jewish wedding ceremonies are conducted under a cloth wedding canopy, called the *chuppah,* which is often embroidered or decorated with flowers. A handmade, temporary structure, it is reminiscent of the tents of the Jews' nomadic ancestors. The *chuppah* represents the room in the groom's home where the marriage will be consummated. When the groom receives his bride under the *chuppah,* it is religiously symbolic of God's (the groom's) acceptance of Israel (the bride).

The Processional

The Jewish processional at the beginning of the marriage ceremony is similar to those in Christian churches. It is common practice for each wedding participant of the processional to start walking down the aisle on the right foot.

I have spoken to many Jewish religious leaders about the rites described here. In the United States, Jewish tradition is interpreted by Orthodox Jews with strict adherence to the legal standards of the Bible, but it is interpreted more liberally by Conservative Jews and progressively by Reform Jews. Traditionally, the bride and groom do not see each other before the ceremony on their wedding day, and there are many other customs strictly followed by Orthodox Jews that are not necessarily followed by liberal Conservative or Reform Jews. In very Orthodox weddings, the groom is escorted by the two fathers and the bride by the two mothers—in keeping with the separation of men and women in public. Alternatively, Conservative and Reform Jews often use the following order of the procession:

The rabbi and cantor enter first, followed by the ushers, best man, and ring-bearer(s). The groom follows, unless he has chosen to enter with the rabbi and the best man from a side entrance and to forego a more public entrance up the aisle. The bridesmaids and maid or matron of honor are followed by the flower girl(s) and finally by the bride. In non-Orthodox weddings, traditionally the groom was escorted up the aisle by his parents and the bride by her parents, but today in Reform ceremonies it is acceptable for the bride's mother and the groom's parents to take their seats just before the bride, escorted by her father, comes up the aisle, preceded by her attendants. She steps into the *chuppah* to stand at the right of her groom.

The Ceremony

Traditionally, the flute is played during the religious ceremony. The music is meant to be joyous, yet dignified—and livelier for the recessional.

The cantor begins the ceremony with a short hymn. The rabbi then recites a blessing over the wine and blesses the betrothal. The groom sips some of the wine, hands the cup to the bride, and her attendant lifts her veil so that she can drink, too. By drinking from the same glass, the bride and groom are signifying the beginning of their life of sharing.

The ring ceremony takes place next. The groom places the wedding ring on the bride's right index finger, so that it may be seen easily by the two appointed witnesses and by the guests. There is another reason for placing it on her right index finger. There is an old belief that a vein in the forefinger runs directly to the heart. (There may be a double ring ceremony, with the bride placing her groom's ring on his right index finger.) The ring ceremony is followed by the reading of the marriage contract, then a short talk by the rabbi on the importance of this occasion, and perhaps he makes some brief personal remarks about the couple. Often he incorporates a modern English translation of the seven marriage blessings into his remarks. Then the couple shares the wine again and the groom breaks a small glass wrapped in a napkin with his foot. This is not an easy act to accomplish. It symbolizes that a broken marriage cannot easily be repaired, but it also serves as a reminder of the sorrows of the Jewish people. At the sound of the broken glass, the bride and groom kiss, and the family and friends turn to each other to express their happiness and good wishes for the couple.

The Recessional

At the conclusion of the ceremony, the bride and groom lead the recessional, followed by their parents, the maid or matron of honor and the best man (walking together), then the ushers and bridesmaids walking in mixed pairs, the flower girl(s), ring-bearer(s), the rabbi, and the cantor.

The Reception

The Jewish wedding celebration is almost always a seated meal, with music and sumptuous food. After the wedding party photographs have been taken, a receiving line is formed. Guests go to their assigned tables and dance until there is a pause in the music. This is the signal for the beginning of the meal. The rabbi offers a brief blessing over the challah, and everyone eats without dancing (if there's music, it's for background only). Then the bride and groom cut the wedding cake, share the first piece, and the best man begins the toasting, as well as reads any telegrams that may have arrived. People dance through the rest of the party.

The festivities come to a leisurely end when the bride throws her bouquet to the unmarried women present, the groom tosses her garter to the unmarried men, and they leave to change their clothes and go on their honeymoon.

INTERFAITH MARRIAGES

Fifteen years ago, no one could have predicted that in the 1980s and going into the 1990s there would be such a rash of interfaith marriages, particularly between Jews and Christians. When either set of parents makes a big fuss over this fact, it can ruin the joy that should predominate on this day of days for the two people who really matter—the bride and groom.

An interfaith marriage can be a very complex situation, because people are dealing with any one of these combinations:

- Bride and groom and both sets of parents with no religious faith
- Bride and groom with no religious faith but with parents who are fervent in their respective faiths
- Bride who is very religious and groom who is not
- Groom who is very religious and bride who is not

Only the first category is easy. The other categories may present problems, but as with anything, it works when people are up-front with each other and make an extra effort—not only compromising but keeping the promises they have made. If the bride or the groom is a very religious person, it obviously makes sense for the spouse who is not to make concessions to the one who is. (The spouse who has made the concession can then ask for a concession in return. For example, a friend of mine who won out on the religious question and raised the children in her faith every year thereafter spent her summer vacations on a farm, a concession to her husband's ardent preferences in this area and not her preferred choice at all.)

For the sake of the people to be married, who will get married in spite of what anyone says—with or without the backing of their parents—it is common sense for the bridal couple and their parents to sit down together coolly and rationally and *compromise*. I have witnessed beautiful, peaceful interfaith weddings, with very touching ecumenical services. I have also observed parents before and during the wedding itself fighting a war with each other, using their children as guided attack missiles, with relatives on both sides tugging, crying, threatening, throwing up their hands, and in general being divisive. (Fortunately, I have also seen some of the latter realize that histrionics get them nowhere and that pulling together for the sake of their children is the fair and moral thing to do.) I have also known the bride and the groom to sit down with their upset parents in private to reassure them of a personal devotion to their own religions, customs, and values. For example, the promise of a Christian daughter to her parents that "we will be with you for every Christmas and Easter that we can, you know that," and the promise of a Jewish son to parents that "we will be with you for every Yom Kippur and Passover that we can, you know that," help to soothe a touchy situation.

All of the feelings and worries of the parents, who have been accustomed to a certain religious control of their children, should be aired before the wedding. It is not too much to ask of a bride and groom to relay to their future in-laws their sincere determination to keep relationships pleasant and to acknowledge the religious concerns of a parent.

The raising of the children born of an interfaith marriage should not be an issue at the time of the wedding. No one can predict what will happen—just as we can't predict most things in the future.

The Ecumenical Wedding Service

The bride's family usually is in charge of the wedding arrangements. In an interfaith wedding, the bride's parents are called upon to express kindness, consideration, and tolerance for the groom's faith in the planning for the religious service. The bride's pastor or rabbi should be consulted first, then the groom's clergyman if he is of another faith. In this manner a service can be designed that will be balanced, appropriate, holy, and memorable. More than once, however, I have seen ecumenical services where one representative of a religious faith was not allowed to do anything but just stand there and might as well have not been present. In each case, it made the guests uncomfortable and became the talk of the wedding afterward. (The talk of the wedding should be the bride and groom!)

How much better it is if the couple, their parents, and their clergymen swallow pride, prejudice, and every other negative feeling for the sake of a happy, beautiful wedding! There are many ways in which the clergy of two faiths can co-celebrate the ceremony—one officiating for half the service and the other officiating for the second half, one doing the homily and the other saying the blessing, or both giving joint blessings.

Both members of the clergy should be invited to the rehearsal dinner the night before the wedding; they should be seated with equal rank at any bridal tables. At one very lovely interfaith wedding I attended fourteen years ago, at the wedding lunch the Jewish groom's rabbi sat on the Catholic bride's mother's right, and the bride's priest sat on the Jewish groom's mother's right. They all had a wonderful time at the wedding, and now, years later, the bride attends Catholic Mass every Sunday and the groom goes to temple every Friday night. The children alternate services with their parents, and when they go away to college, they will decide what faith to take as their own.

In another very happy marriage, the groom, who cares very much about his Jewish religion, is raising the children as Jews. His wife, of Christian background but not raised to be a devout observer of any faith, agreed to have their children raised as Jews. "I am the recipient of his compromises on many other issues," she said with a smile in talking about her acquiescence on this point. "We've worked it out." (If only all interfaith couples and their parents showed similar wisdom!)

Another Option: Two Ceremonies

On rare occasions couples of different religious beliefs choose to have two separate religious ceremonies on the same or even different days. For example, if the bride is Jewish, the ceremony might be held on Sunday afternoon, followed by a large reception for the wedding party, families, and friends. On the preceding day, Saturday, in the late afternoon (after sunset, at the end of the Jewish Sabbath), the couple would have been married by the bride's family's minister in a Christian service, with just toasts in champagne for the wedding party and the immediate families afterward. If the bride is Christian, the large reception would be held after the late afternoon Saturday services, and the small family champagne gathering would take place after the Jewish Sunday service. The wedding party would wear their bridal finery on both occasions and keep their bouquets in water to keep them fresh for both days; there would be only one cake cut (at the larger reception) and only one bouquet and garter tossed (at the larger reception), but the processionals, recessionals, and the other rituals would remain the same at both services.

If the couple wish both services on the same day, the Jewish service would take place after sundown (five o'clock) on Saturday, and the Christian service could follow at seven o'clock, followed by the large reception. In this case, the Jewish parents would invite their friends to the Jewish ceremony, and the Christian parents would invite their friends to the Christian ceremony. Everyone would be invited to the same reception.

It is *much* simpler (less expensive, too) to have one ecumenical service. Having two services on different or even the same day is costly and exhausting, but there are times when it is the only way out of a parental confrontation. Everything should be done to get the two married and to make the families happy. Nothing is too much trouble or too costly to accomplish this.

WEDDING APPAREL

The Bridal Attendants' Dresses

The bride has a responsibility to select dresses for her attendants that they will really like and that are affordable. Rarely does a bridesmaid's dress emerge from the owner's closet to be worn again after the wedding. (If it looks pretty in the pageantry of the wedding, it serves its purpose.)

The color scheme of the dresses is the bride's decision, and the flowers are usually coordinated with her color decisions. The maid and matron of honor can be dressed in separate colors, while the bridesmaids wear dresses of another color. Or everyone's dress can be in a different shade or hue. Or everyone can wear the exact same color. The wedding may even be entirely in white.

If some of the attendants don't fit the standard sizes in which the dress comes, the bride can give a sample dress to a dressmaker and have it copied to the measurements of any extra tall or heavy bridesmaid.

The bride should take the season as well as color preferences and price into account in selecting her dresses. Velvet and satin dresses look heavy in the heat; cotton dresses look unsuitable in winter cold. The dresses can be any style—long or short, with hats or without, with flowers in the hair or not, with shoes that match or contrast. The bridesmaids' dresses should not be overly sexy, with deep cleavages and low-cut backs, out of respect for the house of worship.

Some recent brides have chosen to dress attendants in black—a flouting of tradition, in that black is the symbolic color of mourning. I personally feel this is unfortunate, first because wedding guests might feel the bridesmaids are in mourning over their friend's choice of a groom, but also because black dresses look gloomy at a wedding—they are appropriate for funerals!

• If a bridesmaid is having a tough time financially, and cannot afford to buy her dress and shoes—much less pay for the airfare to the wedding—the bride might approach someone in her family (who can afford it) to help pay for these expenses quietly and make it possible for the bridesmaid to serve.

The Apparel of the Groomsmen

The groom's best man and ushers are dressed in rented finery, and the men should be fast and efficient in sending their measurements to the rental place (as instructed by the best man) and in showing up for a fitting when they are supposed to. Call me conservative, but I feel strongly about how great the groom and his attendants look in dark classic styles, and how inappropriate they look in colored suits or suits with colored piping and frilly shirts. (The latter styles look fine when worn by members of the orchestra, but not by members of the wedding party.)

The groom may be dressed slightly differently from his attendants (in terms of fabric weight and the kind of stripe in his trousers, for example), but the rest of the group should be identically dressed. *It is a good idea if the groom buys the ties for the best man and ushers so that they are the right kind.*

FOR A DAYTIME WEDDING

• *Informal for summer or resort only.* Appropriate wear would be all-white suits with white shirts, shoes, and socks; or dark blazers with either gray flannels or white trousers, worn with white shirts (French cuffs), conservative four-in-hand ties, and black shoes and socks.

• *Informal.* For an informal morning or early afternoon wedding, particularly if the bride wears a street-length dress or suit, the groom and his attendants would wear dark business suits in black, dark blue, or dark gray, with white shirts (French cuffs) and four-in-hand gray or gray-striped ties.

• *More formal.* Appropriate wear would be single-breasted gray or black *strollers*, gray vests, and striped trousers. The men should also wear gray or striped gray ties.

• *Most formal.* The men wear dark gray or black *cutaways*, gray vests, gray striped trousers, and a wing-collar shirt with gray ascot or a starched fold collar and a striped or checked four-in-hand gray tie.

FOR AN EVENING WEDDING

• *Informal.* For an informal evening wedding (after six o'clock), groomsmen wear a black dinner jacket and trousers (a white jacket is correct for hot weather, but black is always better). A single- or double-breasted black vest or black cummerbund may be worn with this. A black bow tie and white pleated dinner shirt with pearl, gold, or onyx studs and cufflinks are proper (no colored stones).

• *Formal.* For an eight o'clock wedding, men would appear in a full-dress black tailcoat with white piqué or waffle-weave waistcoat and bow tie, starched white shirt with wing collar, and wearing white pearl studs and cufflinks.

GLOVES

The groom at a formal wedding may decide to have his men wear gloves (gray for cutaways, white for tailcoats). The men should remove the glove on the right hand, of course, when shaking hands, and both gloves must be removed for eating and drinking. The groom and the best man would also remove their right gloves at the point in the wedding service where the best man hands the groom the wedding ring to place on the bride's finger.

The glove should be tucked in a pocket when not in use. The groom can always hand his right glove to his best man when he is placing the ring on the bride's finger.

SHOES AND SOCKS

Except when wearing all-white summer suits, the men in the wedding party should wear plain undecorated black shoes and black dress socks. For a black tie or white tie evening wedding, they should wear black patent leather shoes and black socks.

How the Guests Should Dress

THE MEN

• *For a winter daytime wedding,* male guests should wear a dark suit (navy, black, or dark gray) with a daytime dress shirt, a four-in-hand or bow tie, and dark shoes and socks.

• *For a summer daytime wedding in the city,* male guests should wear lightweight dark suits, with the same accessories that would be worn for a winter daytime wedding.

• *For a summer resort daytime wedding,* which is more casual than a city wedding, a dark blazer and contrasting trousers of a "quiet" color are appropriate. A white, beige, or cream-colored summer suit (of linen, poplin, or other lightweight fabric) is also appropriate. Khaki trousers or jeans with a blazer are just too informal for a wedding.

- *At a very informal summer wedding,* a man may wear a summer sports coat (of a bright color or a plaid) with white or contrasting color trousers.

- *For a wedding at six o'clock or later, when the invitation reads "Black Tie,"* a man should wear a winter-weight black dinner suit with a white or cream dress shirt (pleats are nice, but no ruffles, please), cufflinks, black hose, and black patent leather pumps or laced black patent leather shoes. He may wear a colored bow tie and matching cummerbund, if he wishes, but black is always right.

In the summer, a white dinner jacket with black trousers is correct for a black tie wedding, but a lightweight black dinner suit still looks best.

- *For that very rare invitation to a "White Tie Wedding"*—held only in wintertime in the city—a male guest would rent from a formal evening wear shop a suit of tails, complete with white piqué vest and white tie. Black silk hose and black patent leather shoes are de rigueur for this kind of outfit, as are tiny jeweled, onyx, or mother-of-pearl studs with large cufflinks. White gloves are optional. In the old days, the guest would have worn a top hat with this outfit, but today it might look silly— alas.

The men in the wedding party, including the fathers of the bride and groom, often wear white tie and tails at a wedding held after eight o'clock in the evening, but usually the invitation to that kind of wedding reads "Black Tie." This means that the men guests wear black dinner suits.

THE WOMEN

- *For a winter daytime wedding,* a woman would wear a dress or a dress suit (a soft, not a man-tailored suit). She should *not* wear something as informal as a blouse and skirt or sweater and skirt, and, in my opinion, pants are not at all proper. A micro-mini on a woman guest, even if she has great legs, is inappropriate—too flashy and sexy. (It's not a guest's but the bride's day to shine and be the cynosure of all eyes.)

- *It's advisable for a woman guest to refrain from wearing an all-white costume.* If she does, it may seem to others that she's trying to compete with the bride, even though she may be totally unconscious of this impression.

- *For a late afternoon winter wedding (after four o'clock),* the woman guest's dress length would still be short, unless the invitation reads "Black Tie." It is appropriate to wear a "little black dress" late in the afternoon, which might look wrong earlier. (Black prints are fine for a wedding at any hour—it's the solid black dress that looks too much like mourning when the sun shines brightly.) From late afternoon on, the woman guest can wear a dress or suit of any dressy fabric (for example, brocades, lamés, velvets). Glittery sequins and paillettes, however, are right only after six o'clock, not before.

• *For a six o'clock (or after) "Black Tie" wedding,* she would wear a theater suit or a short, three-quarter or floor-length evening dress appropriate to the season, whether winter, summer, or resort. Her shoes would be dressy sandals or pumps, and her handbag a small evening purse. This formal attire can be anything from a clinging crêpe sheath to a bouffant satin ballgown. If the invitation says "Black Tie," she can wear her favorite evening dress. (This is the time for her to wear her real or costume jewelry, too.)

• *A "White Tie Wedding," seldom seen these days, calls for everyone to be dressed in their most formal.* A woman would wear a décolleté ballgown, not a covered-up sheath. She would properly wear long white gloves.

THE WEDDING RING

The bride may opt not to have an engagement ring, but instead to have an impressive band of diamonds or colored stones with diamonds as her wedding ring. Or she may want to have the traditional wedding band to wear in conjunction with an engagement stone ring. (The wedding ring should be made of the same metal as her engagement ring—yellow gold, white gold, or platinum.)

The bride does not wear her engagement ring to the ceremony on her wedding day—the groom places the wedding ring on her bare finger. Later, she will put her engagement ring back on outside her wedding ring.

Perhaps the bride will be given one or two guard rings (slim bands of small diamonds or colored stones) for future anniversary or birthday presents. The guard rings would be worn outside and inside the engagement ring.

If the groom will wear a wedding ring, it does not have to match the bride's, but it should be of the same color metal. The bride should order it in his proper ring size and have it engraved on the inside—as hers will be—with both sets of initials and the wedding date.

ANNOUNCEMENT IN THE NEWSPAPER

If you wish to have your wedding announcement published in the local newspapers (often the day after the wedding), you will have greater success if you organize yourself accordingly far enough in advance of the wedding date. In large cities, the space for featuring brides and engaged girls is so small in comparison to the numbers being married that newspapers become selective in publishing the announcements. Often they will consider only a bride or groom who comes from an illustrious or socially prominent family, or who is a success story him- or herself. Sometimes a wedding will make it into the newspaper of a major city if the groom's grandfather was a famous general or author, or if the bride's great-grandfather founded a well-known company. If the bride or groom is personally successful in the health, education, business, sports, or entertainment world, the wedding announcement will probably be published. (A celebrity bride or groom, of course, means that the news desk will cover the wedding, whether the couple wishes it or not.)

Sometimes there will be room for the announcement but not for the bride's picture. Sometimes an announcement makes it only because a bride whose photograph was sent in with her announcement was so beautiful that the editors couldn't resist using it. You never know. What can help your chances, however, is to send in a perfectly typed, properly spelled announcement, written in the style of the paper, giving the information the paper generally prints in its wedding section. If the newspaper is going to publish the announcement, an editor will call the bride, her mother, and often the groom to double-check the information. (Always put your home and office telephone numbers on anything you send in to the paper.)

Some local newspapers give a full account of the wedding, including the names of the entire wedding party, a description of the bride's dress, and a description of what kind of reception was held and where. For a newspaper like the *New York Times,* only the "bare bones" information is published. For that coverage the bride's family should send in a glossy photograph (head shot only, whereas most other papers publish anything from a half-shot to a full-length portrait of the bride in her dress and headdress) with the following kind of information:

The Marriage of Cameron Edson Delaney and Edward Lee Grant, 3/19/92:

Cameron Edson Delaney, a daughter of Mr. and Mrs. David Edson Delaney of New Canaan, Connecticut, was married yesterday to Edward Lee Grant, a son of Mrs. Jonathan Wright and Frederick Grant of this city. The Reverend Andrew C. Smith performed the ceremony at Saint James Episcopal Church in New York.

Mrs. Grant, a graduate of the Spence School in New York and Kenyon College in Gambier, Ohio, is a credit analyst in the private banking and securities industries division of the Manufacturers Hanover Trust Company in New York. Her father is the chairman of the Delaney Manufacturing Company in Bridgeport, Connecticut.

The bridegroom, a graduate of the Collegiate School in New York and Princeton University, expects to receive a J.D. degree in May from Harvard Law School. His father is on the editorial staff of *New York* magazine, and his mother is with the real estate firm of Stribling Associates. The bridegroom is the grandson of the late George H. Grant, Jr., the founder of the Grant Advertising Agency in Chicago.

MOMENTARY WEDDING DISASTERS

Almost every bride—and her parents, too—experiences feelings of panic and attacks of nerves as the big day approaches. It is common for a bride to have certain crises of feelings (fortunately, very temporary ones) about the man she is about to marry. Understanding and patience on everyone's part, including the groom's, usually solve this problem. Then certain brides begin to feel something akin to stagefright, feelings of inadequacy, and a dread that they simply can't go through with all of the machinations of a wedding. Suddenly the bride may find she no longer wishes to be the center of everyone's attention during endless rituals and a long schedule of events. Suddenly she finds she can't accept the requirement that she look fabulously put together and dewey-eyed, too, when her feet hurt. And she may find that being unremittingly nice to everyone when she doesn't feel like it is too heavy a task.

These feelings are something of a natural defense mechanism to steel the bride against disappointing anyone during the wedding festivities. Fortunately, they disappear as the beautiful and romantic drama of her wedding unfolds. She *is* the center of attention, and almost always discovers she loves it. And almost everyone agrees that she is more beautiful on this day than on any other day in her life.

The bride's mother has other anxieties: Will the "horrible" new wife of her ex-husband, the father of the bride, try to steal center stage? Will Uncle Louie forget to fetch Grandma from the train station? Will it rain and ruin the garden wedding? Might the caterer have prepared inadequately for the crowds expected? This is not a tranquil time around the house, but in the vast majority of weddings, regardless of the minor slip-ups or even major disasters that loom on the horizon, the bride's and groom's happiness manages to cast light on everything and everyone around them. Problems find their solutions. Disasters become minor nuisances. The show goes on—and it's a fine show indeed.

If you are feeling panicky about your wedding, put your mind at ease by considering some of the things that have gone wrong at other people's weddings—weddings that turned out successful and happy nevertheless.

• Two hours before the wedding, just after the florists had completely decorated the interior, lightning struck the church and burned it down. Without blinking an eye, the bride's parents and the minister shifted the services to the school gymnasium next door, with improvised floral arrangements using flowers gathered from the peony and lilac bushes in sympathetic neighbors' yards. The fragrance from these flowers was far more noticeable and beautiful than that from the original flowers that had been put in the church. And the service in temporary quarters seemed far more touching than it would have been in the church.

• The groom broke both legs in an accident on his way home from the rehearsal dinner the night before the wedding, but he managed to make it to the wedding by ambulance with his legs in casts. He was wheeled by ambulance attendants into the church and to the reception on a cot, wearing at least the top part of his wedding suit, with its boutonniere in place. The couple's skiing honeymoon was postponed until a year later, on their first wedding anniversary, at which time the groom won the downhill slalom race, and the hotel management gave the couple a totally free vacation.

• The groom got into a fight at his bachelors' party, broke his arm, and was married with his cutaway coat cut open to allow his cast-encased arm to be carried in a sling.

• At the end of the wedding ceremony, the bride was left at the church by the excited groom as he took off in a limousine for the reception with other members of the family. The bride's absence was noticed about half an hour later. Someone went back to the church to fetch her and found her sitting alone in a pew, wondering if she had made a terrible mistake. Later, relaxed and forgiving, she made a wedding toast to her groom, claiming that although she had perfect grounds for annulment of the marriage, she would give him one more chance.

• The bride at the reception following a Conservative Jewish wedding, while joyously borne aloft in a chair by male members of the wedding party—along with her groom in another chair—was tilted so badly that she fell out. She went to the hospital to have her sprained wrist attended to but made it back to the reception in record time.

• The caterer made a mistake and sent the wedding reception food to a bank's golf-outing picnic. The picnic food went to the wedding reception. The hosts were so busy receiving guests that they did not realize the mistake until the guests were all serving themselves egg salad, hot dogs, kosher pickles, and potato chips. The golfers in the meantime greatly enjoyed the reception food, particularly the wedding cake, though thinking it a little odd as the choice for their dessert. They had demolished three quarters of it by the time the caterer's truck pulled up to rescue it. The remaining piece was brought to the wedding reception, and the bride and groom laughingly cut into the small piece with their beautifully decorated cake knife. Everyone at the party had a tiny piece of it, and the entire crowd really had a good laugh when, following a drum roll, the bride announced at the microphone that the golfing group had placed a wedding present for them inside the remaining piece of cake. She held it up—a shiny new golf ball!

• The father of the bride slugged the mother of the bride's newest husband at the reception after a few glasses of champagne. Everyone witnessed it. The bride's father helped revive his victim and then took over the microphone to say, "I apologize, Don, for that uncalled-for show of aggression. You happen to be a great guy. I want you all to join me in a special toast to a very fine person, someone who has made the bride's mother a very happy woman. I drink to Don!" (His toast fixed things up, believe it or not.)

• As the procession was about to start in the back of the church, the bride noticed her athletic four-year-old nephew ring-bearer was without his pillow (which had her wedding ring sewn onto it). It had been given to him fifteen minutes before, and he had managed to lose it somewhere between the house, the car, and the church.

The bride lost none of her composure. "Geoffrey will still walk down the aisle in his proper place without the pillow," she said, noting his face was a thunderstorm about to break. "It doesn't matter, Geoffrey." Then she commanded one of her bridesmaids to take off her own wedding ring at the altar and to give it at once to the best man to use in the ceremony. The groom looked nonplussed when he tried to get the ring on the bride's finger and found it was too small to pass her knuckle. "It's okay," the bride whispered, "I'll tell you later." Later at the reception she asked her nephew what he thought had happened to the ring pillow. His older sister, aged eight, answered for him. "Oh, he threw it out the window of the car." It was the only hitch in an otherwise perfect wedding, and as the jeweler later made a new engraved wedding ring for the bride—gratis—it wasn't even a hitch.

• The outdoor tent, laden with the weight of too much rain, collapsed early on in the reception. No one was hurt, but everyone was covered with water and plastic. A group started laughing, the laughter spread, and soon the entire wedding party was convulsed as they extricated themselves. The guests didn't seem to mind their ruined clothes and hairdos, and the band resumed playing. The reception lasted four hours beyond its planned length. The caterer brought new food (frozen dishes that they warmed in microwave ovens) and an endless supply of champagne. The latter was the caterer's gift, since it was his tent that had collapsed. The guests, including the entire wedding party, remained completely wet and disheveled. Yet they all stated afterward that it was one of the greatest weddings they had ever attended.

• The father of the bride spent a great deal of money having a thousand balloons blown up to festoon the guy ropes and the tent supports for the reception tent. It was an extremely hot day, and the balloons, scraping against the ropes, began to explode with loud bangs. The thousand balloons popping off over a period of two hours made it sound like war inside the tent. Although that made things difficult for the musicians, it added to the general excitement of the reception.

• A limousine full of bridesmaids bound for the church was hijacked by an escaping thief. The concert of screams from the back seats drove him to desperation, so he chauffeured them to the church—they made it to the service only slightly late. After they got out of the stolen limo, the thief drove off at high speed, only too glad to have the screaming damsels out of his life and into their wedding duties.

• The father of one bride announced on the microphone to the happy, dancing throngs at the reception, "The cars of everyone here who parked on State Street have been towed away by the Police Department and have been impounded across town." Then he put all the couples and families whose cars were involved into the chartered bus that had carried wedding attendants and family from the church to the reception. The bus driver took them to the car pound with the flamenco band from the reception on board, too, playing merrily away throughout the trip. The driver had also been given a large check to be turned over to the police to pay for the release of all the impounded cars. It was an unexpected, unbudgeted expense for the wedding, but it was one the father of the bride felt was important.

Hundreds of receptions regularly run out of food, drink, and ice. Hundreds of neighbors' freezers then contribute to the ice supply. Hundreds of best men, ushers, or bridesmaids have scurried in cars to replenish the food. The merriment at a reception always seems to continue unabated for the guests, most of whom don't know the real story.

Hundreds of best men or grooms have forgotten or lost the bride's wedding ring. (One groom's little brother "lost" the ring for the bride's finger right before the ceremony in the family's large aquarium—where it was swallowed by one of the twenty fish swimming around.) In each case, a friend in the wedding party or in the congregation has lent her wedding ring for the ceremony. . . . Hundreds of brides or bridegrooms faint during the religious ceremony, and all are rehabilitated quickly, in order to let the service proceed. . . . Hundreds of best men or grooms have forgotten to get the bridal couple's passports or air tickets packed into the possessions accompanying them from the reception to the airport, with the result that the bridal couple misses their flight abroad. It is never the end of the world, and often the adventures they have on their alternative wedding night turn out to be far more exciting than flying off on a plane on schedule. . . . Hundreds of stepparents or stepchildren or stepsiblings have let loose with some kind of animosity at some point during the wedding festivities, but these transgressions are quickly forgotten by the protagonist and have no effect on the majority of the guests' enjoyment of the wedding.

In other words, things can go wrong—but nothing should be magnified. Seeing the humor in a situation will get you through anything, and almost nothing is so important that it should ruin the day. Solving the dilemmas that present themselves during weddings requires creativity, kindness, fast action, and humor—always humor!

GIFTS

Wedding Gift Record Book

Every bride should keep careful records of the wedding gifts received in a "Wedding Gift Register." You can purchase a handsome notebook and make your own headings, such as these:

WEDDING GIFTS

Who sent	Address	What Sent	Store	Arrival	Date of Thank-you Note

If the groom writes some of the thank-you notes, his initials should be written in the "Date of Thank-you Note" column.

The Exchange of Gifts Within the Wedding Party

There is a delightful, well-established tradition of gifts involving members of the wedding party. There is, for example:

- *The engagement ring* given to the woman by her fiancé.
- *Her engagement present to him*—usually a personal gift such as a new photograph of herself in a handsome frame, or a pair of cufflinks.
- *The groom's wedding ring for his bride.*
- *Her wedding ring (optional) for her husband.* (Advice to the

bride: Don't make your husband wear a wedding ring if he really doesn't wish to.) If a two-ring ceremony is decided upon, the bride's and groom's rings should be the same color of metal, but they do not have to be the exact same design.

o *His or his family's gift of jewelry to his bride* for their wedding—for example, a watch, string of pearls, gold pin, silver bracelet, heirloom locket on a chain.

o *Her gift to her husband for their wedding*—for example, a watch, set of studs for his black tie, gold tie-clip, leather desk set.

o *The bridesmaids' gift to the bride*—often a joint gift, such as an engraved piece of silver or an etched piece of crystal, with each bridesmaid's initials, plus those of the bride and groom, and the wedding date.

o *The bride's gift to her attendants*—perhaps a silver picture frame that will eventually hold a photograph of the wedding party, engraved with the wedding date, or a leather one, embossed in gold; a charm for a bracelet; an engraved silver pen, mirror, or compact; or something in crystal, such as a water pitcher, etched with the wedding date and the bride's and groom's initials.

o *The attendants' gift to the groom*—such as a small silver tray engraved with their signatures and the wedding date, something for his car (like a tape deck or a telephone), a briefcase, a set of bar glasses etched with the initial of his last name.

o *The groom's gift to his attendants*—a silver or leather frame, like the one the bride gives her attendants; a leather stud box with his initials, the wedding date, and the usher's initials; a silver pen engraved with the initials of the recipient; an engraved silver jigger for measuring liquor for drinks; a wallet with the recipient's initials embossed in gold.

Gifts from Family and Friends to the Bride and Groom

Family members and friends who send wedding gifts most often use these points as their guides:

o How close they are to the bride or groom
o How much they have to spend
o How much the bride and groom need help in furnishing their household

No one should overspend on a wedding present, no matter how much affection there may be for the couple. The note accompanying the wedding present is often as important as the gift itself—a note carefully written by hand, in which the donor expresses his or her love for the couple and very special wishes for their future.

BRIDAL REGISTRY

It is very useful for everyone if the bride registers—not in many stores, but in one or two that are easy to reach. Bridal registries have become so sophisticated today that if you call some large stores and ask if a certain bride is registered there, the operator may say, "Yes. Would you like to be connected to the department where she is registered in crystal, silver, china, appliances, or kitchenware?" In smaller stores, there is only one registry in which the bride has listed everything she would like in that store.

A bride can register for certain useful items that are expensive in the hopes that a group of her relatives or friends may group together to buy one of them. But she would be wise to list items she really needs and that are not out of the ballpark, costwise. If she registers for her silver pattern and expensive plates or something like a VCR or a microwave oven, she, her family, and her friends should be briefed to inform anyone who asks that she has registered for certain things that would have to be the gift of several people, or that she would appreciate the gift of just one fork or one spoon or plate in her pattern.

THE GIFT OF MONEY

Money from a relative or close friend is always an acceptable gift. At many weddings, particularly ethnic ones, it is traditional to give money as the wedding present—and to slip it in an envelope to the bride or groom (most often the groom) at the reception. The money may pay for the honeymoon or be used for a car, household furnishings, or other needs.

It is best not to give cash—it is too easily lost or stolen. Before the couple leaves on the honeymoon, the should both endorse the checks, assuming they have a new joint account, and a member of the family or wedding party should deposit the checks, with a properly filled-out deposit slip, at the next available banking hour.

In thanking for money, the bride and groom should express their thanks for "the generous check," without stipulating the amount. It is much more tasteful if neither the donor, the bridal couple, nor the couple's families publicly state how much any one person gave the couple.

RETURNING AND EXCHANGING GIFTS

It can really hurt feelings if the donor finds out you have exchanged his or her present for something else. (Duplicates, of course, can be exchanged for something else; so can items of which you have more than one, such as a water pitcher or a salad bowl.) Often a family member will have a prized family possession that he or she gives the couple as a very sentimental gesture, such as Great Aunt Mary's silver cake knife. If it is a "hidiosity," as one recent bride described her grandmother's Victorian lamp, it must be kept and displayed when that family member comes to their home. I kept certain of my own "hidiosity" wedding presents (from 1963) in the back of a closet; they have since become rather chic again, so I now use or display them.

Couples should keep in mind the disappointment someone they truly love may suffer when he or she comes into their home and finds that wedding present nowhere in sight. Out of respect and affection for the donor, the couple can always keep "Aunt Mabel's bowl" for a year or two, and then the bowl can quietly be put away or "retired" to a thrift shop.

THANK-YOU NOTES

In the past, it was the bride's chore to write all the thank-you notes, not only because most of the presents came from her side of the family, but also because she was at home. Today, when often the bride and groom work equally hard, the groom should write thank-you notes, too—if not half the load, at least those to his relatives and his parents' friends.

• *Thank-you notes to people who gave parties for your wedding* should be written *the day after.* You should also send flowers to your hosts, but what you say in your letter is what counts most of all. A sample note:

> Dear Aunt Midge, Uncle Bob, and Aunt Nancy,
> You will never know how grateful Jim and I are for the incredible rehearsal dinner you gave us last night. Everyone in the wedding party had the best time—and you should have heard them all extolling the virtues of the great cuisine, the lovely flowers in the center of the tables, and not only the quality of the champagne, but the endless amounts of it!
> You are the most generous aunts and uncle in this world. Jim and I will never forget your toasts to us, either, and I only hope that someday we can become the great uncle and aunt to our nieces and nephews that you have been to us.
> It is the morning of our wedding day, and I must hurry to get dressed, but I wanted you to know that as far as I'm concerned, you've already made this wedding a success!
>
> Affectionately,

• *Thank-you notes for wedding gifts* should be written within two weeks preferably—at the outside maximum, within two months. I know of couples who have taken six months to write their thank-you notes, which leaves many people wondering if their presents ever arrived, and others wondering why they spent so much time and money selecting that wedding gift! I remember a spunky woman who rang the doorbell of the bride and groom's home one day and announced that, since she had heard nothing for nine months from the day she'd sent her gift, it obviously was not appreciated. And since the gift had cost her an infinite amount of trouble and a great amount of money to buy, she then proceeded to ask where it was and took it back home with her! (I am sure a lot of other wedding present donors would like to do the same thing, but don't have the nerve.)

• *Thank-you notes should be written on good-quality stationery, by hand.* If the bride can afford it, she uses notepaper engraved with her new monogram (not to be used, however, until *after* the wedding ceremony). If she writes her thank-you notes for the presents as they arrive, weeks before the wedding, she thanks for them on her social stationery (paper engraved with her maiden name or monogram). If engraved stationery is not within the bride's budget, she should purchase good-quality plain notepaper (single sheets or folded notes) with matching envelopes—in any color and with any color border.

The groom should use for his stationery either plain notepaper or, after the wedding, he may use jointly with the bride social stationery engraved only with their home address (and perhaps home telephone number) at the top of the sheets.

If the bride or groom has unintelligible handwriting, he or she may type the thank-you note on social stationery (or use a word processor).

What is unacceptable is a printed card that says "Thank you" on it, to which the bride simply signs her and her groom's names with no written message. I've seen that several times lately. Help!

• *An unacceptable thank-you note from the bride:*

Dear Mrs. Castro,
　　George and I really like your wedding present. Thank you so much, and I hope we'll see you soon.

　　　　　　　　　　　　　　　　　　　　　Sincerely,
　　　　　　　　　　　　　　　　　　　　　Susan

For all anyone knows with this kind of letter, Mrs. Castro could have sent George and Susan a lawnmower or champagne glasses. Such a note is better than sending nothing at all, but only slightly better!

• *An acceptable thank-you note from the bride:*

Dear Mrs. Castro,
　　George and I are absolutely delighted with the beautiful place mats and napkins from you and Mr. Castro. The pale blue is such a perfect color, we have decided to repaint the walls of our dining area a pale blue, too. What a compliment to the place

mats! [You would say this only if you *were* painting the walls blue.]

We have already used them at dinner for my parents, and we will use them again when my boss comes to dinner next week. We really appreciate this useful, wonderful present, and I hope the Castros will be coming to Topeka some day soon, so we can have *you* to dinner, using the blue place mats.

Sincerely,
Susan

P.S. Married life is terrific!

• *An acceptable thank-you note from the groom:*

Dear Mrs. Castro,

Susan and I really appreciate the Castros' gift. We have already used those blue place mats for a special dinner for my in-laws, and somehow they even made our food look better! They are really great.

Susan is at her night class in business school as I write this. We are both very happy and very busy—and your place mats and napkins are making our lives easier, too, when we entertain. You gave us just the right present.

Sincerely,
George

POSTPONING THE WEDDING

It happens. Sometimes the wedding must be postponed. There may be a death in the immediate family. The groom may be quarantined. The bride may be in a body cast from an auto accident. There may have been a fire in the bride's home, where the wedding was to take place. The groom may have been asked to serve on a three months' commission inside the People's Republic of China—an assignment all-important to his career.

If the invitations have already gone out but there is plenty of time to get postponement announcements printed and into the mail, then the parents of the bride would send a printed announcement like this, in the same typeface as the original invitation:

> *Mr. and Mrs. Duncan Forsythe Teston*
> *announce that the marriage of their daughter*
> *Suzanne MacDonald*
> *to*
> *Mr. Henry Foscue Cavalchini*
> *has been postponed from*
> *Saturday, the ninth of June*
> *until*
> *Saturday, the sixth of September*
> *at five o'clock*
> *Saint Barnabas Church*
> *Boston*

If the postponement decision is because of the death of a member of the family, that may certainly be included in the announcement:

> *Mr. and Mrs. Duncan Forsythe Teston*
> *announce that because of the death*
> *of their son Geoffrey*
> *the marriage of their daughter*
> *Suzanne MacDonald*
> *to Mr. Henry Foscue Cavalchini*
> *has been postponed*
> *etc.*

If the postponement decision does not leave enough time to have these cards printed and mailed, send the same message in a Mailgram to each of your guests, and be prepared for a host of worried telephone calls from all your friends wondering why the postponement, if you did not mention the reason in the mailing. In fact, instruct whoever answers the telephone at your office and at your home to explain quickly the reason for the postponement. People's curiosities know no bounds.

CALLING OFF THE WEDDING

Sadly, it also happens that a decision is made not to go on with the wedding. It is a very difficult time for everyone. Again, a formal printed announcement may be mailed—if there is time to give people enough advance warning to change their plans with ease. (Out-of-town guests should either be called or sent Mailgrams.) This is not the kind of message you would fax to someone's machine, unless you had less than twenty-four hours in which to get in touch with people:

Mr. and Mrs. Thatcher William Gray
announce the marriage of their daughter
Ruth Leigh

to

Mr. Saxton William Baines
by mutual agreement
will not take place

This is a time for face-saving and compassion. Anyone connected with the wedding should say whenever the cancellation is discussed, "Both decided it was the best thing to do . . . Both equally agreed that the wedding should be called off." Of course, it is almost never a mutually agreed-upon decision, but for the sake of saving the injured person's pride, everyone should play his or her part. With time, the sadness and perhaps even the humiliation suffered by the woman or the man will subside.

The woman should return her financé's ring, and he should return any of her gifts to him. He may refuse to take back the engagement ring if he is the one to call off the wedding, but she would probably not wish to wear it again anyway. (I do know of some cases where the spurned fiancée has managed to exchange her engagement ring successfully for a beautiful substitute piece of jewelry.)

All wedding presents should be carefully wrapped and returned directly to the donor with a short note announcing the wedding is off and expressing the couple's thanks "for your beautiful, generous present." That's all that has to be said.

PRENUPTIAL AGREEMENTS

Thanks to the proliferation of divorce in this country, the prenuptial agreement has become common. It has also sadly become a common topic of conversation among friends, like hanging out the family's dirty laundry on the line for anyone to see. Prenuptial agreements used to be considered relevant only for billionaires, movie stars, and highly paid athletes. Today they are prevalent enough to inspire many states to adopt the "Uniform Premarital Agreement Act"—the benchmark legislation for marital contracts. This act greatly assists someone with an agreement who moves to another state and then worries about the validity of the agreement under the new state's laws.

Prenuptial agreements make the most sense for people with children who remarry and wish to protect their assets in the future. They make sense, too, for a very rich person marrying for the first time. However, for a young couple marrying for the first time, with limited assets, a prenuptial agreement puts a sour note into what should be an exhilarating, optimistic experience. It is almost asking for trouble in the marriage. A great deal of misunderstanding and hurt feelings can result from the premise upon which these agreements are based—that one person will try to cheat the other in case of a breakup. Some people talk about their agreements the way others talk about what their psychiatrists told them this week. It suddenly all becomes very distasteful!

From the point of view of etiquette, it's important to keep this in mind:

- o Don't discuss the financial and legal ramifications of your marriage contract.
- o If anyone asks if you have a prenuptial agreement, mention that the subject is a private matter.
- o Never discuss the details of it with anyone except your spouse and your lawyer.

A good agreement strikes a happy medium between preserving your marital relationship and protecting your property.

THE NEW MANNERS WHEN YOU MARRY
MORE THAN ONCE

Second and third marriages have become so common, that by the time they reach the age of forty-five, many people are attending more of their friends' remarriages than they are of their friends' children's marriages.

When you marry for the second time, the protocol is fairly rigid, but you can choose not to follow it, and many brides do not follow it! In this section I will lay on the table what is proper and in good taste in the conventional sense, guaranteed to ward off any criticism behind your back. Of course, you are free to accept it or not.

The religious ceremony, whether you have it in a church, temple, your home, a club, or a hotel, should be small and include only family and the very closest friends. The participation of your more extended circle of friends should be centered on the wedding reception, which can be anything you wish—with no limitations as to number of guests invited or lavishness of food and entertainment.

Who Does the Inviting?

Usually the small number of people who are to attend the ceremony itself are invited by the bride or groom by personal note or telephone call. As for the reception, if the bride is very young, her parents once again invite the guests to the reception. If the bride and groom are in their thirties or older, usually they themselves extend the invitation to their reception:

Agatha (or optionally, Mrs. Agatha) Henley Freeman
and
Chapman (or Mr. Chapman) Delano Blaine
request the pleasure of your company
at dinner
following their wedding
on Thursday, March third
at seven o'clock
Colony Club
New York City

R.S.V.P.   *Black Tie*

000/000-0000

It is important, in the case of a second or third marriage, to disseminate as many announcements as possible to all friends of the bride and groom, because friends will want to be aware of the news.

Changes in the Ritual

When a woman remarries, tradition decrees a change in her clothing and in certain symbolic aspects of the wedding ritual. Of course, you are free to go against tradition and repeat the whole ceremony once again—long white dress, being "given away" by your father, and tossing your bridal bouquet at an unmarried bridesmaid. Some women who eloped or who didn't have the money to be married with all the fuss the first time, long to do it up right the second time. A woman certainly may and you certainly may. But if you wish to remarry according to traditional etiquette, there are certain things you do *not* do.

These are among the things you would avoid:

• *You would avoid having an official announcement party.* Instead, you and your fiancé call and write all family members and friends with your very happy news. If someone wants to give you a party, great—but call it "a party for us," not an "engagement party." A woman who is remarrying does not go through an "engagement period." She just gets married.

• *You would avoid wearing a long white bridal dress with a train and a veil.*

• *You would avoid having a galaxy of bridesmaids.* Instead, you and your groom have one attendant each. Yours may be a married or unmarried friend or relative. You and the groom may wish as your attendants one of your own children—hopefully thirteen or older and mature enough to understand the solemn significance of the marriage vows.

How You Dress

A man always dresses to match his bride. If you are in a long, flowing white dress and veil as a first-time bride at a large formal afternoon wedding, he would wear a cutaway. Or after six, he would wear a black tie. There is no symbolism in *his* clothes, as there is in the bride's.

THE BRIDE

Your second wedding may be a daytime (informal or formal) affair, or a black tie evening affair. If you wish to get married after six in a floor-length gown with your groom in a black dinner suit, then the invitations should spell it out to the guests by including the words "Black tie"—

meaning the guests are to come attired in evening dresses and tuxedos. (This is no time for that odious phrase "Black Tie Optional"!)

When a bride is being married for the second time, a full-fledged formal white tie wedding, held at eight o'clock or later, is simply never held.

For a very informal daytime wedding, you would wear a street-length silk dress or dressy suit (a strictly man-tailored style of suit is not appropriate) in an off-white or pastel color (not red or black).

For a more formal, larger afternoon wedding, you might wear a dress of a rather formal fabric (silk, crêpe, chiffon, organza, velvet, brocade, or whatever, according to the season) and in any length you desire, including floor length. For a six-o'clock-or-after wedding, you would wear a long evening dress.

You may carry a bouquet of the flowers of your choice—or a white prayer book with flowered ribbon streamers. You may wear a hat, bandeau, bow, or flowers in your hair, but forget the veil. It is a nice touch if your shoes match your dress. What is inappropriate is to be married in a house of worship wearing a backless dress that is cut extremely low in front, even if you have a great shape and the dress bears the label of the number one dress designer.

Although the wardrobe departments of Hollywood and TV-land often don't seem to realize it, a woman marrying even for the fourth time should exude a sense of dignity appropriate to the occasion.

THE GROOM

His wedding attire matches his bride's, according to the time of day. He would wear a dark business suit for an informal daytime wedding, perhaps a stroller and gray striped trousers for a more formal daytime wedding, and a black tuxedo for an evening wedding. For a daytime wedding in hot weather, the groom would be dressed in a dark blazer and gray flannel or white trousers.

THEIR ATTENDANTS

The groom's attendant would be dressed as the groom is. They may wear identical or slightly different boutonnieres. If the bride's and groom's children from previous marriages attend their parents, they should be dressed in their best clothes. (I attended one wedding recently where the groom's attendant was his small, nine-year-old son, dressed up in a tuxedo. It looked ludicrous rather than right.)

The bride's attendant would be dressed in a coordinating style. If the bride is wearing a long chiffon gown, for example, the bridesmaid might wear a chiffon dress, too, of an identical or different color but in a harmonious design. For a daytime wedding, the bride might wear a long dress and her attendant a short one of the same kind of fabric. For a very informal wedding, the single attendant may wear any dressy daytime dress (not a suit) as long as it is not white, red, or black, and as long as the pattern in the fabric (if there is one) is not a strong one. She could wear a hat, flowers or a bow in her hair, or nothing. She should not be dressed more elaborately than the bride.

The Ceremony

There is no processional or recessional in your second wedding. There may be organ music (or any kind of church music), but preferably not the traditional "Here Comes the Bride" or the wedding march from *Lohengrin*. You are not "given away" by your father, since you were already given away at your first wedding. There are no ushers seating people. There is no runner and no satin ribbons to pull through the posts of the pews. Your two families simply sit down in the front rows, with your closest friends behind them.

At the musical signal that the wedding is to begin, your attendant precedes you as you walk unescorted from the vestry door at the side of the front of the church to join your groom and his attendant at the foot of the altar. (A very young bride the second time around may wish her father to escort her to the groom's side, and that is perfectly fine, but he does not give her away again.) The ceremony should be brief and is almost always, in this kind of intimate and personal environment, very touching and memorable.

Parties and the Second Wedding

Showers for a second-time bride are simply not appropriate. You had that kind of festivity the first time and supposedly became equipped with what you and your husband needed for your household. If your husband absconded with all of the household possessions at the time of the divorce, then your friends might give a shower kind of party to help out, but it wouldn't be labeled a "kitchen shower." It would just be referred to as a "party to fix up Mamie's kitchen."

There would not be a rehearsal dinner as such, given by the groom's family the night before the wedding, but the latter might give a dinner "in honor of" the bride and groom to fete the occasion. (There usually doesn't have to be a rehearsal of the simple wedding ceremony—just a talk with the clergyman during the week before the ceremony.)

Gifts the Second Time Around

Do you give a wedding gift the second time around? Yes! When you love, or even like, a person, no matter how many times he or she is married, you should want to bless the union with your good wishes. You do not have to give a friend to whom you gave an expensive present the first time an equally lavish gift the second or third time around. If you attend the wedding, you should send a modest gift. Even if you were not invited to the small wedding, if one of the pair is a good friend of yours, hearing about the wedding or receiving their wedding announcement should move you to send a little something to show you are delighted with the news.

The note that accompanies your gift is as important as the gift. You wouldn't write a note like this one, recently received by a friend of mine who was being married for the third time:

Dear Nancy, I hope this time it will finally work! Love,

Instead, you might write a warm word like this on the gift enclosure:

Nancy, along with this small present goes a multitude of good wishes for you and Hank. You deserve great happiness, and you make a wonderful pair. This is going to be a terrific year for you two!

Stepchildren, Stepparents, and Grandparents

When a man or woman with children from a former marriage remarries, a sizeable emotional problem presents itself, one that requires every bit of tact, compassion, and self-sacrifice humanly possible for its solution.

The following scenarios, for example, are repeated all over the world when a divorced parent plans another wedding:

• The wife has been deserted by her husband for another woman, and he wants his children to attend the wedding to his new young wife. Or the husband has been deserted by his wife for another man, and she wants the children to participate in her wedding to a new husband. In both cases, the wronged partner is ready to declare war.

• The children of a parent about to be remarried are upset by the advent of a new stepparent and stepbrothers and sisters coming to live in their household. They fear they will no longer dominate the scene in their own house and feel they must now fight for their turf.

• The grandparents of the children whose mother has been divorced by their son feel that now that their son has abandoned his home, their grandchildren will not longer be available to them. They feel that their ex-daughter-in-law will keep the children away from them for spite.

• The children who will accompany the parent who has remarried and move after the wedding into his or her spouse's home have a new stepparent to contend with. In addition they feel inordinately threatened by their stepsiblings, who already call that house "home."

• The new stepfather or stepmother worries about how to gain the acceptance of the new stepchildren, plus worries about how his or her own children are going to accept this disruption.

In short, *everyone* is under great emotional pressure as the wedding day approaches. When the wedding of people who have children from prior marriages takes place, it's a wise moment for all persons involved—adult and child alike—to take a deep breath, and to say to themselves, "This is happening. It will not go away. I will therefore do my best to make it happen with the least amount of pain to the people I love. I will do my part to make it a good day for everyone involved."

If ever strong character and self-sacrifice were needed, it is now. The generations of family involved with each other should talk it out calmly, be frank in expressing how they feel, and discuss the emotional ramifications of the wedding for the sake of protecting the feelings of the children, who are always the ones who suffer most. It's a question of each person's calling upon his or her personal strength—an extra measure of emotional adrenaline—to help get through the wedding period with flying colors, behaving in such a kind and gracious manner that he or she will be a pace setter. One person's brave behavior alone might help smooth the path of harmony for many months to come. A wedding involving upset ex-husbands and ex-wives, widowed parents, and new stepparents and stepchildren is an opportunity for any individual to become a leader and a star in the complicated family firmament. For example:

• The deserted wife swallows hard and tells her children that of course she wants them to attend their father's wedding; or the deserted husband tells his children that of course they should attend their mother's wedding—with his blessing. It helps if the deserted one has planned a lovely treat for herself or himself (like a wonderful trip) to think about during the actual wedding.

• The children on both sides of the family are taught to approach their new stepsiblings with enthusiasm, because after the petty little problems are ironed out (mostly questions of turf and seniority, not questions of who is the most or the least loved), they will have *much to gain* from each other.

• The new spouse writes a letter from the heart, telling the deserted one how much it means to her or him to have the stepchildren present at the wedding. The new spouse expresses her or his love and admiration for the children, compliments the deserted spouse on the way the children were brought up, and pledges to do everything possible to keep peace and harmony in the family.

• The deserted spouse refrains from talking against the new spouse who has taken his or her place—either to the children or to friends. The deserted one knows that expressed criticism and bitterness solve nothing but do make it hurt worse for everyone.

- The deserted spouse makes sure that the newly married spouse has constant access to the children, and that the grandparents do, too. A deprivation of access completely ruins a child's sense of well-being.
- The newly married spouse takes very seriously the times of visitation to the divorced spouse's household, being careful never to cancel an appointment with the children. He or she never talks against the former spouse in front of their children. Instead he or she praises the ex-spouse to them.
- The widow who remarries invites her late husband's parents to her wedding. She is careful to explain that no one will take the place of their son in her heart, but that she is now walking down a new path. She is careful to maintain their relationships with their grandchildren.

The above scenarios are a reflection of an ideal world, which, of course, this world is not. But everyone should make a supreme effort for the children's sakes at the time of the emotional shock of a parent's wedding to someone else. The one who gives the most ultimately gains the most.

* * *

Of all the rites of passage, a wedding is certainly the biggest production of them all—the most expensive, the most emotional, and offering the most potential for frayed tempers and possible disagreements. If all those involved will only keep telling themselves to act in a concerted manner to stay calm, think of the happiness of the bride and groom and not pursue their own agendas, and think positively about all the arrangements, the wedding will be a monumental success. And if the prepared script isn't quite followed here and there during the proceedings, what does it matter? A year later, the rough spots will have been forgotten; only the rosy memories will remain. If you personally had a hand in helping someone else at the wedding forget a rough spot, you can take personal satisfaction in the happiness of the couple who celebrate the anniversary of their marriage.

13

Pregnancy, Birth, and Other Rites of Passage That Welcome a Child into the World

When we attend a rite of passage of a good friend or of a child, we feel blessed to be present at this kind of celebration—except, of course, for the ultimate rite, a funeral. Until that last rite is performed, there is a sense of joy when a family comes together, when there's a reunion of good friends, and when everyone present partakes of each great step forward in the maturation and development of a beloved person's life.

THE HAPPIEST EVENT OF ALL:
THE BIRTH OF A BABY

Polite Pregnancy at Work

If you can manage it—and this requires a lot of willpower—it's very wise not to tell anyone at work until you actually show, even in loose-fitting dresses or suits (this could be as late as the fourth or even fifth month). Once the fact is known, there will be much conversation about your condition, with many questions asked (including overly personal, prying ones) and many stares. That is why it is much better to put off the inevitable holding of center stage in your workplace as long as you can.

• *Keep yourself productive—and the others around you, too.* Be courteous in your answers, but cut off any pregnancy conversation amiably and turn it back to your work:

> Q. "Are you having that nausea that most women have the early months?"
> A. "Oh, I feel just fine—none of that. What worries me is where is that statistical report from the Budget Division that we need for Monday's meeting? Has anyone seen it?"

> Q. "Has the baby begun to kick and move around yet? Is that a twitch I just saw?"
> A. "This is a good baby—it never moves when I'm at work. Tell me, Agnes, how are we doing with the new Antco account? Are they happy with our work?"

> Q. "Have you looked into that new kind of life insurance for the baby, that dates from the hour of its birth?"
> A. "Maybe you could tell me about it when we take the bus home tonight. I'd be interested in getting information on it when I have the time to think about it."

In other words, in deference to the people who are paying your salary, show everyone that you are absolutely delighted about the baby but are not going to let baby conversation overtake your productivity at work.

Returning to Work After the Baby Is Born

The less complaining any woman who works during her pregnancy does about fatigue and the fewer comments made about the baby's progress within her, the better. (Such subjects as gas pains, swollen ankles, and frequent urination should not become part of the daily office agenda.)

If she plans on returning to work after a hiatus of several weeks or months, she should inform her office and stick to her promise of when she is to return. During those weeks at home, she should read all the informative material circulated at work that she can get her hands on. (Maybe a friend will bring her a packet once a week.) She should make some calls to her colleagues in the office from time to time, asking them how this or that is proceeding, so they know she is interested in her work. Perhaps she should keep in touch with her regular clients or customers. She should drop into the office once every three or four weeks (without the baby), looking well dressed, as she would for an important meeting. These occasional drop-ins to say hello to everyone (members of senior management, too) and to be informally briefed on what is happening are very helpful to the aura of professionalism she wants to exude. Her appearances remind her colleagues that she is keeping up and will soon be back in their midst.

The new mother should be able to sneak the time at least to skim the trade journals she normally would see if she were in the office. She should keep informed not only on the work of the office but on the gossip, too. (Short office visits are well worth the cost of paying for a baby-sitter's services at home.)

A company that holds a woman's job for her and that grants her a decent maternity leave has the right to ask that she keep in touch with her work. It is paramount in earning the respect of colleagues and superiors.

Nursing the Baby

There are some young women who not only feel it is a woman's right to nurse her baby anywhere at any time, but they take it as their moral obligation to do so in public whenever they can. That is one school of thought, but the other school, to which the vast majority of men and women belong, feels that nursing a baby is a private, beautiful act that should be done away from the public eye.

I personally feel that a woman nursing a baby in a public place is trying to draw attention to herself. She is asking for people to look at her.

As for nursing the baby at the office, it is distracting and out of place, except in the restroom. A woman who cares about the direction of her career is not going to breast-feed in front of her bosses.

THE BIRTH ANNOUNCEMENT

There are many ways to ånounce the birth of a baby. One happy father had a skywriter announce it in puffs of white in a bright blue sky over his town's busiest section at noon. Another one hired an actor, dressed him up as an eighteenth-century colonial town crier, handed him a proclamation written on a piece of parchment, and had him ring his bell all over town, shouting, "Hear Ye, Hear Ye" followed by the name, weight, and hour of birth of a baby girl. New York parents have advertised their babies' arrivals on giant billboards in Times Square on more than one occasion. But there are more conservative ways of doing it!

For example: Mail announcements. You can buy pretty pink or blue ones at gift card shops, with lines on which to fill in the information. Or you can have announcement cards printed or even engraved. Quality stationers usually provide engraved cards, bordered in pink or pale blue, for those who can afford to have them custom made. The information on these cards is engraved in black in a classic typeface; the baby's own tiny calling card is attached to the larger announcement card by means of a pale pink or pale blue satin ribbon bow.

Some proud parents enclose a snapshot of the baby in their Christmas card by way of announcing the birth; others have the baby's photo printed on a card that becomes their Christmas card. Many use their baby's footprint made for the hospital's records for the birth announcement. One rather overenthusiastic couple had their three-week-old baby's portrait painted in oils by a well-known artist; the colored photograph of the oil painting was then mailed as an announcement card to all their friends.

The cleverest announcement I've ever seen (or rather heard) was a cassette tape that arrived one day in the mail, with absolutely no information on it and no return address. I naturally played it out of curiosity, thinking it was probably going to be something cheap and tawdry. Instead I heard ten seconds of a baby's cry. Then the father's voice was heard saying, "The lusty squall you just heard came from the seven-day-old lungs of a future tight end for the Chicago Bears. His name is Matt." Not only did I love it, but that cassette was played for everyone who came into the office that day; everyone smiled, then laughed and felt good about the state of the world.

The full information that should be imparted on a birth announcement is:

- o Full name of the baby
- o Birth date
- o Parents' name
- o Parents' address

Optional additional information:

- o Hour of birth
- o Name of hospital
- o Birth weight

(A birth announcement printing the number of hours the mother was in labor is too much!)

It's much nicer, of course, when one of the parents personalizes a printed announcement with a little sentence or two written by hand, anything from "He's so sweet, we can't believe he's here" to "She's the longest baby! She'll be an Olympic basketball player, there's no doubt." When the father pens a note on a birth announcement, he inevitably says, "The baby, of course, looks just like me," and the mother inevitably agrees and writes, "She looks just like her father." I have a feeling this is a concerted campaign to make the father feel he had more to do with the baby's birth than just help with the breathing exercises. (The truth is, of course, that a newborn doesn't look like anyone!)

How to React to a Birth Announcement

When a good friend mails you a birth announcement, or you hear via the grapevine that their baby was born, react right away—with a letter, telephone call, Mailgram, or gift with a note. Such happy news should not go unacknowledged—particularly if it's a couple's first baby. (By the time the sixth child arrives in that family, you can be a little more blasé about it!)

NICE THINGS TO DO FOR A FRIEND WHEN A BABY IS BORN

Presents for the Parents

The baby receives so much attention that the parents often rate hardly a glance. Therefore, if you are close to the parents of a newborn, it's amusing, gracious, and appreciated to give *them* a gift rather than give one to the baby. One of the things my husband and I most appreciated when our first was born was a case of wine, with a card from friends that read, "You are *really* going to need this within a short time, so enjoy!" I also will never forget receiving a gift certificate in the mail from a friend to avail myself of a "Miracle Morning" at Elizabeth Arden. It arrived a week after Clare was born and presented a glorious opportunity to get my tired, misshapen body out of the house and into a salon to have my hair done and take advantage of other options, including a massage, facial, pedicure, manicure, sauna, paraffin wax bath, and general pampering. The baby received nothing from the donor, but I loved my friend for thinking of me, the one who needed it most! My husband will always treasure the present he received from Vincent Price when our first was born, because "the father never receives anything, and he deserves everything."

Presents for the Baby

The first-born inevitably receives a raft of presents, the second child a token amount, and the third almost nothing. So one of the nicest things to do is to be sure to give presents to the subsequent children when they are born. Even an inexpensive little book (the baby's first book for his library) is a symbolic and important note of welcome.

When a second child comes along, it is very thoughtful to give a small present to the first child, too, because the first one, having lost center stage, usually feels threatened by the newcomer and wishes it would go away. (Our daughter tried to make her little brother go away by standing over his crib when he was ten days old and grinding fresh pepper into his face with the pepper mill.) When a brother or sister receives a little gift, too, somehow that gesture makes having the baby in the house not quite so hard to take.

Studio Cards

Even if you are not particularly close to a new mother who works with you or whom you know through your church or synagogue, your tennis group, your volunteer team or other connection, the arrival of a baby is important enough to commemorate with a studio card or a note. If you decide on a studio card, remember that the little message you write by hand is as important as the card. Something as short and innocuous as the following, penned on the bottom of the card, will sufficiently personalize it: "We were all so thrilled to hear about Bobby, and can hardly wait to view your new creation. Congratulations!"

Letters of Congratulation

A well-written letter congratulating the parents—or the baby itself— is usually reread several times by the entire family and often is placed in a scrapbook, where it will be saved for the baby's own family to enjoy someday. A good letter is really appreciated by the family receiving it. When Maurice and Joan Tobin of Washington had a little girl, Alexis, after several years of marriage, many of their friends wrote them, including my late brother, Mac Baldrige, who at that time was Secretary of Commerce in the Reagan administration. This is the kind of letter that gets saved:

> Dear Alexis,
>
> While presently you are probably shorter than your name of Alexis Dorette Bouffleur Tobin, you will soon outgrow that and enter a fascinating life with your mother and father. They are two special people, and it will be a lot of fun for you to grow up and help educate them.
>
> Of course, they will give you a lot of advice—I'll let them do that. But I have some of my own, also. My advice would be: Don't study too hard if it interferes with your playtime; be sure to play in the mud whenever you can or you will miss a lot of enjoyment, no matter what your mother says about your new dress; and learn to hit back if a boy hits you first.
>
> Best regards from your special friend,
> /s/ Mac Baldrige

Don't forget to make a scrapbook of the letters and congratulatory messages sent to you or your baby at the time of the birth. That book will mean a lot to him or her thirty years later.

TRADITIONAL CHRISTIAN CEREMONIES MARKING THE CHILD'S ARRIVAL AND MATURATION

The Christening

The first invitation you could ever receive involving another person is to his or her christening. Catholic children are often baptized within the first six weeks of life, in fact, often by two weeks of age. Protestants (except Baptists) are usually baptized by six months of age, but it is not unusual to have the ceremony later. When unbaptized adults convert to the Christian faith, they go through the same religious ritual the baby does, except that they can do what a baby can not—select their own godparents and stand up through the ceremony.

In most Protestant faiths, the pastor prefers that the godparents of the baby be of the same religion as the parents, but it is not obligatory; in the Catholic faith, the godfather and godmother must be Catholics, although co-godparents do not have to be.

It is a great honor to be chosen a godparent, but it isn't just an amusing gesture. It is a serious responsibility. The godparents should be very close friends or relatives (like an aunt or uncle or an older cousin). The main duty of godparents is to oversee the spiritual education of the child, particularly if the parents are deceased. Sometimes godparents are made legal guardians of the child by its parents; in case the parents are killed in an accident, the godparent then takes over the raising and education of his or her godchild.

A godparent who is unable to attend the baptismal ceremony may have a proxy stand in for him or her. The godparents separately or jointly give the baby a present. If there are financial problems in the family, they would give the baby something practical, like a complete layette, a stroller, or a freshly opened savings account in the baby's name. If there are no financial problems, they might give a piece of sterling silver engraved with the child's name and birth date (like a frame, small cup, baby spoon, or silver teething ring). If possible, a godparent should send the child a present every Christmas or birthday until he or she becomes an adult.

I have attended several weddings where the father of the bride was deceased; the bride walked up the aisle on her godfather's arm. Godparents and godchildren can have a very strong, meaningful relationship throughout their lives. They become surrogate parents and children for each other.

THE CHRISTENING PARTY

Generally, only the godparents, family, and perhaps a couple of very close friends attend the actual christening service in the church. (Protestants sometimes have their christening services at home; ask the minister what he will need other than a silver bowl to use as a font.) Afterward, there is often a reception—which may be an informal, light buffet lunch following a morning christening, an afternoon tea following a two or three o'clock ceremony, or champagne and cocktails following a christening at four or five in the afternoon.

Invitations are usually extended by note or by telephone call, although it is certainly proper to use a fill-in kind of invitation purchased from a store selling stationery and studio cards. It's wonderful to make the christening party a family affair, so that the young members of the family and close friends can help celebrate the happy event.

The baby should be dressed in the prettiest long white lace and ribbon-trimmed dress that can be borrowed from a relative or friend. Except for occasional passes through the party group to be shown off in the arms of a parent or older sibling, the baby should be kept in peace in his or her crib. He or she has already been through a lot on this day—including having a shock of cold water on the head—and has the right to be cranky and fussy in a house full of people and noise.

• *The highlight of the party is when the baby is toasted.* There should be a christening cake (a white cake with white icing, with perhaps the baby's initials and birth date carved in frosting). The first piece is cut by the baby's parents together (shades of cutting their wedding cake!). Then the godfather or godmother should raise a toast to the baby. (The baby should be present at this moment in the proceedings, unless he or she is crying lustily.) There should be wine, punch, or champagne in each guest's glass at this point (soda, of course, for any children or nondrinkers present). After the godparents have had their say, anyone else who has a clever or sentimental thought should make a toast. I'll never forget when a friend toasted our six-week-old son Malcolm at his christening. She made a very sentimental toast as I was holding him. Everyone raised their glasses to him, and his godfather said, "Well, now what do you say to that?" There was a stillness in the room, then Malcolm replied by letting out a large burp—right on cue. Perfect timing.

Everyone has his or her favorite christening stories. The parents should write down all these happenings in the child's baby book, so that he or she can laugh over them many years later. The presents given to the baby should also be recorded in this book. It's also a great idea to have a tape recording made of the toasts so that they can be saved for posterity.

First Communion

When a Catholic child in a Catholic school reaches seven (the "age of reason"), he or she takes a course in Catholic doctrine, and the class makes its First Communion together, usually at a regular Sunday morning Mass. The priest gives a special sermon to the children and gives them the Sacrament of the Eucharist before the others in the congregation receive it. (Non-Catholics guests invited by the family are not supposed to join the others in receiving Holy Communion or in taking the wine—nor do they have to "bob and kneel up and down," as my Protestant father used to describe our Catholic Mass. (If they want to follow the Catholics' "bobbing," they certainly may; if they prefer just sitting in the pew, that is okay, too.)

When a boy or girl is not a student in a Catholic school, he or she takes religious instruction outside—usually once a week for a few months. The child may then be the only one to make a First Communion at a particular Mass. The girls dress in white dresses with white veils for this occasion, the boys in dark blue or gray suits (or white, in summer resort weather), with either long pants or shorts (white knee socks with the latter).

Family members and close friends who are invited to attend the First Communion Mass would go on afterward to a breakfast or a brunch, usually in a public place close by.

As a gift for the occasion, a godparent would give the child something religious—for example, a book on the lives of the saints or a rosary that was blessed by the Pope in Rome. Others would give the child a present along the lines of an amusing book or a game.

Confirmation in the Protestant and Catholic Faiths

The confirmation ceremony signifies that the child has officially become a member of the congregation. Children in the seventh or eighth grades are given instruction in their faith to prepare them for this important day in their lives (they must be able to answer a detailed quiz). It is usually a quiet family occasion, with only the godparents and relatives present. Some very simple gifts are presented, sometimes religious in nature, but usually not. There is almost always a festive lunch held afterward, often hosted by a godparent. The boys and girls are dressed in their festive best.

TRADITIONAL JEWISH CEREMONIES FOR "THE COMING OF AGE"

B'rith Milah

Eight days after a Jewish baby boy is born, he is circumcised, given his name, and given godparents. This ceremony can take place in his parents' home or in a special room in the hospital. Only a few family members and close relatives attend the ceremony. Gifts for the baby are sometimes presented on this occasion.

A girl is given her name on the first Sabbath after she is born (in a service in the temple). Her father is called up to the Torah, where he recites a short prayer and states his daughter's name. The rabbi then recites a special blessing. Afterward, there is a small reception hosted by the baby's mother.

In the Reform congregation, the child's name is given and a prayer is said at the earliest religious service that both parents can attend after the baby's birth.

Bar and Bat Mitzvah

The celebration of the Bar Mitzvah takes place when a thirteen-year-old boy student of the Talmud traditionally comes of age and hears the thrilling message from the rabbi during the service, "You are now entering the Congregation of Israel." It is one of the most important events in a Jewish man's life.

In the Reform congregation the women's movement has sparked the custom of holding a similar ceremony for girls, called a Bas or Bat Mitzvah. This ceremony also takes place when the girl is thirteen. It is not permitted in Orthodox congregations. (Before the 1970s, girls were usually confirmed at the age of sixteen, when they graduated from religious school, and some families still prefer to have their daughters confirmed only—particularly in the Conservative congregation.)

The Bar or Bat Mitzvah is a most touching and impressive ceremony, lasting three hours in the Orthodox temple, one and a half to two hours in the Conservative temple, and just about an hour in the Reform temple. The young person has studied, practiced, and rehearsed long and hard for this great day in his or her life. After the indoctrination into the Congregation of Israel on the Sabbath, the immediate family may gather in a private room at the temple to talk with any members of the congregation who wish to offer their congratulations. This is often followed by a seated luncheon or dinner in a temple reception room, hotel, restaurant, or banquet hall. There is often dancing, beautiful flowers, and decorated tables. Sometimes the child will change from his conservative temple clothing to more dressy clothes for the party following the ceremony. Guests often attend in formal dress.

It is not appreciated when friends who were invited to a Bar or Bat Mitzvah attend the usually lavish party following the service, but not the service itself. In the family's eyes, to miss the child's reading of the lesson, which has been practiced for months and months, is to miss everything.

GIFTS

Gifts for the boy or girl should not be brought to the temple. In fact, it is better to send them to the child's home, rather than bring them to the reception.

Presents are very important to young people on the occasion of their Bar or Bat Mitzvah. For many years, it was traditional to give a young man a fountain pen, so there is an old Jewish joke that the boy says, "Today I am a fountain pen" (instead of "Today I am a man"). The children naturally like gifts but also appreciate checks, and the latter often range from $100 to $500. My old friend from my Kennedy White House days, lawyer Mike Feldman, a devout Reform Jew, does not believe in giving money. He gives every young person a year's subscription to the Jewish Publication Society in Philadelphia. The young person then receives for one year one or two excellent books every month on Jewish life and traditions—a very appropriate gift for this solemn religious occasion, to reinforce his faith.

Confirmation

Confirmation in a temple, for a boy or girl, usually takes place at the age of sixteen, seven weeks after the second day of Passover (on "The Feast of Weeks"). Children attending Hebrew school are confirmed as a group.

In Conservative congregations, some rabbis confirm both boys and girls, while others will Bar Mitzvah the boys only at age thirteen, and confirm the girls only at age sixteen.

DEBUTANTES

Today's "deb," who comes out after graduating from high school or after completing her first year of college, is a far cry from the glamour girls who preceded her before 1965. The youth rebellion and the women's movement of the mid-sixties all but sabotaged the tradition of the debutante year for young women of social standing who traditionally, by virtue of making their debuts, were now ready to be married off.

The days of the lavish single parties—dinner dances and private balls given for one young debutante alone—are over. Most young women come out in a group at one or two large, beautifully produced benefit dances. Their parents make a donation to the charity sponsoring the party.

Today's deb usually goes to three or four large parties, besides the ball at which she officially comes out. She wears a white dress to her own ball, and perhaps dresses of different colors to her friends' balls. She may have two or three escorts. She may use her brothers as her escorts. No one is looking at her escorts as possible husband material, which they used to, in the good old deb days, when all a young woman had on her mind was going to the next party, sleeping through the day to prepare for it.

There are many churches today, particularly in the black community, that sponsor debutante balls as fund-raisers.

If you are a relative or a very close friend of the debutante's family, it is nice to give her a personal gift (like real or costume jewelry, makeup, or a handbag), but it is no longer common practice.

* * *

Manners come into play from the time a child is born until that child is released into adulthood and independence. They are important in all the rites of passage that mark the stages of a child's development into that special adult that every parent hopes his or her child will become. Hopefully, we teach kindness, grace, and manners from the heart all the way.

14

The Last Rite of Passage: Funerals

It is a custom, in some forthright families where good relations abound, to discuss death and funeral plans frankly and honestly—but not ghoulishly—with elderly or ailing relatives while they are still living and able to make decisions. Usually, it is that person who wants such a discussion, to make sure that his or her wishes are carried out. The tenor of all such discussions should be loving, with deference demonstrated to those wishes.

No matter whether a family is prepared ahead of time or death catches them by surprise, the procedures described in this chapter will help anyone go through this last rite of passage more easily and in the proper manner.

TAKING CHARGE OF THE ARRANGEMENTS

When a relative or a close friend dies, someone should immediately shoulder the responsibility of ensuring that the bereaved family members are being helped and that immediate steps are taken to plan the funeral. There is much to be done—quite apart from trying to console the family affected by the death. A relative or close friend of the deceased (such as a brother-in-law, a business partner, or an adult sister of the deceased) should offer to serve as "director of funeral events." As such he or she will be responsible for the overall smooth coordination of the funeral and interment, and also for helping the surviving family in every possible way. The person acting as director of the funeral would be there most of the day with the family for two or three days, or until the funeral events are finished.

He or she should first make a checklist of what has to be done and appoint the logical volunteers to get these various chores done responsibly. He or she should also make sure that everyone is doing what they promised to do and that every action represents the wishes of the deceased's spouse, parent, sibling, or child—whoever is the major survivor.

The person in charge must do the following:

- *Find someone to take charge of the small children,* if there are any—to feed them, play with them, and keep them occupied. This may necessitate taking the very little ones home to the friend's house to stay with the friend's own children.

- *Find a person to be in charge of the telephone* at the home of the deceased, to make sure that there is a capable adult (working in shifts, if necessary) handling the constantly ringing telephone. That person should also make sure that

  o All family members and close friends of the deceased are notified by telephone of the death and the funeral arrangements
  o The deceased's boss and place of employment are notified of the death and, if necessary, that the grieving survivor's boss is notified.
  o All queries as to when the services will be held are answered correctly

- *Immediately notify the lawyer of the deceased.*
- *Notify the funeral home* and deal with its director in terms of

  o Possibly arranging a viewing or wake to be held there prior to the funeral services
  o Selecting the casket and arranging for it to be open or closed during the viewing
  o Deciding on the burial clothing and getting it into the hands of the undertaker
  o Coordinating burial plans with the church and the cemetery (or crematorium)

- *See that someone is put in charge of getting food on the table for everyone staying in the house* during the funeral period.
- *See that someone is in charge of the logistics and invitations for the lunch, tea, cocktails, or supper to be served immediately following*

the interment. This gathering is held either at the home of the bereaved, at the house of a close friend or relative of the bereaved, or in a hotel private dining room or a private club. The mourners invited to this gathering after the burial would include

- o Members of the family
- o The minister or priest in charge of the service
- o Ushers and honorary pallbearers, if there were any
- o Close social and business friends
- o Family retainers (the housekeeper, baby-sitter, gardener, or cook)
- o Anyone who came from out of town for the services

• *See that someone at the house is in charge of listing all incoming messages,* with carefully noted names and addresses, so that thank-you notes may easily be mailed later. These might include

- o Telegrams and Mailgrams
- o Telephone messages of sympathy
- o Hand-delivered letters of condolence
- o Mass cards—for a deceased Catholic only. (A person of any religion may arrange with a Catholic priest anywhere to have a Mass said for the soul of the deceased. When this is arranged, a card to this effect is mailed to the family, giving the priest's name and parish, and sometimes giving the date of the special Mass. The person who ordered the Mass said—or the "novena of prayers," another option—usually makes a gift of anywhere from $5 to $25 to the priest or the church, according to what he or she wishes to pay. A payment, however, is not obligatory.)
- o Condolence cards, which may be purchased from a stationer or greeting card shop. (Don't just sign a name; write a sentence or two by hand at the bottom of the message printed on the card.)
- o Flowers. (In my opinion, the best time to send them is a few weeks *after* the funeral, when the surviving family is really feeling blue and let down.)
- o Gifts of food for the family

• *Make sure that someone is at the house to assume charge of all out-of-towners* coming for the funeral:

- o Getting them hotel reservations, if necessary
- o Meeting their planes, trains, or buses
- o Providing them with transportation during the one or two days they are in town
- o Making sure their meals are taken care of

• *Appoint someone to call the local newspapers and have a paid death notice* put in the earliest possible edition of the local newspapers. (See below.)

Preparing the Death Notice

• *If the deceased was a prominent person, appoint someone to prepare his or her obituary.* Be sure to check the facts in the obituary with the spouse, parent, or sibling of the deceased. The obituary should be hand-delivered as soon as it is ready to the Metropolitan Desk of the local newspapers (as well as sent later to the alumni magazines of the deceased's schools or to the journal of any organization to which he or she belonged). An obituary for a prominent person would contain the following information:

- o Name and address of the person
- o Date and place where he or she died
- o Cause of death
- o Name of spouse
- o City of birth
- o Name of his or her company or place of work and title
- o Education, including both earned and honorary degrees
- o Military service, if any
- o Corporate directorships
- o Any major awards received
- o Titles of published works, films, or plays and names of museums where his or her art is exhibited or major theaters where he or she may have sung or danced
- o Names of survivors and their relationship to the deceased
- o Details of the funeral services and interment
- o Name and telephone number of the person to be called in case further information is needed by the newspaper

Here is a sample death notice for a newspaper:

JONES, Jacqueline Teaman. On June 29, 1991, age 38. Beloved wife of Hamilton, devoted mother of Geoffrey, James, and Alana. Sister of Marian Berquist and Geoffrey Teaman. Friends may call at Frank E. Campbell, 1076 Madison Ave. at 81 St., Sunday 2–5 P.M. Mass of Christian burial at St. Thomas More Church, 65 E. 89 St., Monday 10 A.M. Interment at St. Mary's Cemetery, Yonkers, NY.

• *It is not necessary to include age* of the deceased in the death notice—only if it is a personal preference.

• *If the family does not wish people to go to the cemetery,* they omit the interment notice. If the family does not wish anyone at either the service or the interment, they put "Funeral private" in the paid death notice.

• *If the family wishes to designate where contributions may be sent* in the name of the deceased, the information is included at the end of the paid notice. For example: "Contributions may be made to the American Cancer Society" or whatever the charity may be.

Some families put in the death notice, "Contributions may be made to the donor's favorite charity."

THE PROPRIETIES IN CONNECTION WITH A FUNERAL

What Do You Say?

People are usually at a loss for words when it comes time to talk to the family of someone who has just died.

All you have to do is tell the survivor in just a few words

- How sorry you were to learn of this sad news.
- How much the deceased will be missed by friends and colleagues.
- How much you loved this person and what a personal loss you feel.
- How much you grieve for the person who is left behind.
- What a wonderful person the deceased was. (Recount warm, loving anecdotes about your late departed friend, and laud his or her accomplishments.)

Sending Flowers

There are options on where to send flowers:

- To the home of the bereaved
- To the funeral home
- To the church
- To the gravesite

The family will state its preference or choice of the last three categories.

Flowers sent to the funeral home are usually transferred to the gravesite on the day of the interment.

Flowers are never sent for an Orthodox Jewish funeral.

In a Catholic church, only a spray of flowers for the top of the casket (from the family) and perhaps one other bouquet of flowers for the altar are permitted. In Protestant churches, flowers are permitted on and near the altar.

THE CARD FOR FUNERAL FLOWERS

The white envelope, containing the card, would be addressed as follows:

The Funeral of Anthony Stedwell Creighton
[Address of the funeral home or gravesite]

The envelope should also contain the name and mailing address of the donor of the flowers.

The white card, on which the message is written in black ink, should state simply something like this: "With deepest sympathy from the Reynolds Family"; or, if sent by colleagues from the office: "With deepest sympathy from the Granger Insurance Company."

Attire for Funerals

• *The widow* should be in a discreetly quiet dress or suit. The days are past when she had to wear a black dress, hat, and veil to the services, but she still looks more dignified in a solid-color costume—on the dark side.

• *The young daughters* of the deceased should wear their best dresses and party shoes, out of respect for their late parent. *Young sons* should be in gray shorts with gray or white knee socks, or gray slacks, with a navy blazer, white shirt, and tie and well-polished shoes.

• *Teenagers and grown children* should wear appropriately quiet clothing. Young men and grown sons should dress as the ushers and pallbearers do, in dark suits, white shirt, dark tie, and dark shoes.

• *Honorary pallbearers and ushers* would wear dark suits, white shirts, black four-in-hand ties, and black shoes and socks.

• *Friends and colleagues* attending the services would be dressed in quiet clothing—the women in modest dresses or suits of a solid color (or at least, a print that is not too colorful and flashy), and the men in dark suits.

CEREMONIES FOR OR HONORING THE DECEASED

A Viewing or Wake

A viewing or wake is often held at the funeral home the day before the funeral or, if the person was prominent, on two successive days before the funeral. Usually it is about two hours long, and it is often held late in the afternoon or early evening, so that people who work will be able to come. Everyone who comes signs in the book that is at the entrance to the main rooms. The casket is present (open or closed), often all of the flowers sent to the home are on display, and the family stands together in a kind of receiving line if there are large numbers of people coming. Otherwise, it is informal, without a receiving line.

Everyone greets—and perhaps hugs or kisses—the grieving family members, whispering words of comfort.

The Christian Funeral Service

At a large funeral of an important and prominent person, there may be honorary pallbearers and ushers, all of whom are chosen by the family of the deceased. It is a great honor to be asked to serve in this capacity, and although traditionally pallbearers have been men, today a woman may also be asked to serve.

• *Ushers* help seat the attendees. They are young men and women friends or relatives of the deceased—perhaps office colleagues, nephews and nieces, or godchildren. They direct people to their seats, filling the front of the church first. (The very front pews, however, are reserved and marked for the family on the right side, and for the honorary pallbearers and the ushers on the left side.)

• *The pallbearers,* employees of the funeral home, actually handle and carry the casket in and out of the church.

• *Honorary pallbearers,* usually from four to ten in number—the men in dark suits, the women in dark dresses—precede the casket in and out of the church, walking two by two in a procession. If the casket should already be in place at the altar at the start of the services (in Protestant churches, it is often covered with a blanket of flowers), the honorary pallbearers march in just before the service begins and take the front left pews, opposite the family. (The ushers have already seated themselves to the left, behind where the pallbearers are to sit.)

An honorary pallbearer is a distinguished person, someone who is known and respected in the community but also a good friend of the deceased. He or she may have been a business associate or someone like the deceased's doctor or lawyer. This person may have been active with the deceased in some civic or political activity or may just have been an old golfing buddy.

• *The family of the deceased enters from the vestry and family members take their seats in the front right-hand pews.* The service is now ready to begin.

THE MUSIC

The music for a Christian funeral is usually organ music. The church music director confers in advance with the family of the deceased to see if they have any special wishes; if not, there is almost always a repertoire of appropriate music ready for this sad occasion. Other music groups, such as chamber music groups, a harpist, or brass quintets may also be asked to provide the music.

There is often a soloist—hopefully, a professional singer who freelances for church funerals. It is better to dissuade an amateur, whether a relative or friend of the deceased, from singing. (I remember the sister-in-law of the deceased at one funeral I attended who insisted on singing; she was so flat the entire time that the congregation had all it could do to keep from laughing, despite their sorrow. Her performance flawed an otherwise dignified and moving service.)

THE EULOGY

For the funeral service (or for a later memorial service), this is usually given by the minister and by a relative or close friend of the deceased. The family decides who may speak other than the clergy person; if three or more will speak, a sheet showing the order is given to each person, so that he or she will approach the pulpit or podium at the right moment. Sometimes a teenage (or older) son and daughter will speak about his or her late parent. A brother or sister of the deceased might say something. There are no rules about who speaks from the pulpit or how many do it, but if you are going to give a eulogy, there are rules to help keep the service from dragging:

• Get in and out of the pulpit quickly. If you go slowly from your pew up to the pulpit when it's your turn to speak, the interval between speakers may take several minutes, and the service will seem to drag interminably.

• Speak for no longer than seven minutes. Three minutes is all right, too, and five minutes is just about perfect.

• If you should completely choke up while you're talking, don't try to continue. (Perhaps the toughest time of all to speak is when it concerns the death of a child.) If you're sobbing and out of control, just say, "I'm sorry," and step down. Everyone will understand.

• Be respectful and affectionate; tell a nice, sweet, humorous story that will make those present smile with fond remembrance. If you worked in the same office as the deceased, mention how much he or she was loved and respected by everyone in the company. If you sailed or played tennis with the deceased, mention some humorous incidents involving his or her skills in the sport. Always end on a note of high praise—for example, mentioning how much he loved his family and what a great legacy he has left them.

A FUNERAL SERVICE PROGRAM

A funeral service program to distribute to each person who attends the services is a nice touch. This is often a double-fold pamphlet, printed in black on heavy white paper. It sometimes includes a headshot photo of the deceased, banded in black (so that it looks like a black frame), with a special prayer printed beneath the picture. The order of events, the names of the clergy and the speakers, and the order of the hymns (as well as the words, so that all can join in) are included in the program. Often special prayers are printed in the leaflet, too. It is a very nice memento of the service and helps people follow the clergy in saying the prayers and singing the hymns.

A Cremation

A cremation, which is not acceptable to the Jewish faith and only recently acceptable for Catholics, is preceded by a funeral service in a church. Afterward only a few relatives and close friends go to the crematorium, where another brief service is held. The ashes are then given to the family and dispersed by them in a place the deceased stipulated in his or her will. Sometimes they are placed in a container, often an urn, which is then placed in the family burial plot. (The care and disposal of the ashes is regulated in some states by law.)

Jewish Services

Orthodox, Conservative, and Reform Jews have different customs for funeral services. Attention is given to the bereaved family, the members of which stay home in mourning for a set period of days. In the Orthodox congregation, for example, following the burial of the deceased (within twenty-four hours after his or her death), the family remains in the home for seven days, "sitting Shivah." Neighbors bring them food, but they do not have any social contact with the outside world, nor do they conduct business, take telephone calls, or do any kind of work. Every evening, close friends may come to the home to participate in a religious service.

Reform Jews often have one brief religious service with a rabbi in their home right after the burial. They spend from one to three days at home, refraining from social and business contacts following the death of a loved one. In the evening, they light one or two Sabbath candles, and an adult in the family says the blessing. All Jews try to visit the graves of their parents once a year—between Rosh Hashanah and Yom Kippur. Devout Jews do not miss a year, even though the graves may be far away from where they live.

Memorial Service

A memorial service is held to honor a much loved or famous person after the deceased has already been interred. It can be held in a funeral home, a church, a community auditorium, a school auditorium, or other similar setting. A memorial service is best held within two months of a person's death, but it may be held later than that. If the person was prominent, there might be two or three memorial services held in the different cities in which he or she was well known.

A clergyman may lead the service, but often it is a lay person with close connections to the deceased who presides, if the ceremony is held outside a church setting.

The person in charge of organizing the service arranges ahead of time for persons close to the deceased—as few as two, but often many more—to give eulogies at the ceremony (and asks that they be kept brief). At the time of the service these people are called upon to come forward and speak.

There may be prayers and hymns or other appropriate music before, during, and after the service.

I remember one memorial service for a beloved patriarch of an entire town, held on the great lawn of his estate with most of the town in attendance. He was of Scottish descent and had many Scottish connections, so in honor of this a bagpiper stepped forward after the eulogies. Silence fell as he began piping his way toward the water at the lawn's end, playing "The Flowers of the Forest." The volume of the music lowered with each step the piper took, until it faded away altogether at the water's edge and the ceremony was over.

Following the service, the family may receive in a nearby room in the church or auditorium, and coffee and cakes may be served. Or the family may simply stand outside on the steps or sidewalk afterward, to talk to those who came and thank them for their support.

There may be lunch or cocktails served in a nearby house or public place after the service.

Often, there is a book on a table in the vestibule of the place where the service is held, in which you sign, so that the family will know you attended the service.

AFTER THE FUNERAL OR MEMORIAL

The Survivor Writes His or Her Thank-you

After the sadness of the funeral period is over, when the main surviving members of the family feel strong enough to tackle the job, one of them should write a personal note of thanks to

- o The relative or friend who served as director of all the proceedings
- o The clergy person who handled the services
- o The honorary pallbearers and ushers

o The people who gave eulogies. (It is not necessary to write family members, but it is a nice touch to do so.)

o Everyone who sent a telegram, condolence card, Mass card, condolence letter, or flowers

o Everyone who gave a charitable contribution in memory of the deceased

The family of a prominent person whose death created a large outpouring of sympathy (and on whose behalf hundreds of acknowledgments must be sent) should order from a good stationer white cards edged in black, engraved with a message of thanks from the family. The wording is simple, something like this:

> *The family of Gregory Johnson Caldwell*
> *greatly appreciates your kind expression of sympathy.*

However, it is nice to personalize these cards. A handwritten word by a family member at the bottom makes the card a strong personal statement of appreciation from the family.

The task of writing and addressing thank-you notes and acknowledgments should be apportioned out to all family members. (In other words, one person should not be saddled with the entire job.)

If you plan to acknowledge expressions of sympathy toward a deceased member of your family on notepaper, buy boxes of good white stationery—either single sheet or fold-over notes or correspondence cards. After you express your thanks in your note, write something like, "Dad always loved you, I hope you know that," or "We will miss her terribly, and we particularly appreciated your sending those lovely roses—because they were her favorite flowers."

Showing Continuing Support

When someone has died, there is a lot of rallying around his or her family at the time of the funeral. Everyone seems to be calling, writing, offering sympathy. But when the support *really* matters is when a surviving spouse or child is left alone afterward. Two, four, eight months later—that is when your support is most needed. Call your friend. Invite him or her for dinner; include him or her in your leisure activities. That's when friends really stand up and are counted!

Remember your late friend each year by getting in touch with the family of the deceased on his or her birthday—a happy memory—rather than on the anniversary of the death.

* * *

There is nothing more difficult to accept nor more absolute than death. It's the time when heart counts more than anything else in this world. It's not the cost of the huge bouquet someone sent to the funeral that matters to the grieving family; it's the warmth of your arms around their collective shoulders that counts, and your promise to "be around to help—always."

PART IV
ENTERTAINING AND GIFT GIVING

15

ENTERTAINING TODAY'S WAY

This section contains my point of view about entertaining—its human side—and is based on the theory that if your heart's in the right place, *your event will always be a success.*

Americans are entertaining less and less in their homes these days. There are repetitive excuses given for this sad state of affairs, none of which, in my opinion, hold up:

• *"I'm so busy and pressured; I work too hard."* Rebuttal: *Everyone* is busy and pressured. Entertaining fits into your life simply by making it one of your priorities—like the two Chicago ad agency executives, a married couple who each work a sixty-hour week, have two teenage children, and give a buffet supper for friends mixed with clients the first Sunday evening of every month in the year, August included!

• *"We can't entertain until the children are grown."* Rebuttal: Again, if you want to, you can arrange to give time and thought to "having people over" several times a year. You just fit things into your schedule and arrange for baby-sitting help. You work on getting your party ready a little at a time, several nights before or the weekend before, when small members of the household are asleep.

- *"My apartment is too small."* Rebuttal: No apartment is too small for staging a dinner party for four or six. People do miraculous things in small spaces by borrowing folding bridge tables and collapsible chairs, keeping the ice in the bathtub and putting a board over it to use as a bar, and sliding trays of dirty dishes temporarily under the bed because there's no room in the sink!

- *"We can't get any proper help."* Rebuttal: Yes you can, with a little effort. There's always someone who needs extra cash who will come to help make your party a success—like that teenager in the neighborhood or in the apartment house who is always asking if he or she can wash your car or mow your lawn or baby-sit.

- *"I don't have a clue to how to make up a guest list."* Rebuttal: Composing a guest list is a stimulating exercise, totally creative. Who but you would have thought of seating your children's lovely-looking young gym teacher next to your overweight bank executive friend who's trying to slim down, and who becomes so inspired by his dinner partner that he resolves to start an exercise program the next morning? Who but you would have thought to seat your recently widowed best friend as a surprise next to your old friend from college days (himself also recently widowed), who you heard was visiting in your city? The best guest list of all is a mixture of people you know, and bringing together unexpected combinations is the key to success.

- *"I really am not a cook."* Rebuttal: You don't have to be. There are frozen foods in the supermarket that can be enhanced by adding fresh vegetables. There are gourmet food takeout places that will do the major part of the work for you, such as preparing your chicken pot pie and dessert, so all you have to do is rustle up a green salad. (Or, if you can afford it, the caterer will do the entire job for you.)

- *"I don't have the proper table accoutrements."* Rebuttal: A poor excuse. That's what friends are for—to borrow from!

- *"I can't cope when things go wrong*—like the guest of honor doesn't show up, or something's wrong with my food, or people don't seem to be having a good time." Rebuttal: Those things don't always happen, and when they do, you can turn it into a plus (like my fancy roast beef dinner, at which I discovered, just before the guests arrived, that I had never turned on the oven for the roast; we ate delivered cheeseburgers and it was one of the best parties we gave).

The rewards of personal satisfaction you receive for entertaining will far outweigh any efforts you make to psych yourself into becoming a host. "Entertaining" is a general term covering all kinds of efforts, small and big, that you make for other people. You're entertaining when you invite a lonely elderly neighbor for a cup of tea, as well as when you invite twenty-four people important to you in business for a seated dinner. You're entertaining if you're a woman serving three other ladies a cold chicken salad lunch on a hot summer's day or if you're a man serving "a bunch of the guys" hot corned beef and cabbage after a poker game on a cold winter's night. In all these cases, you have taken the time and trouble to invite people to your home—or perhaps out to a restaurant for a meal.

When you host people just for the sake of pleasing them—to give them a good time and make them feel happy and glad—you're reaching out to them and thinking outside, not inside. All the pleasure and contentment you give them will come back to you, multiplied.

So do it. Call people and ask them to come be your guests. And while you're at it, go on the record—send them a reminder by mail, so that they won't forget the logistical details communicated in the telephone conversation!

I'm not going to tell you very much in this book about what to serve or how to cook it. That's up to you—and those many books out there on the subject. I'm going to give you all the *reasons why* you should want to have people over, why you should make an effort, why entertaining is a worthy priority on your list of activities. I'm going to tell you what makes a good host and guest, which today is a far cry from all the ludicrous, anachronistic formalities of yesteryear's entertaining. There are, however, some traditional tried and true ways of doing things, everything from knowing where you put a fork on the table, to being aware that one serves from the left and picks up from the right of the guest. I'm going to teach you how a dinner should properly be served, so that if you have someone serving who doesn't know how to do it, you can help him or her. (That person serving may be your own teenager.) These rules are not capricious or foppish; they have evolved from experience through the years; they represent the most efficient way to do something.

I'm not going to tell you what wines to buy, but rather how to serve them. I'm not going to advise you what flowers to put in the center of the table, because you may want to put beach pebbles and shells there instead. My job is just to give you a few ideas that will stimulate your own imagination. I won't agonize over how many courses you will serve at your meal, because that's your choice, but I will advise you to serve very few—two or three—and to use your energies instead on making what is simple and easy taste good and on serving it properly. I won't sympathize with you over your fear of breaking someone's wineglass in his house or spilling food on his table. Instead, I'll tell you how to clean up whatever mess you may have made, and how to apologize so nicely that your host won't give a second thought to what you consider a disaster.

The important thing to remember is that whatever position you are in, that of a host or of a guest, you have responsibilities and creative possibilities. As one individual you have the capacity to make or break a party. That sober thought should instill in you a feeling of power!

This chapter is all about making a party successful. And to me, two people make a party, as well as two thousand. What a wonderful feeling it is to serve a meal or to host an event the guests will talk about with admiration for months to come. And what fun it is to be a guest at someone else's party that is worthy of remembering for months to come.

It's all up to you. No one else makes you into a consummate host or a consummate guest. You do. And remember, too, that in order to break the rules of entertaining with verve and panache, you have to know them in the first place!

HOW ENTERTAINING BRINGS FRIENDS INTO YOUR LIFE

People's motives for entertaining—or, let me correct that, the reasons people *should* be motivated to entertain—encompass a variety of considerations. The most important one, of course, is that people need to be with people. Loneliness is a common ailment; humans need to get out of their homes and to interact with other humans once in a while. The most effective way to answer the need for human companionship is through entertaining. If you really don't have the proper home in which to entertain, take your guests out—to a restaurant, hotel, or club. The truth is, however, that many people who think their homes aren't worthy to serve as a backdrop for receiving guests are "copping out." I have a young friend who entertains all the time in a small, ugly apartment (his description) in New York (it's all he can afford). He says, "My friends are the decoration around here. I have beautiful friends who make my apartment beautiful." Another friend who also hates her apartment (it's all she can afford) lights her dinner parties only with candlelight, so that no one can see what her apartment looks like! Too many people use the excuse of an insufficiently grand home as justification for never entertaining.

If you're entertaining on business or at charity events, which is the nature of most entertaining these days, it usually takes place in hotels and restaurants and is often cold, without a vestige of warmth from a personal touch. But you can change all that—you can make it warm, personal, and individually exciting. I'll tell you how.

Perhaps you will find yourself in one of these categories.

- *You owe someone who has entertained you.* Bachelors of the world, this means you, too. Just because you're single men and in demand does not mean that you can continue being constantly feted, without ever repaying your social obligations!
- *You meet someone who interests you,* and you'd like to get to know that person better.
- *You feel a great need to enlarge your social circle;* you're stuck in the circle you are part of now, and it's not getting any better.

o *You're new in town and are starting from scratch socially.*
o *You want to rekindle an old romance.*
o *You want to ignite a new one.*
o *You feel compassion for someone who's lonely.*
o *You want to help a friend or relative of a good friend* who wrote, asking you to help this person.
o *You realize your hosting expertise will help expand your business contacts.*
o *You want to show your gratitude to a person or a group* for what they did for you personally, or for what they did for one of your favorite causes.
o *You want to go to work on someone in a compatible environment,* so that he or she will offer you a job, lend you money, help you run for office, write you an important letter of reference, get you on a board, invest in your company, maybe even want to marry you!
o *You feel invitationless* and conclude that maybe if you start to entertain, others will entertain you back.
o *You want to honor a special person,* to make him or her feel very good, either because that person has done something extraordinary and deserves the honor, or because he or she is sad and depressed.
o *You want to mark a special occasion*—an anniversary, the opening of something, the honoring of someone, the awarding of something to a person or an institution.
o *You just want to please someone.*
o *You have a sudden desire to shake yourself up and do something totally out of character.*

THE KINDS OF ENTERTAINING PEOPLE LOVE

If you're wondering about the kinds of occasions in which people love to be included, have a conversation with those whom you'd like to invite along any of the following lines:

o "Come on over after church to join us for a big family breakfast."
o "I'm giving a breakfast for the organizing committee of our big benefit a week from Monday, the seventh, at eight A.M. It should be a productive meeting, and I'm also a very good omelet and waffle maker!"
o "Come for lunch on Saturday, the twentieth. It will be a surprise birthday party for Leslie, so don't say a word to her."
o "We'd like to invite you to an open house to inaugurate our newly

redecorated house on Sunday the second, from noon to five o'clock. This time it's for adults only."

- "We're new in the neighborhood, so we're having an open house for all our neighbors, children included, the Saturday before Thanksgiving, from four P.M. to seven-thirty P.M. It would be nice to get to know your family, so do drop by."
- "Why don't you come by for a cup of tea Saturday at four o'clock? I haven't seen you in such a long time, and I want to catch up."
- "We'd like to invite you two for dinner Friday, the twenty-fifth, at seven o'clock. We'll sit down at the table at seven-forty-five." (There are no rules about where your dinner must be served. It can be in the house or the garden, in the kitchen, on the patio, by the pool, on the back porch, in the gazebo, out in the yard, up in the treehouse, on the dock or at the beach. Don't forget the bedroom, either.)
- "Do stop by for 'a drink and a bite' " (before or after the concert, play, art exhibition, movie, or your children's piano recital).
- "Come for supper at eight-thirty, before the club's big Leap Year Dance."
- "Join us for one of our regular Sunday evening chili suppers on the thirtieth at six o'clock."
- "I'd like to invite you to my 'Singles Only' party—with after-dinner drinks and dessert ('Bubbles and Sweets'), on Wednesday, April fifteenth, at nine o'clock."
- "Remember the date—a week from Saturday, for a cocktail-buffet at our apartment. We'll have lots of food, so you won't need dinner afterward!"
- "We're organizing a big family picnic for the first Sunday in July. We're coping with the games and athletic equipment. I'm counting on each family to bring one dish—enough to feed the entire gang. Would you be able to bring the salad?"
- "Join us after the theater—we have some of the other benefit attendees coming by our house to collapse, talk about the play, and have a glass of champagne."
- "We'll have hot food waiting to warm you up after Sunday afternoon's football game at the stadium."
- "Our gourmet club is meeting at my house this month. It's Spanish Night. Hope you can join us on the thirtieth for a little *Olé*-ing."
- "We're starting a book club, because we all feel we could use some intellectual stimulation. Two weeks before we meet we will all start reading the same book, and then we'll discuss it at dinner. This first session is at our apartment. I hope you both can join us, Friday the first, at seven."

- o "It will be your choice, whether you want hot chocolate or soup at four after ice-skating Sunday afternoon. Come to our house, and we'll warm up watching the Winter Olympics skating finals on television."
- o "Yes, we'd like your whole family to join us for a pool party on July fourth, from eleven A.M. to four P.M. Just bring your own bathing suits and towels. We'll supply the rest!"
- o "I'm *finally* having a dinner party, so would you both be able to come for dinner at the Palm Restaurant on Thursday the fifth, at seven-thirty? I thought it would be fun to dress up for a change, so I'm making it black tie. I'm inviting ten close pals to say thanks for being so nice to me since Jeffrey died, and you are at the top of my list."
- o "Yes, come see me tomorrow morning at ten-thirty with the baby. We can put her in Jennifer's old pen, and she can play with Jennifer's old toys. You and I can have some coffee and some sinful Danish that is waiting for us in the freezer. We'll have a long, much-needed chat."

Any kind of invitation can be very meaningful to the person who receives it. And by extending such an invitation, the host gives the recipient much more pleasure than he or she probably realizes.

Every kind of invitation—formal or informal, to a big event or to one with only one guest—requires thought, planning, and, to be really successful, a caring and kind heart.

EXTENDING INVITATIONS

*T*he invitation is what makes people come to your party.* If you are anxious to have people come to whatever you're planning, concentrate on extending the best possible invitation for that event, and use the most effective method for extending it. Perhaps it's the warmth of your own voice and the excitement and enthusiasm you convey over the telephone that will make a potential guest eager to come to your party. Or perhaps it's your handwritten note or the look of the distinguished or amusing printed piece that you mail that will entice your guests to come.

There is a wealth of creativity in the field of invitations today, and your options are numerous. (As the late Elsa Maxwell, a legendary party-giver, once said in an interview, "Make them *die* with anticipation to come to your party because of the invitation, and once you get them there, don't let them down!")

How Far Ahead Do You Extend an Invitation?

An invitation extended well in advance is more appreciated than one extended a week or less before the date. If someone calls you on the telephone and invites you for dinner at their house in three weeks' time, you feel very differently about that evening than if your host invites you two days before.

If you plan to have invitations printed for a large party, remember it can take from two to four weeks. (Count on at least four weeks to have them engraved.) Then you must also address the envelopes and hand-stamp them. Add five days from between the day you mail them and the day they reach their destinations.

Naturally, there are many invitations for get-togethers that are last-minute and spur-of-the-moment and turn out to be great fun. However, most social planning involves mailing invitations, and your invitations should arrive well in advance of your event.

• If you have a choice on your entertaining timetable, follow this rule of thumb for mailing or telephoning your invitations. *Put your invitations in the mailbox:*

  o Two to three weeks before a business or social lunch
  o Three weeks before a cocktail party
  o Four weeks before an important business or social dinner
  o Three weeks before an informal dinner
  o Six to eight weeks before a wedding
  o Six to eight weeks before a dance
  o Two to three months before a weekend in your home

• *Don't be insulted if you receive a last-minute invitation.* Some people organize their dinners at the last minute. Don't be insulted if you're invited only a couple of days before or even on the morning of the party. And don't be miffed if you know you weren't on the host's original guest list but are part of the last-minute fill-ins for drop-outs. When I'm asked if someone will lose face in accepting an invitation where he or she is obviously a last-minute substitute for a guest who dropped out, I say "no." The invitee should readily accept this kind of invitation—because he or she will probably have a great time (which turns out to be true more often than not). It is also a golden opportunity for the last-minute guest to prove so attractive and such good company that he or she will land on the host's first list the next time a party is given in that house.

Save-the-Date Cards

A "save-the-date card" is sent usually three or four months in advance for a very large and important event, which could be anything from a corporate centennial celebration to a large fund-raising event such as a charity auction or a benefit ball.

The save-the-date card, which may be a simple printed postcard or a specially designed printed card with matching envelope, is the first news a potential guest has of the event. Therefore, it should be well designed and well executed—a hastily scrawled postcard is not going to make much of an impression.

A sample text follows for a card announcing a forthcoming private function. The hosts' names in this case are at the bottom:

PLEASE SAVE THIS DATE
Thursday, September 28, 1993
for a black tie dinner dance
in honor of our parents' fiftieth anniversary
at the David Browns' farm
corner of Spring Lake and Ransome roads
Omaha
Invitations will be forthcoming
The David Browns; Susan Brown; The Richard Tysons

A sample hold-the-date card for a fund-raising benefit:

HOLD THIS DATE
Saturday, June 15th
Black Tie Gala
8 o'clock to midnight
in celebration of the opening of
Il Mondo Chic store
The World Mall
Newport, California
A benefit for the Institute of International Education
Invitations to follow
(For information, call 000/000-0000)

Parts of a Formal Invitation

A formal invitation should follow the traditional form simply because over the decades it has proven to communicate the information most efficiently.

For example, this invitation, in eight parts, is a good form to use for your own social functions—adapted, of course, to your own needs. You might wish to substitute your dress instructions ("Black Tie") in the lower right-hand corner for "Valet Parking." You might wish to change what is written in the lower left of this invitation, where the RSVP information is given, according to whether you wish to furnish only a telephone number or only an address, or whether you wish to say "RSVP card enclosed" or whether you wish to put nothing in that corner (an enclosed, self-addressed RSVP card is, after all, self-explanatory).

STANDARD FORM FOR A FORMAL INVITATION

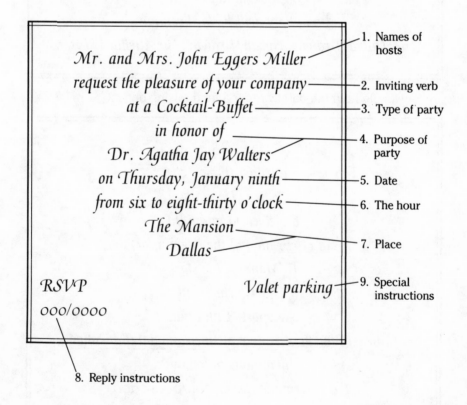

Mr. and Mrs. John Eggers Miller — 1. Names of hosts

request the pleasure of your company — 2. Inviting verb

at a Cocktail-Buffet — 3. Type of party

in honor of — 4. Purpose of party
Dr. Agatha Jay Walters

on Thursday, January ninth — 5. Date

from six to eight-thirty o'clock — 6. The hour

The Mansion
Dallas — 7. Place

RSVP   *Valet parking* — 9. Special instructions

ooo/oooo

8. Reply instructions

Who Does the Inviting?

It's important always to have a host on your invitation, not just to use a corporate name. In other words, an invitation that reads "The Corner Stores, Inc. invites you to . . ." or "Miggs National Bank cordially invites you to . . ." does not sound right. A human being or a group of human beings should always do the inviting, and proper names are best. At least a human title should be present on the invitation, if for some reason you don't wish to list names—for example: "The Chairman of The Corner Stores, Inc. cordially invites you to . . ." or "The Board of Directors of the Miggs National Bank requests the pleasure of your company . . ."

- When there is more than one host:

  - You may list their names vertically or horizontally; your graphic artist may wish to list the names as part of a special design scheme of the invitation.
  - List the names alphabetically if the hosts are on a par in age and importance; otherwise, list the senior people first.
  - If the party is being given in someone's home, list that couple's name first, the other co-hosts after.
  - Use a uniform system of listing names if there are many, such as on a benefit committee. In this case, it is preferable to list people by their given and surnames, without titles, as shown in the column on the left, and not with a hodge-podge of titles, as shown in the column on the right:

Correct Listing	*Incorrect Listing*
Marilyn Acorn	Mrs. John Acorn
John Agnew	Mr. John Agnew
Evelyn Andrew	Mrs. Evelyn Andrew
Victoria Arthur	Mrs. Tazewell Arthur
Benjamin Barnwell	Benjamin Barnwell, Esq.
Barbara Berson	Ms. Barbara Berson
Jennifer Bierwirth	Miss Jennifer Bierwirth
etc.	etc.

Invitationese (The Language of Invitations)

OPTIONS FOR THE INVITING VERB PHRASE

FORMAL

> *Mr. and Mrs. Seamus O'Brien*
> *request the pleasure of your company*
> *at dinner, etc.*

INFORMAL

> *Mr. and Mrs. Seamus O'Brien*
> *invite you to*
> (*or*, cordially invite you to)
> *a dinner*

• Also formal: A calligrapher or someone with a fine hand writes in the names of the guests right on the printed or engraved invitation:

> *Mr. and Mrs. Seamus O'Brien*
> *request the pleasure of*
> *Mr. and Mrs. Hiram Hoguets'*
> (this line written by calligrapher)
> *company at dinner*
> *etc.*

OPTIONS FOR STATING THE PURPOSE

Much the same phrasing is used for either a formal or informal invitation, except that for a formal invitation the English version of "honor" ("honour") and "favor" ("favour") is always used.

The honored guests' names or the reason the party is being given is placed either:

- In the upper left-hand corner of the invitation, where it may be written by hand, or
- On the line below the description of the kind of party being given

MORE FORMAL

George A. Stephenson
President of Markton, Inc.
requests the pleasure of your company
at a luncheon
in honour of Samuel R. Magill
Monday, the eighth of February
etc.

LESS FORMAL

In honor of Samuel R. Magill
George A. Stephenson
President of Markton, Inc.
cordially invites you to
a lunch
Monday, February 8th
etc.

How the Date Is Written

○ On a formal invitation, the date is written out:

on Sunday, the eighteenth of September

○ On an informal invitation, numbers may be used:

on Sunday, September 18th

How the Time Is Written

○ On a formal invitation, the hours are spelled out and "o'clock" is used:

at seven-thirty o'clock

○ On an informal invitation, numbers and "A.M." and "P.M." may be used, such as on this cocktail party invitation:

. . . Cocktails
from 5 to 7 P.M.

How the Address Is Written

On a formal invitation, there are no abbreviations. For example, "Washington, D.C." and "2000 Mason St. NW" would be incorrect. "Washington, District of Columbia" and "2000 Mason Street, Northwest" would be correct.

However, there is an exception to this rule. For the sake of space considerations, the address *under your RSVP* in the lower left-hand corner of the invitation may have words like "Street," "Northwest," and "District of Columbia" abbreviated. Also, ZIP codes are listed with the two-letter abbreviations for the states.

Reminder Cards

These cards are used for two purposes:

○ For people who have accepted your invitation by telephone but have nothing on the record to help remind them of the what, when, and where of your party
○ For people who were sent invitations four or five months ago for your very special occasion and need to have their memories jogged

These are the kinds of reminders you can send:

• *You might write a simple postcard* reminding your guest:

Dear Sally and Mark,
　　We're delighted you can come! Dinner is Thursday, November 2nd, 7:30 P.M. at our house (132 Ridgewood Terrace).
　　　　　　　　　　　　　　　　　　　　　The Griersons

• *You might send that same message in a Mailgram or Express Letter, if you have invited people only a few days before the event and a mailed reminder might not get there in time.*

• *You might have your own reminder cards printed for a large party and mailed ten days before—with a text like this:*

This is to remind you that
Mr. and Mrs. Jean-Jacques LeGuay
expect you for dinner
on Wednesday, the sixth of October
at eight o'clock
The Hunters Club
1900 Georgetown Street
Washington, D.C. 00000

• If you entertain regularly and need reminder cards on a continuing basis, it is easier and less expensive to buy them by the box from a stationer. *These are engraved fill-in reminder cards* (you fill in the blank spaces by hand *in black ink*). The text already engraved on the cards reads as follows:

To remind that
(write in host's name here)
is expecting you
for (write in lunch, dinner, or cocktails)
on (the date is written here)
at (give hour) *o'clock*

RSVP

000-000-0000

Your name
Street address
City, State ZIP

Kinds of Invitations

When you decide to have a party, you have many options for how you will invite your guests. In taking the hypothetical case of Betty Knowlton, for example, who is giving a dinner party in honor of her husband's fortieth birthday, the hostess might do any of the following:

- *Write notes on her good personal stationery:*

Dear Rose,

I'm asking a few friends for Sunday supper, July 23rd, at 7 P.M., at our house (1420 First Avenue), to celebrate Bob's fortieth birthday. I do hope you can come. Please call me at home (000-0000) or at the office (000-0000).

Cordially,
/s/ Betty Knowlton

- *Send Mailgrams* to all invitees, if she does not have time to call or write them regular letters:

PLEASE COME TO OUR HOUSE (1420 FIRST AVENUE) FOR DINNER SUNDAY JULY 23RD AT 7 PM TO CELEBRATE BOB'S 40TH BIRTHDAY, RSVP HOME (000-0000) OR OFFICE (000-0000)

BETTY KNOWLTON

- *Design her own invitations:* She has fifty copies made of a five-by seven-inch black and white photo made of Bob Knowlton when he was a baby, and on the back of each she hand-writes the invitation to the fortieth birthday party for her husband.
- *Purchase fill-in invitations at a card shop or stationery store;* perhaps amusing invitations that resemble greeting or studio cards.
- *Buy engraved fill-in cards from a stationer* (as in the illustration).
- *Order from a stationer her invitation text printed, thermographed, or engraved on cards* (as in the illustration).
- *Telephone the recipients:* This is the least expensive method of all, but if she has many people to call, it is very time-consuming. Also, if she leaves a message with someone in a person's home or on a person's answering machine, she cannot be certain that the message will be properly relayed. This is why she should send a reminder card.

Mrs. Robert Knowlton
requests the pleasure of the company of
Mr. and Mrs. Thomas Wheeling
at *Robert Knowlton's Fortieth Birthday Dinner*
on *Sunday, the twenty-third of July*
at *Seven o'clock*

R.S.V.P.
000-0000

*1420 First Avenue
Fort Worth, TX 00000*

An engraved fill-in invitation.

Betty Knowlton
hopes you will join her
for dinner
to celebrate with gusto Bob's 40th
and to make him feel 20 again
Sunday, July 23rd at 7 p.m.
at home, 1420 First Avenue
Fort Worth

RSVP

000-0000

An invitation with the full text printed.

CREATIVE POSSIBILITIES

If you want to be creative, look at what other people do. People love receiving invitations that reflect the host's own poetic spirit. If there's some small different touch about your invitation, it will jump right out at the recipient and impress itself on his or her memory.

- *A wedding anniversary*—for example:

Jamie and Bill Hartman

cordially invite you

to a cocktail dance

in celebration of their 10th wedding anniversary

Saturday, May 7th

5 to 8 p.m.

at the same address, The Octagon Club

1st and Pierce Street

and with the same receiving line

and with the same band, the Fortnighters

as on their wedding day

RSVP

000/000-0000

When the Graebers of Washington, D.C., celebrated their twentieth anniversary, they sent out a little poem, printed in red script, on a vertical white invitation card:

George and Betty Beale Graeber

It would give us the greatest of pleasure
if you would take time off for leisure
and join us on the nineteenth of May
for cavorting at a dance buffet
to celebrate our twenty years of bliss
at the Chevy Chase Club edifice.
Come when it pleases you anytime
between the hours six-thirty to nine.
But for heaven's sake don't bring a gift
your very selves will give us a lift.

RSVP—ooo-oooo

Another couple sent out as an invitation for their thirty-fifth wedding anniversary a card on which was printed a photograph of the bridal pair cutting their cake at their wedding reception. The text did not give the hosts' names—just the date of the anniversary dinner dance, the address of the club, the hour of the party, and a telephone number of the person at the club handling the replies. Some guests who had not known the couple in their youth had trouble identifying them, but eventually everyone figured out who their hosts were. The invitation made the anniversary party just that much more fun.

• *A christening.* One couple handwrote their baby's christening invitations on pieces of pale pink rice paper with matching envelopes, which they had purchased on a visit to Japan and had never had occasion to use. They wrote:

Nothing would give us greater pleasure
than to have you join with us
in the celebration of the beginning of life
of the sweetest, dearest little girl
ever born
Amanda Gilchrist
Born March 12th at St. Joseph's Hospital
Come drink a glass of champagne with us after her
baptism
Sunday, April 3rd at five o'clock
0000 Lake Shore Drive
Chicago, Illinois 00000
And if you can not be with us that day
please say a prayer for her
to wish her a long, happy and blessed life

Ruth and Jeremy Farrell   *000/000-0000*

• *A Valentine's Day thought.* The hostess for the Valentine's Day dinner party for eight, with budget a consideration, cut out a heart for each guest from red file folders purchased at an office supply company. On the back of each heart she wrote her invitation to a "romantic dinner" on February 14, and mailed them in bright red office envelopes, also from the stationery store—just a little extra work that resulted in a very big effect.

Requesting a Reply

• You may request a reply in the lower left-hand corner of your invitation: "R.S.V.P." (or "RSVP" or "R.s.v.p.") with an address or a telephone number on the line below.

• You may enclose an RSVP card with a self-addressed envelope. (Many hosts timidly stamp these envelopes, thinking that this will cause more people to accept the invitation; I feel that the least a guest can do is pay for a stamp and stick it on the envelope!)

The text for an RSVP card (which is engraved if the invitation is engraved, or printed if the invitation is printed) looks like this:

M/M _____

 _____ *will attend*

 _____ *will not attend*

Dinner at Mr. and Mrs. Anson Mooney's on
Saturday, June eighth at eight o'clock

REGRETS ONLY

It is correct to put in the lower left of your invitation "Regrets Only" with a telephone number. However, in my opinion this is a cop-out, so that people can be lazy about replying. It is a negative on the invitation and sticks out like a sore thumb. Of course, a guest should let his or her host know if it is not possible to attend the party, but the guest also should let the host know if it *is* possible to attend the party. Use "Regrets Only" if you wish. I would never use it. I expect my friends to be nice enough to reply to my invitations, regardless of whether they accept or regret.

A REPLY REQUESTED BY A CERTAIN DATE

Many people add at the bottom of their RSVP cards, "Please respond by the (day, month and year)."

You are certainly at liberty to add that phrase or any other, such as this: "The favour of a reply is requested by such-and-such a date." This is yet another reinforcement of social laziness, because people should deem it an honor to be invited to your party and should reply quickly, with pleasure, rather than be threatened with a deadline for the arrival of the reply. However, some people believe the phrase goads recalcitrant guests into making up their minds sooner about attending the party. (My response to that is, "Who needs guests like that?")

"No Gifts" on Invitations

Many people, when they host birthday and anniversary celebrations, are serious about not wanting guests to bring gifts, so they include that fact on their invitations. I think phrases such as "No gifts" or "Please, no gifts" join a phrase like "Regrets Only" in the negative category on an invitation. It is better not to use it. Instead, pass the word around among your friends when you talk to them that you are serious about the policy of no presents. Your guests should respect your wishes.

An Invitation from the White House

Perhaps the most thrilling invitation that could ever arrive in your mailbox is one from the White House to a state dinner. (The sight of that raised gold presidential seal on the top of each piece of White House stationery makes anyone's pulse beat a little faster!) The President's House on Pennsylvania Avenue is, after all, the scene of the most important social functions held in the world. An invitation from the White House is also impressive because it is a command, to be regretted only in the most exceptional circumstances.

White House entertaining follows the highest standards of international protocol. This is evident in:

o Its stationery
o The pomp involved in the way a visiting head of state and spouse are welcomed by the President and his wife at the North Portico
o The playing by the Marine Band of the President's arrival music ("Hail to the Chief") as the hosts and guests of honor proceed into the East Room to join their guests
o The manner in which the guests are organized into a receiving line according to their rank
o The carefully thought-out protocol of seating at the tables in the State Dining Room
o The order of toasts at the conclusion of the dinner

The esthetics of the dinner—the food and wines, flowers, design of the table decorations, and the nature of the entertainment—set the nation's standards of style and talent. Although we cannot duplicate the White House and the scenario for presidential entertaining, we can certainly derive inspiration from it. We can learn from how they do things in the White House and adapt it to the best of our capabilities. For us, it's a matter of simplifying and adapting presidential ways according to our own wishes and resources.

White House social stationery contains the raised, embossed presidential seal in gold at the top. The envelopes and the engraved invitations are lettered with the guests' names in calligraphy performed by experts on staff and supervised by the Social Secretary. We can follow the form of this in our own printed or fill-in invitations, reply cards, table cards, place cards, and menus—without, of course, that gold embossed presidential seal! As for the invitation text, "Mr. and Mrs. John Tadwell Smith request the pleasure of your company . . ." sounds *almost* as good as "The President of the United States and Mrs. Bush request the pleasure of your company . . ."

On the occasion of the visit of

His Excellency

The President of the Republic of Mali

and Mrs. Traore

A separate card (3½ by 4½ inches) announces the purpose of the dinner.

The President and Mrs. Reagan

request the pleasure of the company of

Mr. and Mrs. Hollensteiner

at dinner

on Thursday, October 6, 1988

at 7:30 o'clock

Black Tie

The white invitation card (4½ by 6½ inches) bears the raised, embossed Presidential seal in gold.

DINNER

Honoring His Excellency
The President of the Republic of Mali
and Mrs. Traore

Vegetable Terrine
and Lobster Medallions
Curry Mousseline
Fennel Leaves

Roast Loin of Veal with Wild Mushrooms
Semolina Gnocchis
Sautéed Zucchini

Radicchio and Endive Salad
Bel Paese Cheese

Cold Pumpkin Soufflé
with Candied Ginger
Petits Fours Sec

CHÂTEAU ST. JEAN *Chardonnay 1986*
STERLING WINERY LAKE *Pinot Noir 1986*
SCHRAMSBERG *Crémant Demi Sec 1984*

THE WHITE HOUSE
Thursday, October 6, 1988

A matching menu card (4½ by 7 inches) is at each place. The menu is given in English and French.

This example of White House "social literature" was used for a dinner in honor of the president of Mali, hosted in 1988 by one of our most popular presidential couples, Ronald and Nancy Reagan. Not shown but also part of a White House state dinner invitation are:

- A reply card
- The security clearance card for the gate
- A table card to inform each guest of his or her table number
- A place card

WHEN YOU REPLY TO AN INVITATION

Every invitation should be replied to within the week of its receipt. If you have a pending trip or another reason that might prohibit your attendance, call your hosts and inform them of this. Ask if it is all right if you let them know later. A host deserves to know possible problems with the invited guests' schedules—he or she should not just find out about it at the last minute, when the guest doesn't show up!

Sending a Written Reply

The best possible form, of course, is to send a written reply to an invitation. A formal reply is written by hand (or typed, if your handwriting is as impossible as mine) on a piece of good stationery—personal letter paper, a correspondence card with matching envelope, or folded note-paper. The reply is written and centered on the page in the exact form as the invitation itself.

THE LONG FORM OF ACCEPTANCE

Mr. and Mrs. Walter Lodge
accept with pleasure
the kind invitation of
Mr. and Mrs. Donald Allen Rice
for dinner
Saturday, the eighth of August
at seven-thirty o'clock

. . . or, optionally:

Mr. and Mrs. Walter Lodge
accept with pleasure
Mr. and Mrs. Rice's
kind invitation for dinner
(or whatever the occasion)

THE SHORT FORM OF AN ACCEPTANCE

Mr. and Mrs. Walter Lodge
accept with pleasure
the kind invitation of
Mr. and Mrs. Donald Allen Rice
for Saturday, the eighth of August

THE LONG FORM OF A REGRET

I am of the philosophy that if you are regretting an invitation, even formally by letter, you should explain why. That's why I recommend including a phrase explaining the reason for regretting the invitation, even if it makes the reply less formal. For example:

Mr. and Mrs. Walter Lodge
regret that
because of absence from the city
they will be unable to accept
Mr. and Mrs. Rice's
kind invitation for dinner
Saturday, the eighth of August
at seven-thirty o'clock

Or the reason given could be "because of illness" or "owing to a prior engagement" or "because of Mr. Lodge's speaking engagement on the same evening"—whatever creates a conflict.

THE SHORT FORM OF A REGRET

Mr. and Mrs. Walter Lodge
regret that
owing to absence from the city
they will be unable to accept
Mr. and Mrs. Rice's
kind invitation
for Saturday, the eighth of August

When One Spouse Accepts and the Other Regrets

Let us say hypothetically that Mr. Lodge will be out of town the night of the dinner, but Mrs. Lodge really wants to go to that party. Their reply would look like this:

Mrs. Walter Lodge
accepts with pleasure
the kind invitation of
Mr. and Mrs. Donald Allen Rice
for Saturday, the eighth of August
Mr. Lodge regrets
that owing to absence from the city
he will be unable to attend

A Typed Reply from the Office

When an invitation arrives at the office or at home for an event that is business-oriented, an executive's secretary may type an acceptance or regret on good-quality office letterhead for her boss and his or her spouse.

GET YOURSELF ORGANIZED

It's no secret that entertaining is hard work. Those stories of famous hostesses who manage to organize fabulous parties on the spur of the moment and can throw together a little dinner for twenty on a few hours' notice are all myths. Either they have been working hard for a couple of weeks on their parties and won't admit it, or they have well-trained staffs who are paid high salaries to move fast without advance notice.

The great thing about entertaining often is that you become practiced, skilled, and fine-tuned. In my twenties, by the time I had produced within three months my sixth buffet supper of Beef Burgundy with noodles, string beans, salad, and store-bought coffee ice cream with hot butterscotch sauce, I could do it in my sleep. Since it was so easy to do, I kept on doing it year after year. Then I realized that some friends had been served this same menu so often that they had no trouble predicting it. So I apologized— only to be told that they would gladly have the same menu once a week, if I would just invite them!

The tough part of entertaining—remembering how to get organized and overseeing all of the details and logistics—really does become easier each time. One friend who does all her own work for her parties proudly states, "I have become the best-trained chef and the most experienced butler I know of." Another friend always does her buffet dinners back to back on consecutive nights, so she can use the same wines and liquors, the same flowers, and even the same food. (It's an easier job marketing—buying only once and in a large quantity—for two dinners.)

Another great plus about gaining experience in the entertaining field is that you become immune to the problems that may develop. You realize that in spite of the crises that may be occurring, the party does continue. I once saw one of the waiters in a caterer's retinue become so sloshed that he had to be noisily evicted from the party, but the hosts kept their cool and consoled the head waiter, not themselves. On another occasion, the orchestra's bus broke down out of state en route to a friend's dance. You learn to compensate, substitute, change directions—or just laugh a lot, so that your guests follow suit. At the dance, our host got on the microphone and told everyone what had happened to the band and then added with great enthusiasm, as though she were organizing a cheerleading squad, "What was to have been 'the dance of the year' will become as of now 'the cocktail party of the year!' " Everyone cheered and applauded, resolved to have a good time for the host's sake—and they did. The evening was a great success.

Basics of Good Entertaining Planning

• *Set up a "party notebook"—your manual*—into which every pertinent item will be entered, from the budget to the invitation list, and from the kind of room scent to be purchased to the number of lemons and limes needed for the bar. *Everything* should be in this notebook— all items pending, all names, addresses, telephone numbers—every bit of information. This should be your constant companion during party-preparation time, the ultimate checklist of checklists. Make a habit of recording any kind of party in your party notebook.

• *Make a budget*—always the next step—and if your means are limited, resolve to stick to it. (See pages 380 and 383 for two sample budgets.) Keep referring to it as your bills mount. You may have to cut back on some items if expenses prove to be higher than you estimated. That's all right. You can always find ways to do your party for less. For example, cut back on the number of fresh flowers ordered from the florist and have him substitute more greenery in your arrangements. Drop one course from your menu—perhaps something that should not have been in your budget in the first place, like smoked salmon. (Your guests won't know the difference.) Don't buy less wine than you originally planned; simply buy a less expensive but palatable wine.

• *Set your party date*—one that will not conflict with any of your town's biggest social events or with a night when everyone wants to be home watching television (for example, Academy Awards night).

• *Decide on the type of party you want to give.* Buffet dinner? Small lunch? Family-style beach picnic? Cocktail reception mixing business and social friends? Pizza and beer party for engaged friends before going to the circus? A party for singles only? For people who have been divorced? A Saturday afternoon tea party?

• *Decide on the place and the hours for your party.* The place may be anywhere you choose, as long as it is comfortable and accessible for your guests, and if it is logistically possible to serve food there.

The classic party hours are these:

- o *Breakfast:* 8 A.M. or 9 A.M., according to what it is related to. Lasts an hour usually.
- o *Brunch:* 11 A.M. Lasts an hour to an hour and a half.
- o *Lunch:* 12 noon or 12:30 or 1:00 P.M. Lasts usually one and a half to two hours.
- o *Tea:* 3:30, 4:00, or 4:30. Lasts an hour.
- o *Cocktails:* 5 to 7 P.M.; 5:30 to 7 or 7:30 P.M.; 6 to 8 P.M. Some guests tend to stay much later than they should—unless the host shuts off the bar a half hour after the supposed end of the party. (For a cocktail party from 6 to 8, if the host shuts the bar after 8:30, he or she is acting in an appropriate manner.) Nothing brings a cocktail party to a graceful conclusion more effectively than closing the bar!
- o *Cocktail-buffet:* 6 to 9 P.M. Again, shut the bar down by 9:30 or your hangers-on will never leave.
- o *Dinner:* 7, 7:30, or 8 P.M. Lasts usually three to three and a half hours, unless there is dancing or other entertainment, in which case it could last until midnight or later. Remember, for any kind of evening party, the cocktail hour preceding the meal should not last longer than forty-five minutes to an hour.
- o *After-dinner reception:* 9, 10, or 11 P.M., depending on whether it follows a theater performance, museum opening, or the like. Usually lasts no more than one to one and a half hours. Unless the guests are college students at something like a prom, most people are exhausted after an evening affair followed by an hour-long reception, therefore, this kind of function should consist of the fast service of champagne or wine or whatever food and beverages are to be served, and no one should be made to stay later than he or she wants to.
- o *A dance:* 10 P.M. (Since guests have eaten dinner beforehand, they tend not to arrive until 10:30 or 11. The dance music usually continues until 2 A.M. (A dance can last beyond 2 A.M., provided the host is willing to pay musicians overtime.) A light supper of something like hot pasta, omelets, or chicken hash, with a salad, rolls, and dessert is often served at midnight, along with wine and champagne.

• *Enter in the book the best guest list you can draw up.* First make a big list of possible names and put them in different categories, so that when you come to a final list, it will be varied and an interesting mix (always the best recipe for any kind of a party, large or small).
Some possible categories:

o People you owe
o Newcomers to the city who would appreciate the chance to meet some new people
o Friends you haven't really seen in the past couple of years but would like to touch base with again
o People who have become important to you in the last year—for example, your Congressman (if he or she is a friend), the new pastor, the children's school superintendent.
o One marvelous conversationalist per twelve other guests (insurance against any embarrassing, heavy conversational lulls)
o An important business contact and his or her spouse
o A friend from your extracurricular life: classmate at your art, cooking, or exercise class; a tennis partner; fellow bird-watcher; fellow volunteer at the hospital
o A couple from an older age group, if you're young; a couple from a younger age group if you're middle-aged or older
o A celebrity in town whom you happen to know well—anyone from a local TV news anchor to a star football player
o A foreign business colleague or student (always adds interest to a gathering of Americans)
o A friend who has been having a tough time (has been ill, has just been separated or divorced, lost a job, or in whose family there has been a death)

If you have a mix at your party, whether it's a huge cocktail party or a small dinner, and if you introduce everybody warmly to each other, your party will be a *success!*

• *Your invitation should be noted in your party book.* Put a copy of the invitation in the book, if you had it handwritten, printed, or engraved. If you telephoned your invitations, put a copy of the reminder card sent (to those who accepted) in the book. Or if you just telephoned the invitations, mark that fact down, too, with the date you telephoned and the reply.

• *Keep a beautifully documented guest list* in your party book, with the latest tally of acceptances and regrets so that you'll know exactly where you stand with your quota of guests.

• *Sign up your caterer and/or the extra help needed for a large event,* whether the extra help consists of a cook, bartender baby-sitter, clean-up squad, or someone to mow the lawn before the guests have to wade through your ankle-deep grass. List all names, addresses, and telephone numbers, plus their advance price quotes, and note how they are to be paid. Some caterers, for example, need a percentage of the total bill a week before the party; others might want to be paid all costs at the end of the party itself.

There are several ways to find a caterer:

- o You see one in action first-hand at a party and are impressed by his or her teamwork, service, food, and style.
- o Someone you know recommends a caterer he or she has used.
- o You read about a caterer's success at a party in the lifestyle section of the newspaper, and you can call the editor to find out the caterer's name.
- o You find a list of caterers in the yellow pages of the telephone book, and you call several or all of them to compare prices. You also check their references.

- *Decide on your menu*—all the courses, including the hors d'oeuvres, drinks, and wine. If you use a new recipe for this party, include it in your party notebook, so you can easily find it again if you want to repeat it for another party.

- *Make a list of everything needed for this party.* Write down all items that you must purchase or have on hand, from toothpicks to dishwashing detergent, cocktail napkins to jars of olives, rye bread to diet sodas, sugar cubes to guest bathroom soaps, decaffeinated coffee to arugula, and place cards to cherries for the Cherries Jubilee dessert. Don't forget to list even the most standard items that must be on hand that night—like salt, pepper, paper towels, and soap for the guest bathroom.

- *Order in advance everything you can, well ahead of time,* including soft drinks, wine, liquor, spices for cooking, and so forth. The more you do ahead, the less onerous entertaining chores will seem.

- *Enter detailed descriptions of your table decorations* for that particular event, including the kinds of flowers, the colors of the table linens, and the like. Take snapshots or Polaroids of your decor, so you'll be able to call it to mind easily later—and perhaps repeat it at some party in the future.

- *If you have entertainment at your party, make an entry for it in your book.* Write down the name, address, and telephone number of any entertainer (and later how you felt about his, her, or their performance). Include how much the entertainment costs, the agent's name and telephone number, and what is required logistically for the entertainer (platform, sound system, lectern, special lighting, and the like).

If your party is a seated dinner, it's good to have a record in your party planner of who sat where around the tables. Even for a dinner for eight, an informal sketch is a nice reminder of the evening.

If you are planning to use only your own musical tapes for entertainment, or if you or a guest will play the piano, include that, too. Write down what selection of tapes are to be played (interesting to look back on).

Sample Party Plans—A Potluck Meal

A very pleasant custom is that of a host organizing an informal dinner at home, inviting each guest (or guest couple) to supply part of the meal. It is an American way of entertaining, and a good one at that— easy on everyone's budget and easy on busy people's time schedules.

The host usually supplies the cocktails, main course, and coffee. In asking people what they would prefer to bring, the host also helps decide what dish in that particular category would be appropriate, so that the menu works. For example, to a guest who wants to bring a fruit salad, she might say, "We are having fruit for dessert, so it would be preferable if you brought a mixed green salad. Is that all right with you?"

Each guest or couple should bring the course in a nice-looking container that can go from refrigerator or stove straight onto the buffet table. (In the best of all situations, the hosts insist on washing the containers and delivering them back within a week to their owners, rather than making the guests troop out to the kitchen to wash their own containers and carry them home.)

An entry in a party notebook would be a simple one page, such as this one, showing who is responsible for bringing what:

POTLUCK SUPPER
March 12th at 6:30 p.m.

Hors d'oeuvres: Lucy and Jim McGrath
Liquor: Us
Grilled lemon chicken: Us
Corn soufflé: Joan and Pete Schultz
Baked tomatoes and onions: Gerry and Phil Miller
Mixed green salad and rolls: Ginny and Hans Mittendorf
Mom's apple pie à la mode: Mike and Adrienne Feldman
Wine and beer: Gordon Matson
Coffee and decaff: Us

Sample Plans for a Small Dinner

Everyone's concept of what makes a party big or small is a personal judgment. To me, dinner for six or eight is a small one; a cocktail party for twelve to fifteen people is a small one. However, for those rarities—people with huge houses and domestic staffs—even a dinner for twenty-four is small. (Let's use my numbers—not those of the person with the big house and staff—in this book.)

Preparing a party checklist or a party plan for any size gathering makes sense, and helps you get organized. For example, here are the entries in the party notebook of a couple who have small groups for dinner once a month, and who keep good records:

DINNER FOR EIGHT

Date: Wed., Feb 14   Time: 7:30
    Valentine's Day

Guest List: Gregg and Marge Lee, Ed Reed, Susan Ameson, George
    and Joan Goodman, Us

Invitations: Home-made red hearts, sent out January 22

Menu:

Hors d'oeuvres:	Crudités with yogurt dip
	Wheat crackers
	Edam and extra sharp cheddar cheese cubes
First course:	Cup of hot canned madrilene soup with slice of lemon and a sprig of fresh dill
Second course:	Roast chicken stuffed with herbed rice
	Steamed broccoli
	Mixed green salad
Dessert:	Peppermint ice cream in heart mold with chocolate sauce
	Espresso
Wines:	Soave Bolla

Decor:

Flowers:	Tall arrangement of laurel leaves in foyer
	Low bowl of multi-colored anemones on coffee table
	Dining table: white ceramic container at each place, containing cluster of red and white carnations. Red and white votive candles in ring in center.
Table favors:	Red satin heart box containing chocolate-covered caramels at each place
	Valentine place card at each place

Music: Frank Sinatra love songs throughout evening (on tape)

Budget: $350

Actual costs:

Hors d'oeuvres	$12.00
Soup	5.00
Chicken	12.00
Vegetables and salad	10.00
Ice cream and cookies	11.00
Wines for cocktails and dinner (6 bottles)	42.00
Liquor (new bottle of scotch, gin, vodka)	40.00
Cocktail napkins	2.50
Sodas	20.00
Ice	5.00
Bar items, like lemons and olives	3.00
Baby-sitter for 7 hours, including 2 hours clean-up in kitchen	35.00
Flowers in living room and for table	70.00
8 table favors	80.00
8 Valentine place cards	8.00
TOTAL:	$355.50

THE LOGISTICS OF PLANNING A LARGE DINNER

In organizing a large party, you go through an exercise much like a painter does in facing his canvas: first the rough, broad outlines, and then the minute details are filled in. The party notebook becomes even more crucial. You will want every dollar you spend on such an expensive undertaking to be used to best advantage, to make certain the event accomplishes your goals. It's very easy to throw money away when you're stepping into elaborate entertaining. Therefore, keep your wits about you, write everything down in your notebook, and *stay in control.*

One very accomplished hostess I know, who recently gave a dinner for forty around an Easter spring theme, always keeps careful notes as she goes along. She entertained at four round tables of ten (rented from the caterer), using two in her dining room, one in her living room, and one in the library. Her entries in her notebook were organized in the following manner:

DINNER FOR 40

Date: Easter Saturday night Time: 8 P.M. Dress: Black tie
Caterer: Henderson Caterers In charge: Alexandre
Tel.: 000-0000
Invitation:
    An entire page in her notebook was dedicated to this. She had
    taped an example of her engraved "fill-in" invitation to the page.
    A calligrapher had written in the necessary information.
Guest List:
    She listed on this page guests who had accepted by the names
    that would be written on their place cards by her calligrapher—
    for example, "Mrs. Abernathy, Ambassador Abernathy, Ms. Nel-
    son, Mr. Wyeth." She had a telephone number by each name, in
    case she had to reach anyone quickly. She also made a running
    list of everyone who had regretted.
Table Placement:
    This page contained four circles, representing her four round
    tables. She gave each table a number from 1 to 4, and penciled in
    each guest at his or her proper place at one of the tables. (She
    explained that the names were penciled in because she had to
    keep changing the seating as guests cancelled or new names
    were added to the party list.)
Menu:
    On this page, she wrote what was to be served at the cocktail

hour and for dinner, and what was to be passed after dinner. For example, she had written:

Drinks:

> Peach Bellinis
> Scotch, gin, and vodka
> Dry vermouth, sherry
> White wine
> Tonic water and club soda
> Ginger ale, diet soda

Hors d'Oeuvres:

> Mushroom caps stuffed with pâté
> Figs wrapped in prosciutto
> Tiny grilled cheese sandwiches (Swiss on dark rye)
> One-inch diameter tartelettes filled with egg salad

Dinner:

1st course:	Fresh asparagus with lemon sauce
2nd course:	Roast lamb
	Fresh mint sauce
	New potatoes with butter-herb sauce
	Tiny French green beans
	Endive and arugula salad
3rd course:	Small sorbet balls of different fruit flavors
	Raspberry sauce
	"Dentelles" lace cookies
	Chocolates
	Demitasses
Wines:	Pouilly Fumé
	Cabernet Sauvignon
	Schramsberg Blanc de Blancs
After dinner:	Remy Martin Cognac
	Framboises and Eau de Poire liqueurs
	Glasses of club soda and ice

Decorations:

On this page the details of how she decorated the house were listed for the record.

Front hall table:

> Large crystal bowl with gardenias and white votive
>> candles in crystal holders floating in water

Living room and library:

> Vases of white lilacs, lilies, and very pale pastel tulips
> Tall vases of branches of forsythia and apple blossoms

Dining room centerpieces for tables:

> Lavender and mauve tulips with peach roses in crystal
>> bowls

Mauve and peach tie-died Easter eggs to ring each bowl of
flowers

Tall white candles in crystal candlesticks

Linens:

Four round tables of 10—mauve and peach plaid cotton
cloths to the floor

Mauve napkins (tied with peach satin ribbons)

Entertainment:

On this page she wrote all of the information on the three Hungarian violinists who serenaded the guests after dinner—their names and telephone numbers, their price, and how long she wanted them to play. She made a note that she had instructed them to wear their red gypsy costumes and to "come bursting into the living room, playing loud and lustily, as a surprise—as soon as the guests assembled there for after-dinner coffee."

Budgeting for a Dinner for Forty

Here is a sample budget for the dinner for forty, as entered in the host's party notebook:

DINNER FOR 40

Budget established:	$15,000.00
Actual costs:	
Caterer's charge per person for the meal, gratuities included: $200 × 40	$8,000.00
Caterer's fee for equipment rental (tables, chairs, cloths, trays, glasses, flatware)	600.00
Wines: 9 bottles white & 7 red (@ approx. $10); champagne, 20 bottles (@ approx. $30)	760.00
Liquor: 2 half-gallons Scotch ($40), 1 half-gallon of gin ($15), 1 half-gallon of vodka ($15), 1 bottle sherry & 1 bottle dry vermouth ($15), 1 cognac & 2 sweet liqueurs ($45)	130.00
Sodas, tonic water, sparkling water (10 qts @ .89)	8.90
Cocktail napkins, after-dinner chocolates & sundry	20.00
3 valet car parkers ($10 per hour for 4 hours each)	120.00
Coat checker ($10 per hour for 4 hours)	40.00

Floral designer: 4 arrangements for house	
($300) and 4 table centerpieces ($400)	700.00
Music: 3 musicians playing after dinner @ $650	1,950.00
Menus, place cards & calligrapher to write them	360.00
25 Invitations $75; Postage $10	85.00
Tips for catering staff ($20 for head; $10 each for	
4 waiters and 2 kitchen people)	80.00
TOTAL:	$12,853.90

• When figuring out how much liquor and wine to order, you must take into account the drinking habits of your region of the country. At this party, there were a lot of Scotch drinkers; down South there might be many bourbon drinkers. At some parties your guests might all drink wine instead of liquor. Be ready for any eventuality—in other words, always order more than you think you will need, and ask your liquor store beforehand to agree after the party to accept a return on any *unopened bottles.*

THE COCKTAIL PARTY

A cocktail party is a wonderful way to entertain a large number of people informally and relatively easily. This kind of social event is supposed to have a duration of from one and a half to two hours (although it is expected that some people will stay longer than that). Since alcohol traditionally is not served until after five, a cocktail party's beginning hour is five, five-thirty, or six. (Before five, a get-together should be called a "tea"—see page 391.)

• *Since the only way to have a successful cocktail party come to an end is to shut off the bar,* everything works more smoothly if this is understood by the bartender(s) ahead of time. Let the bar stay open until a half hour after the party was supposed to end. If, for example, your cocktail party hours are from five-thirty to seven thirty, simply instruct your caterer or bartender to shut off the bar at eight, and the hangers-on will get the message.

How Many Bars, How Much Help, and What Supplies Are Needed

BARS NEEDED

Two bars are best for a party of fifty guests, but one efficiently run bar can handle up to sixty guests, particularly since guests will help themselves if the bartender is busy and if the liquor, ice, and glasses are all accessible on the table. For a party of sixty to a hundred, two bars are needed. (The hosts usually help out, too, at an informal party, making sure the guest's glass is filled and that the hors d'oeuvres are being passed around.)

Help Needed

These specified numbers of help needed are based on the premise that a host, or a husband and wife host team, will be working, too, if necessary at the peak hour, to make sure the service goes smoothly.

- *If you have a party for fifty,* a bartender and an assistant waiter or waitress can handle the crowd, particularly since the fifty people arrive at different times during the two-hour period.
- *A group of sixty to eighty* will be immersed in a logjam if you have only one bar and one table full of food. It is better to have drinks served by bartenders at two stations, and to have the hors d'oeuvres passed by a waiter or waitress, rather than make people crowd up against one table to get food. (What happens is that the people in front of the food table begin to socialize and chat with each other, instead of serving themselves and stepping away to allow others to approach.)
- *For a crowd of ninety to one hundred twenty,* three bartenders and two waitresses will be needed. The serving help have more to do than just pass hors d'oeuvres or make drinks; they must carry out glasses, bring in fresh glasses, empty ashtrays, keep the hors d'oeuvres replenished, pick up, clean up, carry ice, and the like.
- *When you're going to have a very crowded party, and you don't have the space for two bars,* you would be wise to have a second bartender making drinks in an out-of-the-way area, such as the kitchen, and then passing through the crowd with guests' orders for drinks on a tray. If the crush gets worse, have this second bartender make tray after tray of assorted drinks, and send them out with a waiter into the crowd, so the guests can simply help themselves from the tray.
- *For a champagne reception,* a special celebration with champagne being served, such as at a christening or an engagement party, you would need two waiters and an additional person to keep passing hors d'oeuvres. There is no need for a bar. Two waiters with trays of champagne can pass constantly through a crowd of up to seventy or eighty; there should always be a few glasses of soda or fruit juice mixed in with the champagne on the tray. You would also need small bowls of nuts, cheese-straws, and other munchies left around within everyone's easy reach, as well as having a few hors d'oeuvres passed.

Checklist of Things Needed for a Cocktail Party at Home

You will need the following items for a cocktail party:

○ Table(s) and cloth(s) for the bar(s)
○ Ice (Keep any bags of ice sent in from the outside in containers, like a roasting pan, so they don't leak all over the floor.)
○ Ice bucket
○ Ice crusher
○ Cutting board
○ Bar knife
○ Lemon and lime wedges (also thinly cut lemon peel "zests" for martinis)
○ Olives and/or cocktail onions
○ Maraschino cherries (if you are serving a fruit drink with rum or vodka)
○ Pitcher with long-handled stirrer for making martinis
○ Large water pitcher
○ One-and-a-half-ounce jigger or shot glass
○ Bar towels
○ Corkscrew
○ Paper cocktail napkins
○ Trays and platters (for carrying glasses and passing hors d'oeuvres)
○ Your selection of liquor, wines, beer, mixers, sodas, fruit juices (If you're having a drink like Bloody Marys, you would be smart to have them premixed, ready for the bartender simply to add vodka and ice. Otherwise, have at the bar the tomato juice and all its paraphernalia, including: lemons, Worcestershire sauce, horseradish, salt and pepper, lemon squeezer, and strainer.)
○ Glasses (any combination of the following):

> Tall *highball glasses* for long drinks, including Scotch, bourbon, or whiskey and soda or water; gin or vodka and tonic; rum and soda or tonic; sodas; beer; and bottled water
> *"Old-fashioned"* glasses for serving wine or wine on the rocks, sherry, aperitifs, martinis on the rocks (*All-purpose wine-glasses* may substitute for old-fashioneds.)

• Delicate crystal, stemmed martini glasses and other specialty glasses are not used for large cocktail parties, simply because of logistical problems. They are better used when a couple of friends come by your house for a drink.

• Don't use plastic glasses indoors either, if you can possibly help it. Borrow or rent your glasses. (Plastic ones are fine for a party held on your deck or patio.)

How Much Wine and Liquor to Order

The advantage in ordering wines and liquors for a cocktail party is that, unlike food, they don't spoil. You can always use what is left over, or you can give the leftover bottles of liquor through the year for holiday and hostess gifts. Most liquor stores where you are known will take back unopened bottles of liquor if you have over-ordered.

I think it's wise always to stock more for a cocktail party than you think you'll need, because you never know what will be the big drink of the hour. The latter changes according to the age of the guests, region of the country, and the time of the year. For example, ten years ago my husband and I gave two business-related cocktail parties for fifty each, back to back. We prepared by laying in a large supply of vodka and tonic, since everyone that hot summer seemed to be drinking it; we decided to purchase only one large (1.75-liter) bottle each of Scotch and bourbon. The guests at our first party surprised us by ordering large amounts of Scotch and bourbon and almost no gin and tonic. The next day I rushed to the liquor store to return most of the vodka and to lay in a supply of Scotch and bourbon for the second party. Our guests surprised us again. Almost everyone ordered white wine, of which we had only two bottles on hand. For the next summer's first cocktail party, we filled our fridge with beautifully chilled bottles of white wine. Only two people asked for it; the majority of drinkers asked for rum. The moral of the story is, don't be surprised. (I might also add that we no longer give cocktail parties!)

If you're watching your budget and want a limited instead of an open bar, decide beforehand on what you are going to offer your guests. If you decide, for example, to have soft drinks, white wine, and only Scotch as your hard liquor, offer guests their choice of those, saying, "What would you like? A soda, white wine, or Scotch?"

It's comforting to realize that today you don't have to offer guests faddish cocktails like Bellinis, or even old standbys like Whiskey Sours and Manhattans. Nor is any host today obliged to have a blender whirring away with all the latest exotic drinks!

- *Always have on hand a good supply of nonalcoholic drinks,* like a variety of sodas, bottled waters, and fruit juices.

Some Suggestions on How to Stock Your Bar

In noting the following suggestions, keep in mind they will be tempered by regional, age, and seasonal differences in drinking habits.

o *If you have the twenty-one- to twenty-seven-year-old set coming to your party,* you might have on hand:

Beer (half of it light)
White wine
Red wine
Soda (half of it the diet variety)

o *For a budget-heedful party for people in their thirties and older:*

White wine
Scotch or bourbon
Vodka or rum in the summer, gin in the winter (again, according
     to your own preference)
Mixers of club soda, tonic water, and ginger ale (which, along
     with your diet sodas, may also serve as your inventory of
     nonalcholic drinks)

o *For a full open-bar party,* you might have on hand:

White wine
Vodka
Gin
Scotch
Bourbon
Rum (dark or light)
Whiskey
Dry vermouth for martinis
Sherry
Mixers, sodas, bottled waters, and a fruit juice
A small quantity of cold beer

• *To determine quantities needed,* use 1.5 ounces as an average
serving of liquor per drink. (Use or have your bartender use a jigger or
shot glass as the standard measure for the drink that is poured into the
glass.) There are about twenty-two drinks in a liter bottle of liquor.

How to Buy Your Beverages

• Particularly for a party for the young, watch the wine sale ads,
and buy a modest-priced wine by the magnum (1.5-liter size, sold six to
a case) or by the 4-liter bottle (sold four to a case).

• Buy your mixers, sodas, and bottled waters by the case at a
special price when they are advertised in your local stores.

• Buy liquor by the large 1.75-liter bottle (you can save money). Do
not buy cheap brands—people can taste the difference.

• *If your cocktail party is in a hotel or some public place,* you may
have an unlimited consumption arrangement with the establishment,
whereby it charges you a flat fee per guest, regardless of how much a
guest does or does not drink. (For example, if the hotel charges $4 per
drink, not including tax and gratuities, and counts on each guest having

three drinks, you would be charged $12 per guest for the liquor, plus tax and gratuities.) Or you may pay for your liquor by the bottle. In that case, keep count of the bottles actually used for your party, and return any unopened bottles to the hotel's inventory.

HORS D'OEUVRES

Serve what you can handle easily. In other words, if you don't have much help, have a menu of at least three cold hors d'oeuvres made ahead of time and only one or two hot ones, so that you are not always dashing into the kitchen to check on what's in the oven.

• *If guests are coming to have an informal drink with you at home,* you only need to have two cold hors d'oeuvres, which might be something as simple as crudités with a dip and cheese and crackers.

• *If you are having a full-fledged cocktail party,* in addition to small bowls of nuts and munchies throughout the entertaining area, you might consider serving:

Three of these	*plus two of these*
Open-faced canapés made with pâté, egg salad, smoked salmon, or the like	Toasted rounds with peanut butter topped with crumbled bacon
Tiny open-face sandwiches of smoked turkey or rare beef on rye with mayonnaise	Miniature pizzas or quiches
Crackers spread with crabmeat and a dash of Worcestershire	Grilled sausages on toothpicks
Endives stuffed with pâté	Miniature hamburgers
Crudités with salt and pepper or a creamy dip	Grilled water chestnuts in bacon on toothpicks
Raw oysters, fresh shrimp, crab claws (very expensive)	Hot cheese or salmon puffs

A Cocktail Buffet

A cocktail buffet signifies a cocktail party that usually lasts from two to three hours (five-thirty to eight-thirty, for example). More food is served here than at a cocktail party. There is a buffet table and at least one hot dish is served. Most guests eat their dinner at this kind of an informal buffet.

There should be a few small tables, each covered with a cloth and perhaps decorated with a small bouquet of flowers in the center, and chairs near the food service area for guests who do not like to eat standing up.

As each group of guests finishes using one of these tables, a waiter should clear it off again for use by the next set of guests who may want to sit down to eat and chat with friends for a short period.

Cocktail Party Manners

- *A guest should not*

  ○ Arrive even one minute before the start of the party, or arrive fifteen minutes before it is supposed to end and then expect to stick around for an hour or so talking to the exhausted hosts and whoever is left.
  ○ Shake hands with a cold wet right hand. (Hold your drink in your left hand.)
  ○ Shake hands with a mayonnaised hand after holding hors d'oeuvres in it. (Either hold hors d'oeuvres in your left hand, or carefully use a cocktail napkin after every drippy bite.)
  ○ Talk to someone while looking over and around that person to see if someone more important has arrived (a common rudeness at cocktail parties).
  ○ Monopolize celebrity guests, so that others can not even get near them.
  ○ Tie up the host in extended serious conversation, as the host has a lot more to do than talk to you all night!
  ○ Monopolize the table with platters of hors d'oeuvres so that other guests cannot even get close to the food.
  ○ Drop cigarette ashes on the rug or use a glass as an ashtray and leave it around for people to gaze upon.

- *A guest should*

  ○ RSVP if that is called for on the invitation.
  ○ Bring a guest only if you call first and get your host's permission.
  ○ Drink only as much as you can hold well.
  ○ Drink beverage from a glass, not from a bottle. (Women look particularly wrong guzzling beer from a bottle.)
  ○ Introduce yourself to newcomers, and carefully introduce newcomers to your friends.
  ○ Write a short thank-you note to your host afterward.

AN INVITATION TO TEA

The tea hour (anytime from three-thirty to five-thirty P.M.) is becoming more and more popular as a business meeting time—presenting the opportunity to get away from the office for a much needed break in the afternoon. You meet a person or a small group in a hotel that specializes in the tea service, and you return to your office, if you care to, greatly refreshed and ready for some more work.

Traditionally, tea was served by the female head of the house for her female friends. It was the highlight of the afternoon visiting hours, when the lady of the house was "at home" to her friends on a specific date. The table was invariably spread with a beautiful white lace or damask cloth, tall sterling candelabra, and a bowl of fresh flowers in the center.

Also on the tea table were:

o A large silver tray on which sat a sterling tea service comprising:

   Teapot, perhaps on an alcohol lamp
   Hot water pot, perhaps on an alcohol lamp
   Milk server
   Sugar bowl with tongs or teaspoon
   Container for artificial sweetener
   Strainer and bowl for used tea leaves
   Small plate of thin slices of lemon, with a small fork

o Porcelain tea cups and saucers, each with a sterling silver tea-spoon
o Porcelain plates for food
o Dessert forks (for pastry)
o Sterling teaspoons for sherbet or strawberries
o Cups of sherbet or bowls of fresh strawberries
o Sterling silver container of cream
o Plates of delicious little sandwiches, cookies, hot buttered scones, fruit cake, brownies, or any sweet
o Dainty white tea napkins (usually trimmed in lace)

Today more people are enjoying tea but, except for certain debutante formal teas still held in the South, the formal tea table has all but disappeared. Today we ask people to come by "for a cup of tea" and give them just that—hot or iced tea in our living room or family room, and perhaps one little sandwich and one dessert item. Having someone over for tea is a wonderful way to give pleasure to friends. It is a warm, friendly custom, and we do not do it often enough.

SETTING AN ATTRACTIVE FORMAL DINNER TABLE

There are several reasons why we set our tables much more informally today than in past generations. Very few people have domestic help; it's a generally more informal world in which easy-care synthetics have been accepted; and everyone seems too busy to give much attention to the formal rituals of life. Vinyl table coverings and paper napkins are here to stay for family meals!

I firmly believe, however, that when you have guests, it's time to make an effort. They deserve better in your home, after all, than paper napkins, paper plates, and plastic glasses. (The latter belong out-of-doors—on the patio, in the yard, at the beach, on a picnic—or a totally informal family meal indoors.)

When you go to an obvious effort to make things attractive and pleasant for those you have invited to your home, the event almost always takes off. People feel festive and pampered—and you become *appreciated.* Wine served in a pretty glass, for example, has a totally different taste from wine served in a paper cup. A piece of meatloaf tastes very different when it's served on a pretty piece of china than when it is presented on a paper plate.

Set a standard in your entertaining, even if it's an old pal or your mother-in-law coming for dinner:

- Serve your food to any guest on handsome plates with a sense of pride, whether it's spaghetti or roast pheasant with truffles.

- If you don't have any nice stemware and flatware to use when you entertain, borrow them from a friend.

The Role of Linens in Table Settings

The table linens you use—whether tablecloths or place mats and napkins—play a starring role in any table setting. They give the zip to the entire scene.

- *Mix patterns and colors without fear, but it helps to know what you're doing!* It's great fun to mix things, but there has to be a logic or a color bond in there somewhere. A plaid mixed with a polka dot fabric makes sense if there is a common color scheme. So does a silky fabric used for a tablecloth, combined with rough-textured napkins.

- Easy-care fabric napkins are not expensive. Make your own if you have a special color or pattern in mind to give your table decor a particularly eye-appealing look. And don't be afraid to give yourself a pat on the back when you do make a special effort for your guests. ("How do you like these napkins? I made them myself last week!") It's not difficult to pamper your guests and simultaneously show off your hosting imagination, ingenuity, and organizational abilities. What an asset!

HANDSOME TABLES

• One of the best-looking tables I ever saw was one that combined oversized navy place mats, thinly striped with white, with crisp white napkins patterned in large navy polka dots. (They were made by our hosts from dish towels!) The hosts also used white china on their table, navy crystal water glasses and wineglasses, and a centerpiece of navy and white porcelain flowers.

• A romantic table setting I once photographed was a "white on white" scheme used by a famous French hostess. Her dining room carpet was white; the Louis XV dining room chairs were upholstered in white satin. She covered her round table to the floor with a cloth made from a heavy white embroidered fabric, and used another shade of white oversized dinner napkins. Her china was of yet another tone of white. White tapers in white porcelain candlesticks flanked the centerpiece. But then came the color! In the center, in a large white *blanc de Chine* porcelain bowl was a mass of bright-colored anemones. Unforgettable!

• Another artfully conceived table setting was one for a recent Maryland wedding reception. The round tables were covered in pale green moiré, with overskirts of sheer pink organdy. Pale pink roses and dark green leaves in baskets formed the centerpieces. The little ballroom chairs at the tables had cushions of pale green moiré, tied at the corners with pink tassles. There were pale green napkins, each one festively tied with a pink sash ribbon. There were little baskets of pink and green mints as table favors at each place. The china was pale pink, green, and white. The bride's mother told me that the table linens provided the theme for the entire table. Working on a budget, she made the table-cloths and napkins herself, and put the bridesmaids to work in making the seat cushion covers. I asked her how she could possibly get all this designed and executed so beautifully when she was already so busy in other projects. She explained, "I just flick the creativity switch in my brain and it takes off. Then I get to the moment of truth—making the creativity conform to a strict budget. That's when the work ethic has to take over!"

Creativity does not depend on spending a great deal of money. I remember what the CEO of a major corporation once told me about the few really successful managers on his team. "There are those who go by the book and are excellent robots," he explained, "and then there are those who take the time to think how something can be done better, faster and cheaper—whether it's a question pertaining to paper clips or important documents. They find creative solutions to their everyday job problems to help all of us work better. They are the ones who really contribute to our profits, and they are the pool from whom my successor will be chosen."

Creativity plays a very big role—in corporate planning or in entertaining. It's that same old philosophy again—caring, thinking of others, making an effort for someone or something else.

Decorating the Tables

Setting a party table or a group of tables is the moment to let your imagination soar to new heights. Just plunking down a florist's arrangement of flowers in the center of the table, flanked by four candlesticks, is what our mothers and grandmothers used to do—on an all-white tablecloth at that. But the scope of our imaginations and the age in which we live have carried us far beyond that pedestrian kind of decor, and we expect the centerpieces we face during a meal at our host's home to amuse, delight, or challenge our esthetic eye.

The way you learn to use your imagination in such matters as table decor is first to inspire it, which is accomplished by an exercise such as one of these:

- o Carefully peruse the photographs of table settings in the decorating and home publications. (Even the china, silver, and glassware in manufacturers' ads can give you inspiration.)
- o Attend table setting demonstrations given in your local department or fine jewelry store.
- o Listen to descriptions of beautifully decorated tables at parties given around town.
- o Check through the photographs in books on entertaining.
- o Make notes of particularly striking table decorations at private parties and benefits you have attended or heard described by your local newspaper "Lifestyle" reporter.
- o Experiment yourself with flowers and fruits of the season, mixing them in different containers and judging them with your table linens for maximum visual effect.

Ways to Experiment

The more you experiment, the easier it becomes to be creative in your table settings. You never have to use the same table setting twice, because linens mix and match with different pieces of china, different growing things go on the table according to the season, and you can look at your possessions from a different perspective each time. For example, one day you might want to use your favorite crystal bowl to serve ice cream for dessert; for the next party you might want to fill it with silver Christmas tree ornaments for the centerpiece; and for a Sunday lunch, you might want to use it as a centerpiece filled to the brim with colorful lettuces and chopped vegetables to be consumed by the guests during the latter part of the meal.

• *When you remember something beautiful that pleases you, do it on your table.* I remember my mother saying that her favorite flower combination was lilies-of-the-valley with small pale pink roses. It gives me such pleasure to repeat her favorite combination on my own table— and its fragrances evoke very special memories. I remember a friend of mine saying that she thought fresh asparagus is a thing of beauty when it arrives in the marketplace in the spring. One night she neatly laid several fat bunches of asparagus tied amusingly with yellow satin ribbons on a long, oval platter, so that the centerpiece looked like a barge carrying a precious cargo. (She also ringed the base of the cargo of asparagus with thin round slices of lemon.)

I will also never forget a friend on Nantucket who remembered my having said that the most romantically beautiful thing about Nantucket for me was the sight of the incredible blues of the hydrangea bushes blooming against the weathered gray shingled houses. When I next came to spend a summer weekend with her, she gave a dinner party with a rough-textured shingle-gray cloth on the table. The centerpiece was a large gray stone container holding a mass of different shades of blue hydrangeas. That's called using the imagination, but it's also called a great act of kindness, in that she paid homage to my treasured memories of Nantucket colors and textures.

• *Use whatever it is you collect on your table*—like putting your collection of toy soldiers in battle positions (or your collection of porcelain figurines) in and around a cluster of small plants and votive candles in the center of the table. I have a friend who has a collection of antique porcelain carnations. She often uses them in the center of her table, with different combinations of fragrant leaves or some smaller fresh flowers.

• *Make an enchanted burning white forest with white candles in a variety of candleholders down the center of your table.* Keep your dining area dark to make the light from the candles really dramatic. The candleholders (single ones will do, as well as pairs) may be of crystal, silver, pewter, tole, porcelain, wood—anything. (Borrow your friends' candlesticks, if you don't have a collection of your own.) It's even more effective if they are of varying heights. Some hosts prefer to make "enchanted burning forests of flowers" in the center of their tables, interweaving crystal candlestick holders with tall, slender crystal champagne flutes, each holding one beautiful flower.

• *Take items in the same color family and mix them with contrast-*

ing shades of green leaves, such as green pears and matching green grapes with contrasting dark green leaves tucked into the centerpiece bowl arrangement, or eggplant and black grapes with dark red geraniums held in little glass orchid vials that you get from a florist, tucked in securely.

• *Go against traditional color taboos and put clashing flower colors together in the center of your table*—such as a bowlful of red carnations, orange lilies, and purple violets, perhaps on the smashing background of a black linen tablecloth.

• *Surprise your guests with unusual combinations in a porcelain or silver cup, mug, or glass at each place.* For example:

  o Place a mass of snow-white carnations around a center cluster of fresh green parsley in a silver cup (something former Ambassadress Evangeline Bruce likes to do).

  o Mix sprigs of pussy-willow branches with delicate little cymbidia orchids, which the late Clare Boothe Luce used to do.

  o Put a small, beautiful crystal perfume bottle containing a few little sprigs of fragrant lily-of-the-valley on the table close to your guest of honor's place.

  o Build a pyramid of lemons for a centerpiece and tuck an occasional white gardenia into the sides.

One of my favorite hostesses will do anything to please her guests— such as when she was giving a dinner party in mid-May in Camden, South Carolina. The morning of her party, she was still visiting a friend outside Hartford, Connecticut. The air was cool on this early spring day, so she picked several beautiful brilliant yellow forsythia branches from her host's bushes, wrapped them in wet paper and flew home with them. Late that same afternoon (it was now hot and muggy in South Carolina), she picked fresh white peonies from her own bushes. Then she combined the peonies and forsythia in tall, graceful arrangements in her house for the dinner party. Not only did they knock our eyes out with their beauty, but we knew what she had done for us—managed to sample the fresh flowering offerings of Mother Nature in two different climates and environments in the same day.

• *Make table favors out of your centerpiece.* You might make an eye-catching arrangement of small flowering plants in the center of the table, for example, and then ask each guest at the end of dinner to select his or her own plant to take home (in a tote bag supplied by you).

Table favors, in fact, always make a tremendous impact on guests. Men and women become equally enthusiastic to find an amusingly wrapped "goodie" at their place at table (just as they become equally bored by the same old loot bags of commercial product samples handed out at benefit balls).

During the Christmas holidays your table favor might be

o Chocolate Santas
o Miniature gingerbread houses
o Mini fruitcakes
o Christmas tree ornaments wrapped in colorful tissue
o A miniature frame containing a snapped head shot of a member of that guest's family

At Easter, it might be

o A candy Easter egg inside an egg-shaped box encircled with ribbon
o Six freshly baked cookies shaped like bunnies or lambs and charmingly gift-wrapped

On Valentine's Day, it might be a

o Chocolate heart
o Giant chocolate Hershey Kiss
o A small book of love poetry

Even when it's not a special holiday, you as host can always celebrate *something* with a table favor. One host announced to us that "this dinner is in celebration of 'Don't-Be-Late Day,' " which none of us particularly understood—until we opened the festive little boxes at our places and found travel alarm clocks inside.

• *Develop your "own thing," to be reinterpreted each time*—as my sister-in-law Nancy Baldridge has done. Whenever she needs table decorations, she finds in her yard tall, handsomely shaped branches (such as those from a privet hedge). She makes a centerpiece for each round table out of these branches. She cuts away any excess offshoots (and green leaves, if there are any) from the branch, stabilizes it in a florist's oasis in a small container of water, covers the base with flowers, and then hangs wonderfully decorative things from it.

o At Christmastime she hangs crystal icicles or little ornaments from the branches, and covers the base with bright red carnations and holly.
o For Easter she hangs dyed Easter eggs from the branches and covers the base with hyacinths and daffodils.
o For a child's birthday, she hangs lollipops or little baskets of candy from the branches and covers the base with gumdrops.

Place Cards

Place cards make sense when you have eight or more people coming to lunch or dinner. When dinner is ready and guests go to the table, the host or hostess may be occupied picking up the cocktail glasses and ashtrays in the living room and tidying up, or he or she may be putting finishing touches on the first course about to be served to their guests. The host may not be near the table at the moment some of the guests take their place. That is why the place cards are efficient. People can see where they are supposed to sit at the table. Here are some guidelines concerning place cards:

- *The fanciest kind of place cards are made of thick white stock, thinly bordered in silver, gold, or a color,* and measure approximately two inches by three and a quarter inches. (They may be any variation of that size.) These are sold in packages (usually of fifty or one hundred) at stationers or in the stationery section of large department stores.

- *Place cards may be single cards meant to lie flat on the table, or they may be folded "tent" cards,* which stand up on the table.

- *For informal dinners in your home, you can make your own cards out of letter-writing paper.* (Many is the time I have made last-minute place cards cut out of manila file folders!)

- *If you're really trying to "put on the dog," you can order from the stationer place cards engraved with your monogram in gold or in a color.* A rarified few have their cards engraved with a legitimate family crest at the top; some social climbers go to the extreme of fabricating a family crest that everyone knows is fake, so it doesn't serve its purpose!

- *The place card is set on the table in any one of several places:* on top of a napkin set in the middle of the plate; on the table above the forks at the upper left of the place setting; leaning against the stem of a water or wineglass or just above the middle of the plate in the place setting.

- *The cards are handwritten in black ink* (hopefully by someone with a good hand), or they may be typed (jumbo type, please) for a business meal. The most posh way is to have them written by a calligrapher.

WHAT YOU WRITE ON A PLACE CARD

- *For an informal party of friends who know each other,* all you need on the place cards are first names ("Pat," "Joanie," and so on). However, if you have two Bobs or two Nancys, put both first and last names of the people with duplicate given names.

- *For an informal party when the guests don't know each other,* put both names, so each guest can glance at his or her dinner partner's card and be reminded exactly who this person is ("Jim Grierson," "Annie Keogh," or whoever).

- *For a formal dinner party,* such as a business dinner or a corporate function for a foreign guest—or any meal at which there will be people of rank—you use only the surnames on the cards ("Mr.

Carruthers," "Ms. Smyth," "Dr. Anson"). If you have two "Mrs. Jones" or two "Mr. Martins," you must use their full names on their cards—for example, "Mrs. Keith Jones," "Mrs. Ronald Jones"; "Mr. Henry Martin," "Mr. George Martin." It is proper to use only a title and the person's surname, but since guests often need to know both names, more and more often the proper way gives way to the more efficient way, and each person's first and last names are given on the place card.

• A person who has held political office, or a military officer of rank, or someone who holds a high appointed office is called by that rank or title on his or her place card, regardless of whether he or she still holds that office or rank. For example, your mayor would be "The Mayor" on his place card. When he is no longer mayor, as a courtesy he is called "Mayor Johnson" on his place card. The present governor of your state is called simply "The Governor" on his card. When he is no longer governor, he is still called "Governor Stuyvesant" on his card.

Once an ambassador, one holds that rank always. "Ambassador Reynolds" is "Ambassador Reynolds" all through his or her life, just as a retired military officer is still called by his or her rank forever—again, as a courtesy.

Menu Cards

Menu cards are a nifty extra touch—a detail that immediately transforms what may be a very simple meal into a special event. Menu cards may be handwritten in black ink, typed (very suitable for a business meal), or, most posh of all, written by a calligrapher. The menu card may lean against a glass or rest flat on the table to the left of the forks. You can provide one for each plate or one for every two guests.

It's fun for guests to know in advance what they're eating. It also helps them judge how much they will eat. A vegetarian, for example, will know he can serve himself two helpings of the salad or vegetable courses, to compensate for the meat course he will not eat. Someone on a diet will decide to skip the Yorkshire pudding when it is passed and go heavy on the fresh fruit compote when that is passed.

It is proper to use a mixture of English, French, Italian, German, and other foreign terms for specialties on your menus. If you are familiar with the proper foreign term for a particular dish you are having served, use it without fear of being called pretentious. For example, *Pasta Primavera* sounds a lot more exciting written on the menu than "Noodles with Vegetables." I learned many of my French words as a child during the Depression years of the 1930s, when my parents would bring home the dinner party menus (which was common practice in those days). I understood *Glace vanille* (what child wouldn't be able to translate vanilla ice cream?), but the *Sauce Fraises* written on the menu beneath the *Glace* would throw me. *"Fraises* means strawberries,"

Mother would say, and I would brag to my friends, "I know how to say 'strawberry sundae' in French!"

The two menus illustrated here are examples of a very informal meal with one simple wine, and a very formal dinner with two wines and a champagne. Both show a mixture of foreign and English dish titles, and both show the reason for the party (written at the top). Guests often like to take their menu cards home with them as a souvenir of a very special occasion. At a White House state dinner, for example, you will often see an entire table of ten people signing the back of each other's menus, so that when they take theirs home, they will have a record not only of what was served at the White House, but of who sat at their table.

Déjeuner du Vendredi 9 juin 1989

Menu

Tartare de Saumon
Mignons de Veau aux Truffes
Salade
Fromages
Ile Flottante

Auxey. Duresses 1983
Château Batailley 1983
Mumm Cordon Rouge

A White House menu card.

• *It's okay to be creative for informal affairs.* I really admire a friend who lives in the country, is a great cook, and gives informal Sunday night suppers for six or eight right in her kitchen. We sit down around an old refectory table, on old French chairs with rough straw seats (protected by red and white checked cushions that match the table-cloth), and eat wonderful things like stew, bouillabaisse, cous-cous, or Indian curried chicken. She has a blackboard on an artist's standing easel, which she pulls up to the table. The menu and wine are written on the blackboard in white chalk. As she knows full well, people sit by their telephones, waiting for an invitation from her.

In *Honor of Ellen's 26th Birthday*

DINNER

June 14, 1995

Hearts of Palm Salad

Beef Bourguignon
Herbed Rice

Butter Pecan Sundaes
Gâteau Anniversaire
Demitasses

Brolio Chianti Classico
1988

A simple birthday dinner menu card.

KNOWING THE RULES FOR CONTEMPORARY TABLE SETTINGS

What's on the Table at the Start of the Meal?

The rules of table settings hinge upon what is logical and efficient. If you are going to hold your fork in your left hand and your knife in your right for cutting food, then it's logical that the fork be placed on the left side of the plate and the knife on the right side. Since most of us are right-handed and reach for our glasses with our right hands, then it's logical to place all glasses in the upper right portion of the place setting.

As you approach it, a table set for guests should contain:

- Centerpiece decoration, including candles *if* your party is an evening one (however, candles are not appropriate for lunch)

The table is set for soup, a main course of meat, and dessert—for a family meal. A little extra effort in making the table look pretty makes the food taste better. The glassware is simple—just a water glass.

- Either a bare place or a plate ready to receive food or your first course already served on a plate
- Butter plate and butter knife (optional)
- Napkin
- Flatware
- Glasses
- Salts and peppers in place

Although in their ads and sales promotion pieces china companies inevitably show an empty teacup and saucer on the right-hand side of the place setting, that is incorrect. They place it there just to show the item to the customer, which confuses many people into thinking it is supposed to be there from the very beginning.

Some hosts like to place the napkin in an empty water or wineglass, making a pretty fan shape or even a flower motif.

The napkin may also be folded and placed in the center of the plate. Or it
may be folded imaginatively, as shown here, and tied with a bit of ribbon.
Some hosts use decorative napkin rings.

WHERE THE NAPKIN GOES

Napkins may be folded in many ways and placed in a variety of
positions on the table.

If you are an ardent fan of fancy napkin folding, there are good
illustrated books that teach you how to do it.

BUTTER PLATES

These small plates seem to be disappearing from tables in our
weight-conscious society today, but they are still used for formal meals,
and they are certainly the most efficient way to serve your guests rolls,
breadsticks, or bread and butter—or the items from a relish tray. In
setting a butter plate on your table, put it above the forks, to the upper

Some hosts prefer to set the table with the napkin in its traditional place to the left of the forks. It looks best with the outside folds facing left.

left; place the butter knife horizontally across on the top, its blade side facing down. Have one or two small butter pats already in place on each butter plate, although optionally you may pass around the table a small plate containing butter pats (or butter balls, made by rolling the butter between two wooden paddles) and a butter knife for guests to help themselves to as much or as little of the butter as they wish.

You would not use butter plates unless you were serving some kind of bread, muffins, popovers, or rolls, or a food requiring buttering—such as corn on the cob or baked potato.

• *If you don't own butter plates,* you can always pass around a butter knife together with a pretty porcelain dish containing pats of butter, a small container filled to the top with butter, or a pretty round container into which you have slipped a plastic tub of margarine. Guest should each serve themselves the desired amount of butter on the side of their plate and pass it on around the table.

SALTS AND PEPPERS

If you have enough small pairs of salts and peppers, place one either at the top center of each place setting or at the top, off to one side. If you don't have enough sets to supply each guest, put one set down between every two place settings, or put them at angles to the centerpiece, so that four people can have access to one salt and pepper set. If you have only two sets, put one at each end of the table. Few people add salt to their food these days, which is a compliment to whoever prepared the food, as well as a heeding of health advice. Instead of salt shakers, you might come across a "saltcellar" in someone's home—a very small open receptacle for salt, with a tiny salt spoon lying beside it on the table.

While people are cutting down on their salt intake, they are not necessarily cutting down on their pepper intake. If you provide the table with a large pepper mill at each end, you will probably delight your guests, particularly if you are serving pasta. (The guests should use the pepper mill themselves; the host does not have to go around the table grinding the pepper on their food, like a waiter in a restaurant!)

ASHTRAYS

In today's world, where smokers and nonsmokers seem to be increasing their combativeness, ashtrays are rarely included in the table settings of nonsmoking hosts. (When I grew up, whether you smoked or not, you gave each adult guest an ashtray at the top of his place setting, near the glasses, plus a small crystal or silver urn containing two cigarettes and a small book of gold or silver paper matches.) If you have invited smokers to your home, and if you permit smoking, put an ashtray and matches in front of each person who you know smokes. It is incumbent upon the guest to supply his or her own cigarettes; that is no longer the responsibility of the host. Just hope and pray that your smoking guests have enough manners not to light up until after everyone has finished dessert.

CANDY DISHES

If you have guests for dinner, it is very nice to have a small dish or a pair of dishes containing special candy (for example, chocolate truffles) as part of the decoration on the table. Hopefully, the guests will

Candy looks pretty on your table in a footed compote—or even in a small bowl. Put a pair of them on your table. I always make a bet with my husband as to how many chocolates will be left by the time dessert is served—because our guests invariably eat them during the soup and meat courses, too!

not eat all the candy during the meal but will wait until the proper moment—when the host sees that it is passed around after dessert.

A small bowl of silver, crystal, or porcelain makes a nice candy dish. So does a tall-stemmed wineglass. A footed compote is perhaps the nicest of all, but far more important than the quality of the serving container is the quality of the candy.

Salad Plates and the Service of Salad

The ubiquitous plate that ranges in size from about seven and a half to eight and a half inches in diameter has many uses. It can serve as a

- o Salad plate
- o Dessert plate
- o Underplate for a footed compote or for a soup cup and saucer
- o Server for small cookies, brownies, chocolate truffles, and the like

People eating informally today usually serve their salad right onto their dinner plate, and thus have no need of separate salad plates.

If you have guests, however, it's nice to give them separate plates for salad that is served with the main course. (Give them a separate salad fork, too, in this case, although it's not the end of the world if the guests have to eat their salad with their dinner forks.)

When you serve a separate salad course, between the main course and dessert, it should be more than just a lettuce leaf! Shown here is the plate of a guest who has served herself endive and Boston lettuce salad, some cheese, and crackers.

If you are serving a separate salad and cheese course (on individual salad plates) in between the entrée and dessert courses, supply your guests:

- First with a salad plate in the center of the place setting.
- Then pass the salad bowl.
- Then pass a cheese tray with a cheese knife.
- Follow with an assortment of crackers (preferably warmed).
- Then pass a container of softened butter with a butter knife.

(Each guest will require a salad fork and a small knife among the implements in his or her place setting for a course like this.)

I have long been an ardent opponent of what often happens in restaurants and at hotel banquets: A plain, boring green salad is served as a separate course, giving it an importance equal to the entrée! That's a waste of time and slows up the service for nothing. It's far better to make the salad part of the entrée service and thus permit the guests in the ballroom or restaurant to go home a half hour earlier!

Using the Right Flatware

WHEN YOU'RE A BEWILDERED GUEST

It is not uncommon for a person to sit down at a formal dinner table and confront an inexplicable array of eating utensils, all terrifyingly lined up in battle formation. Panic may ensue, with the guest wondering which to use for what.

Even one guest for dinner (in this case, a fish dinner) merits an extra effort to make the table look pretty. A white wineglass joins the water glass on the table.

It's easy for something to go wrong. The waiter may not have set the table properly. Or one can make a classic error, such as I did at a black tie dinner party when I used a spoon to eat the stuffed avocado first course instead of the tiny fork on the far left that I should have used—with the result that when the creamy dessert was served, I had only a tiny fork left with which to eat it. (To make matters far worse, everyone at my table had followed my lead, thinking I knew what I was doing. I had to SOS the waiter to bring spoons for our entire table.)

The table is set so that *you eat from the outside in*—in other words, you take the outside utensil or utensils for the first course, and then proceed, course by course, selecting the next utensils toward the plate until finally you have used them all up.

DESSERT IMPLEMENTS

Dessert utensils may either be left at the top of the place setting, as shown in the illustration, or the dessert spoon may be placed on the inside right of the place setting. Or the waiter may bring you a plate with the proper utensils on it when dessert is ready to be served.

When special guests—your boss, for example—come for dinner, the table setting becomes more complex, because the menu is, too. There is crabmeat cocktail as a first course, roast beef and Yorkshire pudding for the second, salad and cheese for the next course, and strawberry shortcake for dessert. Both white and red wineglasses join the water glass for this kind of meal.

If you set your table with the dessert implements lying horizontally at the top of your plate, put the spoon on top (its bowl pointing left) and the fork beneath (its tines pointing right). By the way, it's not absolutely necessary to use two implements for the dessert course. It just makes eating a little easier for the guests if they have something to help push the dessert onto their fork or spoon. If you can't supply both a fork and spoon for dessert, but only one of them, don't worry. As long as the implements with which you set the table convey the food to the guests' mouths, you will do very well as a host!

Most of us don't possess a great variety of flatware. You can always improvise. For example,

- o A *salad fork* may be used for fish, salad, or dessert.
- o A *luncheon fork,* smaller than a dinner fork, may be used for the same varied purposes as a salad fork.
- o A *fruit knife* may also be used as a cheese or dessert knife.
- o A *steak knife* may also be used as a dessert knife.
- o A *teaspoon* may be used for dessert if you don't have large dessert spoons.

WHAT TABLE ACCOUTREMENTS MUST YOU BUY FOR ENTERTAINING TODAY?

Some people who can't afford nice things for the table use that as an excuse for not entertaining.

That is *not* a legitimate excuse to avoid entertaining. You can buy nice things slowly, and use what you have in the meantime. You don't have to set a table with lavish objects. Instead, set your table imaginatively, without apology, and make an excellent meal for your guests. The spirit of hospitality you display is far more important than the cost of the table accoutrements you display.

You don't have to buy an entire set of anything. You can mix and match. As a single woman into my mid-thirties, I did not have any of the "loot" brides receive, but I entertained all the time anyway. I bought things slowly on the installment plan, and I borrowed things I really needed from married friends who had an excess of wedding gifts. It's fun to grow with your possessions as you grow in your entertaining skills.

• Learn to use your possessions for more than just one purpose. Your individual wooden salad bowls can make fine dessert servers. Your porcelain teapot can serve as a nice flower container for the table centerpiece. Your extra wineglasses can be used to serve cold soup or dessert—or to hold the mixed nuts you offer guests during the cocktail hours before the meal.

If you don't have demitasse cups, use teacups to serve after-dinner coffee; if you don't have teacups, serve after-dinner coffee in the mugs that you undoubtedly have in your cupboard.

In entertaining, where there's a will, there's a way. Don't be ashamed of what you have. Go ahead, use it all, without apologizing. Have people over for a meal or a party! It's the idea and the effort to please that count.

Buying Your China

A place setting of china consists of:

o Dinner plate
o Dessert or salad plate
o Butter plate
o Cup and saucer

You don't need to buy complete place settings. What if you would like dinner plates in one pattern and dessert plates in another? Buy only the items you need. (Merchants will kill me for saying this!) If you are going to have dinners for six, purchase six dinner plates and six dessert plates and six demitasse cups and saucers from open stock. (You can always drink everyday coffee or tea from everyday mugs.) The dessert plates and demitasses do not have to match the dinner plates. If, when you start out entertaining, you find yourself with an assortment of dinner plates of different patterns, it doesn't matter—have that dinner party anyway. One young friend of mine has twenty-four dinner and twenty-four dessert plates—all different—which she has picked up during her forays in thrift shops. Instead of looking poor, the plates are beautiful—and an enhancement to her frequently held buffet dinners for twenty-four people.

Buying Table Linens

Buy what appeals to your eye. You should like what you buy—don't buy colors or patterns because they are the current fad and considered chic. (One year, it seemed everyone had to buy mirrored place mats; the next year it was flowered chintz tablecloths; the year after that it was bold geometrics.)

Coordinate the colors and patterns of your china and linen, so there's an intelligent approach to your table decor. You may use multi-colored napkins or napkins of different patterns, as long as they color coordinate with your tablecloth or place mats. If you have a tabletop that is scarred or not in good condition, use a tablecloth to cover it instead of place mats. If you can't find or afford nice linens, buy inexpensive

Now the full galaxy of the hostess's table accoutrements is in use for an elaborate dinner of soup, fish, veal, and a chocolate ice-cream praline bombe for dessert. The white wineglass is properly lined up on the far right, then the red, then the water glass, and last, but certainly not least, the champagne goblet in the rear.

fabric and run them up yourself on your own or a borrowed sewing machine.

Buying Flatware

You do not have to be a bride to buy flatware. Many men and women marry late in life, as I did, and you most assuredly don't have to wait until you're married to have nice things on your table.

It's *very nice* to own sterling silver flatware, but in today's era of informality, you can certainly make do with silverplate or stainless steel. If you don't have sterling silver candelabra, you can make do with porcelain, glass, or terra cotta candlesticks.

If you approach a store like Tiffany's to buy sterling silver flatware, the salesperson will ask if you want to buy place settings of luncheon- or dinner-sized flatware. (The only real difference between the two is that the dinner knives and forks are about an inch longer than the luncheon-sized, and are more expensive.) A *place setting* consists of: fork, knife, teaspoon, dessert spoon, salad fork, and butter spreader.

If you're on a strict budget, as I was as a young single working woman, buy what you will need on the installment plan (or time account). Don't buy by the place setting, because that is not the thrifty thing to do. What are you going to do with all those butter spreaders? And you can buy your dessert spoons later—for example, when you get your next promotion.

As with china, buy pieces of flatware according to the number of dinner guests you usually have. If, for example, the maximum number of people you can entertain in your small apartment is six, you will need

- o Six soup spoons
- o Six dinner forks
- o Six dinner knives
- o Six teaspoons
- o Six salad forks

Purchase items like serving pieces, dessert spoons, and luncheon forks and knives when you have the money and as you need them. You can always ask family members to give them to you as Christmas and birthday presents. You can pick up little demitasse spoons reasonably in thrift shops or old silver shops. Perhaps you want to buy them one at a time. As with your china, the coffee spoons do not have to match each other.

Buying Glassware

When you first start to entertain, you need only six all-purpose wineglasses, six old-fashioned, and six water glasses for the table. As your income expands and you entertain more lavishly, you can start to buy the champagne flutes, white wineglasses, liqueur glasses, and brandy snifters. Matching stemware is wonderful, but your glasses do not have to match. Water glasses of one pattern and wineglasses of another pattern look great together on the table. Your guests will care much more about the flow of wine and the quality of the conversation than they will about matching stemware.

THE SERVICE OF THE SEATED MEAL—WITH OR WITHOUT HELP

One of the most important aspects of entertaining gracefully is knowing how to serve the meal—or knowing how to direct whoever is serving it to do so properly. (In today's society, there are all too many untrained waiters and waitresses working at their profession.) If you are using raw recruits for serving your party (your children included), it helps to stage-manage a quick run-through of how things are to be done. If you are paying a lot of money for a catering staff and you fear they are not up to snuff in the art of serving, it helps to give them a quick rehearsal run-through, too. The ritual of proper serving is totally functional—how to get the food on and off the table gracefully and efficiently. Knowledge of the ritual of service helps avoid accidents, collisions, awkwardness, and sloppiness in the service of your meals.

The waiter, when offering a platter of food, serves from the guest's left. One hand is behind his back, the other hand, with his palm up (protected from the heat of the platter by a napkin) offers the platter close to the guest's body. The serving implements should be in position to make it easy for the guest to pick them up and use them.

Who Is Served First?

When there is no help, the person serving the meal—or the host couple, as the case may be—first serves the woman on the host's right (or the man on the hostess's right), who is the guest of honor, and then continues on around the table counter-clockwise. The guest of honor is the most important person present at the table by virtue of age, senior family relationship, or prominence in the community. Or it may be someone who is being honored for another reason—such as a person visiting from another city, someone celebrating a birthday, or a friend who is moving away.

When an important couple is present, the wife sitting next to the male host is served first, rather than the husband sitting to the right of the hostess. After serving the guest of honor, the waiter then passes the bowl or platter around the table counter-clockwise. If the wife of the important couple is served first, then the host beside her would be the last to be served at that table.

How Does the Waiter or Waitress Serve?

One person can handle a table or eight, but with ten or twelve guests to a table, it is more efficient to have two people serving. If two servers for your large table are not in the budget, go with one, but be content with having the service very slow.

The person serving passes the food from the left side of the guest, and removes each finished plate from the right side of the guest. If a serving dish is hot, the waiter places a folded napkin under it to protect the palm of his hand. The wine, of course, is served from the guest's right side, where the wineglasses are in place. (To serve the wine from the guest's left side would require reaching across the guest's face to get to the glass.)

A trained waiter is capable of removing a used plate with the right hand while simultaneously putting down a clean plate with a flourish of his or her left hand. If you are serving your guests yourself, you may not be that dexterous, in which case it is easier first to remove finished plates, one in each hand, and then bring in the plates for the next course, one in each hand, on the way back to the dining table. Even a caterer's so-called trained waiters often must be reminded to take out plates, one in each hand, instead of scraping the remnants of food from several plates onto one plate (in front of everyone) and then carrying out the stack of used plates into the kitchen. It may be a lot speedier to scrape several plates at the table before taking a stack into the kitchen, but it is also a lot noisier and certainly less attractive.

Waiter #1
serves
in this
order:

7. Host

1.Woman guest of honor	Woman guest 6.
2. Man guest	Man guest 5.
3. Woman guest	Woman guest 4.
4. Man guest	Man guest 3.
5. Woman guest	Woman guest 2.
6. Man guest	Man guest of honor 1.

7. Host's wife

Waiter #2
serves in
this order:

When there are more than eight or ten guests, two waiters are needed, as for this dinner for fourteen. Waiter number one begins serving the woman guest of honor; waiter number two begins serving the man guest of honor. Each waiter ends up serving the host or hostess last.

The proper way to remove a guest's finished plate is to remove it from the person's right with the right hand and to clamp down on the fork and knife (or whatever implements are being used) with the right-hand thumb. In this way, the trip is made to the kitchen *safely* and gracefully. (No clattering of fallen plates and flying knives!)

Watch out! If the waiter at your party (or a son or daughter who is helping you out) removes the plates from the table in this fashion in order to bring on the next course, there will inevitably be some unexpected sound effects— and some new bills to pay in a china and glassware store!

Serving a Dinner Party of Six Without Help

It is much more efficient for a small group of six or eight if either the husband or the wife acts as the server for the group. Then one of the two hosts will be in the dining room at all times to keep the conversation going. If both keep getting up and going in and out of the kitchen, the guests are distracted, to put it mildly. If you are single and doing the serving, appoint a friend to act as host when you have to be absent in the process of serving.

A smart host keeps firm control of the service of the meal so that there is a minimum of noise and confusion as it is served. Couples who are skilled at giving dinner parties keep aprons handy in the kitchen— and don them only in the kitchen. As the designated server carries two used plates out into the kitchen, behind a closed door the food is quickly scraped and the plates are rinsed and then stacked into the dishwasher. In this way the kitchen is always tidy and there is enough room to cope with the next set of used dishes.

Should the Guests Help?

If you are like me, you don't particularly want the guests, however well intentioned, meddling in your kitchen. Not only could they ruin your efficient system and create havoc, but they could also spill food and splash water on their party clothes at the same time. The place for guests is in your party area, not in your kitchen. An exception to this rule is, of course, if you have one of those handsome large kitchens where everything, including the dining table is in one vast room. (But even here there is no reason for guests to help.) I could never operate in one of those party kitchens, nor can anyone else like me who needs total concentration and generally makes a terrible mess of the entire kitchen environment while cooking.

Training Young People to Wait on Table

In our world today, with help so difficult to find and expensive to hire, a little imagination and footwork can ease the burden. If you have teenaged children or if there are teenagers in your neighborhood or apartment house, you are all set.

Train these young people in the art of serving a meal. Teach them what to do and have them practice first at a couple of family meals or make-believe dinner parties. Pay them nicely for the services they perform in serving, dishwashing, and cleaning up after your party. What a teenager receives depends upon the part of the country and what the local market will bear, like baby-sitting rates; some parents pay their children $3 an hour, others $5, others $8. Have the boys dress in dark pants, white shirts, and black bow ties; the girls can wear black skirts and white blouses. Your guests will be delighted to have the meal served by attractive young people with smiling faces. Moreover, the training you will have given them will help them earn money in college. There are many functions on college and university campuses in need of trained waiters—particularly parties given by the president, faculty members, and administrators, for whom entertainment is a fact of life.

Advice to Waiters on Serving a Typical Three-Course Meal

- Fill the water glasses three-quarters full. Check the table to make sure that no guest's place is missing anything, such as a fork or a napkin.
- Wait until the guests are seated. Then, if the first course is not served on a plate and already at each place on the table, pass this course to the guests. It should be passed first to the woman on the

host's right; it should then be passed counter-clockwise around the table, with the host served last. Remember, always serve from the left.

• Pass the rolls, crackers, relish tray, or anything that goes with that first course.

• Pour wine into each glass, moving around the table counter-clockwise after first filling the female guest of honor's glass. If a guest puts his or her fingers over the rim of the glass, it is a signal that he or she does not wish to have wine poured in the glass.

• When you notice that all of the guests have finished eating, or when you receive a signal from the host, it's time to remove the plates containing the first course and bring them to the kitchen area. Standing to the right of the guest, remove his or her plate with your right hand and transfer it to your left; then go to the next person on the right and remove that plate with your right hand—so that you can bring two plates into the kitchen at once. If there is a fork and knife or spoon on each plate, hold onto the utensils with your thumb so they don't fall off the plate while you are en route to the kitchen.

• Now that the table is empty of used plates, bring in the clean plates for the next course, one in each hand, and lay each in front of the guest, again from the left side.

• Pass the next course, serving from the left. Then pass anything accompanying the entree (gravy, sauces, vegetables), again from the left. Always readjust the serving utensils if they have been put back on the platter the wrong way, so that the next guest to be served can get at the food easily. If one of the guests has managed to get sauce all over the handle of a serving utensil, wipe the handle with a napkin before putting it back on the platter.

• Pour the next wine on the menu, or refill glasses with the first wine.

• Pass the rolls again (if there are any).

• Pass again anything your host previously instructed you to pass twice—provided, of course, there is a sufficient amount left. If there is very little left of any one item, don't pass it again.

• When it's time for dessert, remove the entrée or salad course plates, being careful to hold onto the eating utensils with your thumbs, so they don't fall. Remove the salts and peppers and any sauce boats or condiments from the table. The table should be devoid of anything having to do with previous courses. If someone has been rude enough to smoke during the meal and has a dirty ashtray, take it to the kitchen, wash it, and return it to the table. (Otherwise, people close to the cigarette butts might not enjoy their dessert.)

If there are butter plates, they must be cleared away from the table, too. Place the butter plates and knives on top of the entrée plates. You

If you don't have a special "crumber," fold a napkin and use the smooth end to push the crumbs from the table onto a small plate.

will now have to cope with a small plate and butter knife, balanced on top of a big plate with a dinner fork and knife.

• Crumb the table, using a folded white napkin to push the crumbs around each place setting onto a plate held just beneath the table top, or use the "crumber" (perhaps a Silent Butler) provided by the host (which you use with a decorative little brush).

• Bring in the dessert plates. If there are to be finger bowls, set down before each guest a finger bowl (three-quarters filled with water) on a doily that has been placed in the middle of the dessert plate.

• Pass the dessert, which may be in two parts—for example, ice cream with a sauce passed afterward, or a soufflé with cookies passed afterward.

• Refill the wineglasses.

• Pass around the dish of special candy or ginger or whatever the host may have provided as a post-dessert treat. If the candy dish (or pair of dishes) has remained on the table through dinner, the guests are supposed to help themselves upon completing their dessert.

In most houses, after-dinner coffee is served from a tray brought to a room other than the one where dinner was served. This permits guests to get up from the table to mix with each other. This tray holds a pot for regular brewed coffee, a pot for decaff, a sugar bowl, a creamer, and a small bowl for sugar substitute.

SERVING COFFEE AFTER DINNER

At dinner parties, coffee should be served in little demitasse cups and saucers, with small accompanying coffee spoons. The host will have instructed you before dinner whether coffee is to be served at the table or in another room.

If coffee is to be served at the table, put down a filled demitasse cup and saucer (the coffee spoon balancing on the right side of the saucer) to the right of each guest's place setting. (Naturally, as with wine or other beverages, you serve this from the right instead of from the usual left.) Then pass to each guest (this time from the left) the tray containing the cream, sugar, and artificial sweetener.

An alternative way of serving coffee at the table is to put in front of the hostess (or host, as the case may be), a large tray containing the coffee cups and saucers, a group of coffee spoons, the coffee pot, a sugar bowl, and creamer. The hostess or host serves each guest separately, pouring the coffee and then passing the guest his or her cup, saucer, and spoon with whatever the guest asked for in the coffee. (NOTE: The spoon is a bother and is often dropped, so it should not even be given to a coffee drinker who drinks his or her coffee black, with nothing added.)

Often the only coffee served these days after dinner is decaff, but a really considerate host makes available to the guest a pot of real coffee *and* decaff.

• *When coffee is served in another room,* the waiter may pass among the guests with a large tray containing already poured cups of coffee, allowing each guest to serve him- or herself from the creamer and sugar bowl. Another option: The hostess may serve the coffee herself while seated on the sofa, with a tray containing the coffee pot, cups, saucers, spoons, sugar bowl, and creamer in front of her on the coffee table. As guests approach her, she asks how they would like their coffee, and then she hands each a properly prepared demitasse.

At the end of the meal, after the demitasses have been served, bring in (or have your server bring in) your prettiest tray set with bottles and decanters of port and liqueurs, plus small liqueur glasses and brandy snifters.

After-Dinner Liqueurs, Drinks, and Glasses of Water

During the after-dinner coffee hour, when everyone has been sipping their coffee, the waiter reappears with a tray bearing a bottle of cognac and one or two sweet liqueurs, plus several brandy snifters and small liqueur glasses. Guests either serve themselves, or the waiter serves them. The tray is too heavy to hold and serve from at the same time, so when the waiter "gets a customer," so to speak, he should put down the tray before attempting to fill the guest's order.

Then the waiter might reappear with a tray of tall glasses of ice water and pass them around the entire group. He should first approach the host or hostess with the tray of glasses of ice water, so the hosts know what is going on. At this point the waiter would also ask a guest who has not taken a brandy, liqueur, or glass of water, "May I bring you something else to drink?" That guest may be longing for a highball (Scotch, ice, and water or soda in a tall glass).

THE ART OF THE SERVICE OF WINE

The service of wine is an art and a mealtime ritual replete with history and romance—and one that is taken seriously by a caring host.

It is wise—and entertaining as well—to educate yourself about wine by

- Reading good books on the subject (there are many)
- Attending wine tastings (and really *listening* to the lecturer, as well as enjoying the sipping)
- Conversing as often as possible with a knowledgeable salesperson at the liquor store (obviously when he or she is not busy)
- Going through a well-established winery in America or Europe to learn how wine is made

Your water glass is filled about two-thirds and a wine-glass only about half-way, as shown here.

Tips on the Service of Wine

- To be correct, fill the wineglass only halfway.
- Whether at home or in a restaurant, show the label to your guests if you are particularly proud of the wine. (A nice guest, sensing that a good wine is about to be served, will ask you, "What is the wine?" thus giving you a good excuse for praising it—just a bit.)
- If you are not particularly proud of the wine, first decant it into a good-looking crystal decanter. (Unlike a wine bottle, a decanter will not mark the table, so does not need to be put on a coaster.)
- Many connoisseurs feel that fortified wine (such as port and sherry to which brandy is added) should properly be decanted. There is an old French saying that a fine red wine *merits* being decanted to allow its real flavor to develop, whereas a humble red wine *needs* to be decanted, to help it along.
- Most red wines should be served at a cool room temperature. If you serve your guests a good red wine that for some reason is too cool, suggest that they hold the bowl of their glasses in their hands, which will quickly warm the wine the necessary few degrees.
- Chill your white wine in the refrigerator at least two hours before the meal, or if you have a wine cooler, chill the white wine in it for

A bottle of white wine is kept cold either in a wine cooler with ice and water or in a cold thermos holder, shown above.

twenty minutes in a bath of ice cubes and ice water. (The finer the white wine, the less chilling it requires.) If you're really in a jam time-wise because you forgot to prechill the wine, stick the bottle in your freezer for fifteen minues. (But whatever you do, don't forget and leave it there!)

• Some people today prefer to drink one wine of their choice all evening. Therefore, a caring host places both a bottle of red and a bottle of white on coasters on his table. A cold thermos holder for a bottle of white wine doesn't look very pretty on the table, but it's a practical assist on a hot summer's night.

• As host, you would serve your guests around the table the first time, going counter-clockwise, starting with the person seated at your right and finishing with yourself. Then you might ask someone at the other end of the table to assume the responsibility for keeping the glasses refilled at that end of the table. If you offer your guests red and white wines at a dinner for eight or more, you should provide two bottles of wine, one white and one red (each on a coaster), at each end of the table.

Put a wine bottle coaster at each end of your dinner table—with a bottle of red in one and white in the other. The host should keep an eye on the bottles, and replace them during the meal when they are empty. In this kind of informal service, guests help themselves to their wine of choice during the meal.

- Never allow a guest to pour a new wine into a glass he or she used previously for another color of wine. It's the principle of good hospitality involved here, not that the taste of a new wine would be altered greatly by having it poured into a used, empty glass.
- Unless you are a true expert, you will probably need a napkin held under the neck of the bottle as you pour wine into guests' glasses. The napkin catches errant drops of wine. The more you twirl the opening of the bottle in an upward motion as you pour, the less wine you will spill, and the less you will need that napkin!
- Occasionally you will see a bottle cradled in (and served from) a basket in almost a horizontal position. This keeps the sediment from mixing into the wine in the bottle.

The Major Categories of Wine and Their Proper Serving Temperatures

Many countries and several states in the United States produce wine today, but the best wines seem to come from California, France, Italy, and Germany, with good wines also available from Spain, Portugal, Australia, and Chile.

There are five main categories of wine.

RED TABLE WINES

The Bordeaux, Burgundy, Beaujolais, Chianti, Barolo, and Rioja wines (from France, Italy, and Spain, respectively) are in this group. So are the varietal wines, such as Cabernet Sauvignon, Pinot Noir, and Zinfandel from America, Australia, and other countries.

These wines should be served at a cool temperature (no higher than 70°). Traditionally, they are served with meat, fowl, and cheese (although today the rules regarding what kind of wine one drinks with any particular food seem to be broken fearlessly).

Rosé wines are known for their lovely pink color and refreshing taste when served well chilled in hot weather. They are not, however, great wines. (*See also* Sparkling wines on the following page.)

WHITE TABLE WINES

These include Burgundy, Chablis, Meursault, Chassagne-Mon-trachet, Muscadet, and Sancerre (all from France); Gavi and Pinot Grigio from Italy; Chardonnay, Sauvignon Blanc, Chenin Blanc, and Chablis from France, the United States, Chile, Australia, and New Zealand, and the sweet Rieslings from Germany.

Dry white table wines should be served chilled, but not to the extent that the flavor and bouquet are altered. Traditionally, white wines were served with light foods such as fish, fruit, veal, and chicken. Today some people use white wine as their preferred predinner cocktail choice, and some prefer to drink it all through the meal (instead of switching to red during the meat entrée).

APPETIZER WINES (APERITIFS)

Aperitifs such as dry or sweet vermouth, red or white Dubonnet, Campari, Cinzano, and Lillet are served as a before-meal drink, usually in a small portion. A lemon zest (a bit of lemon peel) is often added to the wine to add a little zing to the taste. They are served according to your preference—at room temperature in a small glass, or chilled, or in a small old-fashioned glass with ice.

Dry sherry, an important member of the aperitif family, is usually served at room temperature—and in a sherry glass, if possible. (Use a liqueur glass, if you don't have a sherry glass, and if you don't have a liqueur glass either, use any small wineglass or bar glass.) Appetizer wines taste best when there is an accompanying plate of almonds, cheese-straws, or anything in the dry munching category.

DESSERT WINES

For several decades sweet dessert wines like Sauternes (which are served chilled in white wineglasses) went into a decline in popularity, but lately they are coming back into vogue. A glass is put down at your place at the table, and the wine is poured from a decanter after dessert is served. Germany has some fine examples of sweet white wines. Sweet sherry, port, and Madeira are normally consumed after dinner at room temperature.

SPARKLING WINES

The fifth category comprises sparkling rosé wines, such as Italy's Asti Spumante, and the really excellent sparkling wines, such as those from the Schramsberg vineyard in California. (Several prominent houses in the Champagne region of France have started wineries in California, too.) Italy, other parts of France, and Spain also produce large quantities of good sparkling wines at reasonable prices. The queen of this category is, of course, champagne.

Champagne Etiquette

GLASSES

Coupe-shaped champagne glasses are no longer in vogue, for practical reasons. They are difficult to clean, and the champagne grows warm inside the hollow stem—because of the warm fingers clasping the stem. A flute or tulip-shaped champagne glass, usually about seven ounces in capacity, is more desirable. (Pour four ounces into such a glass.)

OPENING THE BOTTLE

First, you must remove the wire enclosure ("bonnet") around the cork. Once you begin this operation, don't stop and change your mind about opening the bottle. (Pressure begins to build up inside and could explode the cork right out of an unattended bottle.) Brace the bottom of the bottle into your abdomen and begin twisting the cork with your fingers. Some people prefer optionally to hold on to the cork while rotating the bottle with their fingers. Whatever you do, take care to aim away from the faces of your friends, as well as nearby crystal pieces, porcelain, or anything fragile. (I will always remember the story told about an English art collector who acquired at auction an "Old Masters" painting of his life's dreams. That evening he invited two close friends to celebrate. One of them opened his gift—a bottle of champagne— carelessly, and the cork put a hole right through the painting.)

Rather than anticipating with joy the sound of a big pop as the champagne cork finally exits the mouth of the bottle, it is better to strive for only a gentle hissing sound as it emerges. A noisy pop encourages the escape of air and disperses the much-desired bubbles.

• *It's important to remember that champagne must be well chilled to be enjoyed to its fullest.* Once you have removed the cork, keep the bottle in a winebucket half full of ice and ice water, or put it back into the fridge until it's time to refill the glasses.

Champagne is the symbol of happiness, celebration, and a special moment in life. That's why it's important to buy a good-quality champagne, to serve it ice cold, and to use beautiful flutes. It's all part of the mystique—the romance and the ritual.

After-Dinner Drinks

When people are enjoying their demitasses after dinner at the table—or when the host moves the guests from the dining area into another room for their after-dinner coffee—it is time to pass after-dinner drinks. Two kinds of glasses are useful here—*brandy snifters* for serving Cognac or Armagnac, and small stemmed glasses to use for *sweet liqueurs*. Port may also be served in a regular wineglass.

The most popular of the after-dinner drinks are these:

- Port.
- Cognac and Armagnac, which come in several price levels, according to the quality and grade. VSOP, for example, is less expensive than a Napoleon Cognac, and vintage-dated Armagnacs are more costly than nonvintage-dated ones.
- Grappa (Italian brandy) is also very popular.
- *Eaux-de-vies*—clear brandies made from distilled fruits. *Poire* (pear) and *framboise* (rasperry) are the most popular ones.
- Green or white crème de menthe (often served over cracked ice).
- Cointreau.
- Cream-finished liqueurs—for example, Irish Cream and crème de cacao.
- Peach-based cordials (and also peach-champagne cocktails).

If you have serving help at your dinner party, the server should pass a tray to each guest (and the host last), containing from two to four bottles of the various after-dinner drinks being offered (brandy must be one of them) and an assortment of empty glasses appropriate for those drinks. The tray may also be placed in a central place in the party area (such as on the coffee table in front of the sofa), where guests will help themselves (at the host's urging) to the drink of their choice.

If you don't have serving help, put down a bottle of brandy plus an optional sweet liqueur on your dinner table as you are finishing coffee, or wherever you wish, and serve your guests. You don't have to be hosting a fancy black tie dinner with waiters in attendance to enjoy an after-dinner drink.

How to Open a Wine Bottle

The best and easiest-to-use bottle opener is a Screwpull. You plunge its Teflon-coated screw into the center of the cork and then squeeze the two arms together around the neck of the bottle; as you turn the top lever, the screw easily extricates the cork from the bottle.

Once you have the cork out, pour a very small amount of wine into the kitchen sink, to remove any bits of floating cork. Also take a clean damp cloth and wipe around the outside and inside of the neck to remove any grime.

A Bad Cork

If you have a bad cork that disintegrates as you try to extract it, you might end up using everything from a screw driver to a letter opener to

The easiest way to open a bottle of wine is to use a Screwpull.

try to get it out. If, as my bad corks always do, your lacerated cork gets pushed down into the bottle of wine, don't despair. Hold a small strainer over a water pitcher and then pour the bottle of wine through it. Now you can transfer the wine from the water pitcher to a decanter that will look attractive on the table.

I have learned by experience from my own dinner parties always to have an extra bottle or two on hand, in case disaster strikes while opening the wine. I would much prefer to give our guests good wine from the bottle, rather than "strained wine" from an embattled bottle. (We drink the latter ourselves the next night.)

If you consume a lot of wine in your household, you would be smart to own—and learn how to use—an "Ah-So" cork remover. This gadget removes fragile corks that crumble when you try to remove them. The Ah-So consists of two flexible prongs which are inserted between the cork and the neck of the bottle; the cork is then jimmied up. It is much better than my system, which requires occasionally straining out the cork from the wine!

Always open your wines gently well in advance of the guests' arrival. Then if there is any cork difficulty, it will have occurred in private and will have been coped with successfully before your guests arrive.

Tasting the Wine at Home

As the host, after you have opened the wine in the kitchen in advance of the guests' arrival, you should taste it immediately to make sure that it is in good condition. The wine sampling should not be done in front of your guests at home—only in a restaurant.

Tasting the Wine in a Good Restaurant

In a good restaurant, it is quite a different story. After you have selected your bottle of wine, the wine steward or captain or waiter will present it to you. (Never, by the way, be embarrassed to solicit his help and advice in making your selection.) When the bottle is brought to your table, you, the host, should then taste it on behalf of your guests. (If you know absolutely nothing about wine or do not drink alcohol, ask one of your guests who you know is familiar with wine to taste it for you.) The sommelier, maître d' or waiter (once he or she has opened the good bottle of wine you ordered) may do any of the following:

- o Hand you the cork, expecting you to sniff it and squeeze it in your fingers to make sure that it is neither dried out nor wet and soggy. (Once you have examined the cork, put it back on the table; it will be removed by the server of the wine.)
- o Pour a small amount into your glass for you to sniff the bouquet and taste it. (Swirl the wine around a bit, finally take a sip, and then give your nod of approval to the wine server.)
- o Upon receiving your approval, move around the table to fill your guests' glasses, serving you last.

RETURNING A BAD BOTTLE

Do not grimace and tell the wine server to "take this bottle back" unless you are on firm grounds and know what you are doing. On a rare occasion, the wine will have turned and taste bitter, in which case the wine server will take a taste of it himself in his own glass. If he agrees that this particular bottle has gone bad, he will bring you another one at once. (In really fine restaurants, the sommelier will already have tasted your bottle in the kitchen, to avoid ever serving a wine that has gone bad.)

It's embarrassing if, when acting from lack of knowledge, you request the wine to be replaced and no one except you finds anything wrong with the bottle. I remember as a young woman on a date being very embarrassed when my host returned an expensive bottle, calling it defective. He was showing off, and everyone in the restaurant was watching us. Then the maître d' noted the clean scent of mouthwash on his breath. My host had just returned from the men's room, where he'd rinsed his mouth with Listerine, which meant that the wine would not taste right, no matter what. After the maître d' gently pointed out this fact, my host apologized and drank from the same bottle fifteen minutes later, now greatly enjoying the taste of the wine.

Wineglasses

A wineglass should be a clear, sparkling stemmed goblet—the thinner the better and the more enjoyable to hold and to drink from.

The bowl of the glass should be larger than the rim, so that the bouquet of the wine can waft up to your nostrils as you drink.

When you need an array of wineglasses on your table to go with the different wines being served, group them on the table chronologically, starting from the outside right as the first wineglass, and going into the center of each person's place setting for the champagne and water goblets. These glasses do not need to be set up in a straight row. They can be informally grouped, but in a manner so that you know which is the next one to use.

Of course, if you are having only a red or only a white wine all through the meal, you can either put down the red or white wineglass— or optionally, an all-purpose wineglass that may be used equally well for either red or white wine. If you don't have champagne glasses and you are going to have a special celebration, borrow some glasses from a friend. (And *never* serve champagne—or wine either—in a plastic or a paper cup inside your house!)

How Much Wine to Buy

If you are having a dinner party, buy your wine by the case—it's usually less expensive that way, and you can always enjoy the rest of the case at a future time.) It's better to have too much on hand than too little, and if you arrange it ahead of time, most liquor stores will take back any unopened and unchilled bottles you have ordered and don't wish to keep.

Never bring a half-gallon or gallon bottle of wine to the table. Instead, decant the wine into a pretty decanter. (The exception to the rule against serving from large bottles at the table is, of course, the larger bottles of champagne, such as the jereboam.)

Normally, you can pour six glasses of wine from a bottle. I always count on two-thirds of a bottle per person for a dinner party. (Some people drink much less than that, some people more, so it averages out.) If some of your guests drink white wine for cocktails, as well as preferring to drink it straight through the meal, you must order more white than red.

- For a dinner party of eight

  o Order three bottles of white wine for the cocktail hour regardless of what other wines are served for the meal.
  o If you will serve only red wine for the meal, order five bottles of red; if you will serve only white, then five more bottles of white.
  o If you will serve both white and red during the meal, order five of each. (Even though your guests will not consume this much, have it on hand—in case they drink more red than you expect or more white than you expect.

Wine Stains

If you spill white wine, be grateful that it's white you have spilled, not red. Just make sure the moisture does not go through the linens to the wooden tabletop, because it will hurt the wood surface. Fortunately, white wine rarely stains linens and will come out in the laundering process. Mop it up with your napkin, or ask the hostess if you can go to her kitchen to get some paper towels (to put between the wet tablecloth and the tabletop).

Spilling red wine is much more serious, and everyone has his or her favorite method of fighting a possible permanent stain situation. If you are the guest who has spilled red wine, or if you are the host at a party where a guest has spilled it, it is worth a momentary interruption of your conversation to cope with the situation. If, as the guest, you hear your host saying, "Stay put, please, I will tend to it," then do just that. If there is a waiter serving, that person will tend to it. Of course, you should apologize, and if there is no serving help, and if your host does not object, rush to the kitchen for some paper towels, clean dish towels, salt, or club soda.

First mop up the wine underneath, blot the stain from on top, and put paper towels underneath the cloth to protect the table surface. You have options on the next step. Some people prefer to energetically rub a great deal of salt on the fresh red wine stain. Others prefer to pour club soda over the spot and then blot it a few times with a clean dish towel. Others prefer to pour white wine over it and then blot. All of these work to a greater or to a lesser degree. If you have spilled red wine on a fabric place mat, soak the place mat in cold water immediately (and use a large napkin in its place at your place setting at the table). Soak your large wine-stained tablecloth overnight in cold water—after the guests have left.

The main thing to remember, if you are the host, is to make the guest who spilled feel that you are not at all upset, indeed that you have already forgotten the incident. If you are the guest who spilled, the main thing to remember is to blot it as best you can, and if the stain is a

There are any number of ways to make room for storing wine in a small house or apartment. One way is to put your bottles in a wine rack on the floor of a closet.

serious one, offer to pick up the linens the next day to take to your city's best dry cleaner.

Wine and Champagne Savers

For people who wish to save and use again their partially consumed bottles of wine, there is a device on the market (available in fine houseware stores) that pumps out up to 95 percent of the oxygen which, if left in an opened bottle, would spoil the wine. This invention consists of a special stopper you place in the unfinished wine bottle, with a pumping device over it with which you pump out the air. This device allows you to conserve the wine for two or three days before oxidation begins. (A new stopper must be used for each bottle; the pumper may be used again.) The device for champagne consists of a reusable stopper and a pumper that puts the sparkle back in the bottle by creating an equilibrium of pressure inside.

Storing Your Wine

There are lavish prebuilt or custom-built wine cellars on the market for wine-lovers with a high income. There are also modestly priced racks that hold anywhere from ten to fifty-six bottles, which are a lot better than my system of storing wine when I held my first job—my wine storage area was any space beneath the sofa that was not already taken with something else. You can buy fancy cellar thermometers and cooling units that keep temperatures in your wine closet or storage area between 53°F to 57°F and the humidity between 60 and 70 percent.

If you're just starting to develop a love for and an understanding of wine, begin slowly in amassing the paraphernalia and storage facilities. Buy a wine cellar book and keep a careful inventory in it of the name of the wine, its winery, how many bottles you purchased and on what date, the price, and the dates on which you consumed the bottles. Also note how you and your guests felt about that particular wine. Put your bottles on a wine rack in the coolest part of your home—preferably not close to throbbing machines such as the clothes or dish washer.

MAKE THE TASTE MEMORABLE

The success of the food you serve at your parties depends on

- o What you serve—the constitution of the menu
- o Having the right quantities of food and drink

- The skill and imagination of the preparation
- The quality and freshness of the ingredients
- The appropriateness of the menu selections for the season and the occasion
- The presentation of the food
- The attractiveness of the serving containers

A good entertainer is a good planner, someone who thinks far ahead and gives great thought to the food being served—even if much of it will not be prepared in his or her kitchen, but picked up at a gourmet shop, made in a hotel kitchen, or prepared by a catering staff.

A noble Italian friend of mine, noted for her inestimable *cucina,* once told me that the secret to her being a good cook—and, she intimated, to *my* one day becoming a good cook—were these four "assets": time, love, a good cookbook, and a good nose.

"There must be enough *time,*" she explained, "to spend experimenting in the kitchen. Think of it as being in *love,* in love!" As she talked, she embraced the concept of her entire kitchen with graceful arms moving in a circle in the air. "A love of cooking," she said with sparkling eyes, "grows more passionate, rather than cools with the passage of time."

She told me I would need an affection for and a trust in one or two *cookbooks*—to have with me always, to know every page, so that it would cover my failings and idiosyncracies ("like that comfy feeling you have for your favorite worn bedroom slippers, Letizia," the Contessa added). Above all, she counseled, I would need *a nose for food.* "A nose for food is the nose of a lover. It draws you into the marketplace. It makes you aware of the sensuousness of fresh foodstuffs. The nose seeks them out—the freshest, the most exquisite tastes and aromas.

"You must have a nose that makes you long for the dry salty taste of prosciutto," she continued, rolling her eyes heavenward, "a taste that curls up the tip of your tongue, but then soothes it with the sweetness of the luscious ripe fig wrapped within its folds. You must have a nose that makes you dream—as you pass by a mountain of fragrant, plump strawberries—of crème fraîche caressing your bowlful of berries like an airy chiffon stole."

The Contessa explained that her nose gave her fantasies about such things as a sauce she would prepare simply because the aroma of different exotic mushrooms in the market stalls had suddenly wafted into her nostrils and reminded her of "past great meals shared with past great loves."

"Remember, it takes you the same amount of time, *cara,*" the Contessa assured me, "to prepare your mind to organize 'chicken with sauce' for your forthcoming party, as it does to prepare your mind for 'chicken with a lemon glaze' on a serving platter garnished with artichoke hearts, stuffed with purée of spinach, and topped with minced egg yolk. Don't forget the small bunches of snow peas, tied with strands of fresh dillweed and tidily piled into tiny potato baskets."

If you really care about cooking for guests, follow the Contessa's advice and you'll see what wonders you create!

Ways to Interest Yourself in Cooking for Guests

• *Try different cookbooks, until you discover the one that suits you perfectly.* The perfect cookbook is something you must seek, like the proverbial treasure-hunter, and once you have found it, as the Contessa advises, "never let it out of your sight."

• *Experiment with the recipes that appeal to you in the gourmet cuisine specialty magazines, as well as the much easier ones in the newspapers.* Make a notebook of great recipes. Paste the cut-out recipes (or duplicated copies of same) on blank notebook pages. Separate the material in the notebook with dividers into any categories you wish— such as hors d'oeuvres, desserts, and vegetable dishes. Take my advice: Put only recipes you have actually made and liked into this notebook. (Don't clutter it up with recipes you would like some day to make, because soon you won't be able to find the ones you *can* make.)

Remember, too, it's wise to practice a dish successfully three times on your family or close pals before you try it on guests for a dinner party.

• *Strive for balance.* When it comes time to settle on your menu, ask yourself:

○ Is there too much starch in this menu?
○ Is there more than one fried item?
○ Is there a green vegetable? (Having one comforts people!)
○ Is the food over-sauced?
○ Are there too many fruity elements? (One dinner I made had fruit in the soup, a fruit sauce with the duck, fruit jam with biscuits, and fresh fruit for dessert. My husband asked, "When do you bring out the fruitcake?")
○ Is there good color content? (Don't do as I did at the American embassy in Rome at an important state dinner, when as social secretary I exasperated my boss, Ambassador Clare Boothe Luce, with an all-white dinner—white creamed soup, white fish in white wine sauce, *blanquette de veau* in white sauce, a white endive salad, and an all-white dessert!)

How Many Courses Should You Serve?

You don't have to have a galaxy of courses when you entertain. Have plenty of what you do serve, but don't try to set a record in the number of dishes prepared. Some menus are given here as examples, to serve only as a guideline to the number and kind of dishes you might prepare for a specific kind of event. Although coffee and decaff are not listed, they should be offered at the end of every meal (or tea, if that is your preference).

The following courses are listed only to jog your imagination into devising your own creative food planning!

• *For a small seated dinner without help,* you can get away with a bountiful main course (meat, vegetable, rice, and salad) plus dessert, with a choice of red or white wine.

• *For a more formal dinner,* you would have a first course in addition (such as hearts of palm, an avocado half stuffed with baby shrimp, soup, or fruit cup), and a choice of red and white wine.

• *For a pull-out-all-the-stops dinner,* you might serve

    o A light soup first
    o A light fish course
    o A main course of meat or fowl
    o Two accompanying vegetables (or one vegetable and potatoes)
    o A salad and cheese course
    o A light dessert
    o Choice of red and white wine
    o Champagne served with dessert

• *For an informal supper, such as one given on a Sunday night,* you might serve

    o One large dish (like a Beef Burgundy with noodles or a hot pasta)
    o Salad
    o Dessert
    o Beer or one kind of wine

• *For a summer lunch,* you need only a cold main course (poached salmon with green sauce, for example, served with small cucumber sandwiches on dark brown bread) and dessert. Serve white wine or iced tea.

• *For a winter lunch,* you need only something like a hot cheese soufflé or a hot pasta dish with a salad and dessert, plus red wine or beer.

• *For a large buffet breakfast party,* you might offer

    o A hot egg dish (shirred eggs, creamed eggs) or an omelet
    o Baked apples
    o Hominy grits (if you're down South) or pancakes
    o Hot biscuits and muffins or sweet rolls
    o Bacon or sausage
    o Fruit juice
    o Cantaloupe or grapefruit

- *For a weekend brunch,* you might offer

  o A hot dish such as creamed turkey, Chicken Tetrazzini, or Seafood Newburg
  o Piping hot grilled cheese sandwiches (made on dark bread)
  o Broiled tomatoes with breadcrumbs on top
  o A mixed green salad
  o A plate of assorted cheeses with crackers
  o Hot baked fruit
  o Wine, or any one of these drinks might be offered to your guests:

    Bloody Marys (basis of tomato juice)
    Bullshots (basis of bouillon)
    Screwdrivers (basis of orange juice)

- *For a cocktail party,* you might serve

  o Two hot hors d'oeuvres
  o Four cold hors d'oeuvres (including crudités with a dip)
  o Small bowls of nibbles and nuts strategically placed all around
  o An open bar plus sodas, bottled water, and fruit juices

- *For a cocktail buffet,* you might serve

  o A pasta
  o A platter of sliced roast meats (such as chicken, roast beef, or turkey)
  o A large basket of assorted breads (rolls, pumpernickel, Scandinavian wafers)
  o A platter of assorted cheeses
  o Crudités with a dip
  o Fresh fruit compote
  o A gooey dessert like chocolate mousse cake

Guests will also usually consume some hors d'oeuvres with their cocktails before seriously attacking the buffet.

- *For an evening reception* (such as after the theater or a museum exhibition opening or a lecture), you might serve

  o Champagne, wine, and sodas
  o Small crustless sandwiches, such as watercress and creamed cheese, chicken salad on whole wheat, rare roast beef and mustard on small pieces of crustless rye bread
  o Sweet things, such as cookies, petits fours, small fruit tarts, chocolates

- *For a postdance supper (midnight or later),* along with champagne or wine, serve

- A hot pep-em-up dish like *Spaghetti alla Carbonara*
- Or Hungarian goulash
- Or piping hot, thin-crusted quiche
- And a green salad
- Ice cream and sherbet
- Small cakes or frosted cookies

- *For a picnic, there should be a big choice.* That's what makes a picnic fun.

  - If the budget can stand it, pack cold cooked shrimp, slices of smoked salmon and pâté into small separate self-sealing plastic sandwich bags, put them all on the picnic table, and let everyone take the bag (or bags) of choice to put on his plate.
  - Serve a variety of small sandwiches, with the crusts removed and cut into four pieces—for example: chopped mushrooms, egg salad, and minced shallots; chicken salad and bacon wrapped in spinach leaves; chopped vegetables with basil on bread brushed with olive oil
  - A salad like coleslaw or a dish like ratatouille
  - Cold *Pasta Primavera* (pasta with vegetables)
  - Slices of roast beef, duck, or any fowl
  - Crudités with an optional dip
  - Dessert: brownies, a fruit pie, cookies, apples, oranges, and bananas

ADVICE FOR MAKING ENTERTAINING EASY, ATTRACTIVE—AND DONE RIGHT, TOO

- *When people call to ask if they can "bring their house guests to your cocktail party"* or "bring along my old college roommate who's in town," if you have enough room, be gracious about it. Your guests will be coming and going at different times—some early, some late—so your empty space will appear to open and close like an accordion. Therefore you can probably accommodate a few more bodies. You can also always count on some guests who have accepted not to arrive, just as you can count on some who didn't respond at all to show up!

- *If you're having a seated dinner party and have a full complement of guests, be firm about not accepting someone else's guest suggestions.* Explain that you have just enough food, chairs, and room at the table for the people already coming, and really can't fit in any more. (It is rude of a guest to try to palm off his friends on you for a seated dinner.) If the person who has called you reacts to this news by saying, "Well, then I won't come either," respond with, "Fine, I'm sorry, but that's the way it has to be." Too many hosts are intimidated by their guests into inviting strangers they shouldn't have to entertain.

• *If you end up with an extra woman or two or three at your dinner party, don't worry about it.* I've noticed that when someone drops out of a dinner party at the last minute, it is invariably a male. It is not the end of the world to have too many women around the table. Women would rather talk to other attractive, intelligent women than be seated between hopelessly unattractive, boring men—so don't scrape the bottom of the barrel trying to balance the sexes at your table.

• *If you're having a large party to which most people will be driving their own cars, make things easy for your guests: Arrange for valet parking.* Unless your own college-aged children can handle it, call on a professional car-parking organization.

In some parts of the country, guests give the young men or women a fifty-cent tip when they get into their car to leave the party, in more expensive areas, a dollar. In a large, expensive city like Washington or a suburb of New York or Los Angeles, guests should give the professional car parkers two dollars. If you are a very kind *and* affluent host, you will pay for all the gratuities yourself and not allow the guests to pay.

• *If you're giving a large party in an apartment house and have coat checking in the lobby or hallway, be sure to have a guard for the fur coats.* A combination guard–coat checking service will also save a lot of confusion for the guests when they leave.

• *If your party is going to run late and you are going to have music and your neighbors live very close,* either invite them to your party or apologize in advance and send them a gift, so they won't hate you as much.

• *Remember the joy of mixing scents at your party, so that people are aware of more than just the smell of your wonderful food.* Add to the ambience of your party: a scented candle burning in the corner of your living room . . . a small cluster of paperwhites next to a guest's chair during cocktails . . . tiny pots of potpourri tucked into the table's floral centerpiece, and into which you add some fresh drops of your favorite perfume before the guests sit down . . .

• *Go easy on the hors d'oeuvres you offer your guests.* People don't want to eat a lot before dinner, and if you have all kinds of tantalizing canapés and things to immerse in rich dips, your guests will probably overindulge and regret it later. Your dinner should be the climax of your guests' anticipation of the evening. If they're no longer hungry, dinner will be a gastronomic let-down—after all your hard work, too!

• *Don't bring people to the table until either the first course is already in place on the table or it is ready to be served the minute the last guest has taken a seat.* People are hungry when they sit down at the table. Too often the hosts get their guests seated and the first course doesn't appear for fifteen minutes. By that time the guests have devoured their rolls, played with their butter, stolen some of the chocolates that are supposed to be eaten at the end of dessert from the candy dish, and are ready to eat their napkins from hunger.

- *If you've noticed that an aggressive guest has changed the place cards on you* to give him- or herself more exciting people to talk to during dinner, don't let him or her get away with it. Simply change the people and their cards back again. (I assure you that guest won't change place cards again at a dinner party.) It helps, too, if you say something like, "I just can't believe you did that, but I'll forgive you—this one time!"

- *If you are having a large party, don't seat husbands and wives, sisters and brothers, or best friends next to each other.* If you are using several tables, put husbands and wives at different ones. Give them a chance to make new friends, to give pleasure to other people, or at least to have a stimulating conversation with someone they don't see all the time.

- *If you're secretly trying to match two people who are die-hard "donwannamarry"* types, it's more subtle to seat them opposite each other at the table. Then they don't feel under any pressure. They can glance at each other through the meal and perhaps long to be seated next to each other, but they will be grateful their hosts haven't tried to force them on each other. (After the meal, watch them get together in a corner!)

- *If you have several sauces to pass around, put them all on one small tray, and then pass it around.* For example, if you have mint jelly and mint sauce for the lamb, or if you are offering a choice of chocolate, strawberry, and butterscotch sauce with the ice cream dessert, put them in little milk jugs or creamers on one tray. Otherwise, each guest will automatically want the sauce someone else has when he's passed a container of sauce.

- *Since the host is in charge of the conversational flow at his or her party, here are some "conversation management ideas."*

A shy guest needs special attention. A host should point out that person to a gregarious guest during the cocktail hour or after dinner— "Jane, I'd *really* appreciate it if you'd go over in the corner and do something about Dick Creedon, sitting over there alone. He's very shy and he needs someone like you to make him join in the conversation."

If the dinner table conversation has descended to depths that are really low—dirty talk—it's the host's responsibility to pull it up again.

If there's a nasty argument, the host must intervene to diffuse it. Politics is one subject about which people begin to feel personally antagonistic. Abortion is another. Foreigners can become very emotional about events in their countries. Another reason dinner parties disintegrate on rare occasions is that one person begins to character-assassi-nate a friend of someone who is present.

In any of these instances, it's time for the host to say something like this: "Look, arguing and getting mad is very bad for the digestive system. Suzy spent hours preparing this lovely dinner for us, and I think that in her honor we should change this downer topic to an up one!" Most likely another guest will pick up his or her wineglass at this moment and say something like, "I'll second that!" and everyone will drink a toast to the ending of the confrontation. Then someone else will gamely start talking about another subject, and within a few minutes, things will be calm and easy again.

• *If the meal is a culinary disaster, which mine have been on more than a few occasions, a sense of humor will save the day.* Laugh about your mistakes. Don't try to hide the fact that the roast is burned. Say something like, "You all get a certificate of good behavior at the end of this meal for eating this meat!" If you have too small an amount of something, joke about it—"I decided you're all so stylishly slim, you weren't going to eat any dessert tonight, so I just made a little." (When children are teased, it's usually terribly difficult for them. When adults are teased, it means that their friends love them, enjoy them, and that they are secure people to be able to take the teasing. When you can tease yourself in front of others, it means you're a winner.)

• *If a guest has had too much to drink, either*

○ Send him or her home in a taxi.
○ Have a guest drive him or her home.
○ Let him or her sleep over in your house.

Under no circumstances let a guest who has had too much to drink have his or her car keys.

THE NEW PARTIES FOR THE NINETIES

There is a lot of creativity in the air. Young Americans have broken out of the mold of doing the tried and true and are trying out new ideas. For example:

The Garage Party

Some people who live in small homes do not have sufficient space in which to entertain. A garage can solve this problem—the room between the garage and driveway can serve as a space for people to dance. The hosts park their cars elsewhere, clean out the garage, decorate it ingeniously (often according to the musical theme of the evening), lay down a rented dance floor (often vinyl) in the driveway, set up a sound system with a disk jockey inside the garage, and put card tables and folding chairs around at random. Each table is covered with a pretty cloth, some flowers, and a candle in a hurricane lamp, or perhaps votive candles in glass cups with flowers around them are used for illumination. The garage party in mild weather solves a big space problem for the owner of a small house. It also means the inside of the house doesn't get all messed up (and the garage gets cleaned up). If it rains, everyone can continue partying inside the decorated garage.

Parties Around Games That Require Using Your Wits

Young careerists in particular seem to love games that require mental agility—perhaps a reaction to this era of television and VCRs. There are parties given today that focus completely on games, puzzles, and treasure hunts.

• *One host invited twenty-four guests for a literary treasure hunt and dinner* and gave them six weeks' warning that they had to do a lot of homework. By party night, they were required to have at least a surface familiarity with all of the books on that week's *New York Times* fiction best-seller list. As the guests arrived, she gave each one a copy of a typed list of 200 clues, based on characters or themes within the books (no names given, of course). There were 200 objects in open view around the first floor of her house (none in the kitchen or baths) that matched these clues. People were given notepads to write down the book each clue represented, and the character, if they remembered it, or the place. The game was difficult, challenging, and everyone raced against the clock. Prizes were awarded to those who finished first and had the most details correct.

When guests arrived that evening, they spent a half hour drinking and meeting each other, then spent a half hour walking around with drinks in hand, clue-searching. The hunt continued for another hour after dinner. The guests kept meeting each other at various points in the house, each trying to divine what the other was looking at. Strangers soon became friends. During dinner no one mentioned the game, because people didn't want to drop hints to competitors as to what they had personally uncovered as clue objects.

The prizes, of course, were wonderful editions of books. One guest, upon saying good-night to her host, admitted that she had not been as mentally exhausted since the days when she had studied for her bar exam.

• *Two brothers gave a fund-raising dinner for their affluent friends, at which guests arrived with a checkbook in hand, knowing they would make a donation for $2000 that evening.* There were thirty guests, and thirty different charities were to be the recipients of those checks, chosen by each person in advance. The host had devised a treasure hunt, and the first one to find the clue that represented their charity received a prize of an additional donation of $2000 to that charity from the host. (There was a donation of $1000 to the second fastest person to find the clue.) After a wonderful dinner, the brothers turned their guests loose in the dark in the yard—first arming them each with a flashlight—to search for their charity's clue. The first winner came rushing into the house with a small doll that had been hidden in a tree trunk—which he felt represented his pet institution, Children's Hospital. The second prize-winner came in with a chocolate heart wrapped in foil, which she found decorating a bush, and which she knew represented her charity, the American Heart Association. The evening began and ended with champagne and a comparing of notes. It was a great success, and a wonderful way to raise such a grand sum.

• *Another couple held a museum party on a Sunday.* The guests were served a buffet lunch at home, then everyone went off to the local museum with a long set of clues printed on paper to compete with one another in a contest. Their task was to work through a series of twenty-five clues on a printed sheet of paper in order to find the painting, statue, or artifact in the museum that fit most perfectly each clue. (Examples: A reference to gold treasures in a page reprinted from an edition of Homer's *Odyssey* turned out to be some Greco-Roman bracelets; a sonnet about a fisherman at sea turned out to be a Winslow Homer painting of a man at sea.) The hosts recorded the exact time each person handed them their finished (and in many cases, unfinished) clue sheets. After an hour and a half in the museum, the party regrouped at the couple's house for tea, petits fours, and the awarding of prizes to those who had finished first and most accurately. The prizes were, appropriately, art books from the museum's bookstore and annual memberships to the museum.

It was a very successful party, and as a result, every single guest present became a proud and knowledgeable supporter of the museum, which previously most of them had known sketchily, if at all.

Parties That Require Exercising Your Body

It is possible, considering America's obsession with health and fitness, to give an imaginative party dedicated to that theme.

• *One young West Coast woman banker invited forty guests to "A Spa Party"* from "six-thirty to ten o'clock" at her house. Her invitations were made with the silhouettes of weights on the outer fold. She ordered guests to come in their "sharpest exercise outfits" and to bring their own towels to use after showering. The invitation also noted that guests would be served their choice of a "500-Calorie Supper" or an "800-Calorie Supper."

When guests arrived, they were offered their choice of a half-hour aerobic dancing class with a beautiful young instructor in the hostess's mirror-lined bedroom, or running in a professionally timed five-mile race. (The participants in the latter were given maps to follow; cars were stationed here and there along the route, with flags on their aerials for identification. The occupants of the cars offered cups of water and helped check on the condition of the runners—and also, as the host explained it, "made sure no one cheated by riding in a taxi for part of the race.")

After their various exploits, the guests were awarded their prizes (which were purchases the host had made in fitness and sporting goods stores). There were consolation prizes for the last racer to arrive and the most hopeless of the aerobic dancers. Guests then had a "cocktail" hour consisting of soft drinks, water, and health drinks (fruit juice shakes, concoctions like Grapefruit Juice Sluicers, and the like). Guests lined up to use the two showers, although not everyone bothered. They ate dinner outdoors at little tables—delicious low-calorie meals that had been prepared by a new young caterer. At ten o'clock the host rang a big schoolbell and told her guests that everyone had to go home and have a healthy night's sleep.

The event was, of course, the hit of the season!

ENTERTAINING OUTSIDE YOUR HOME

Making Your Parties Personal

When you decide to give a lunch or dinner in a club or public place like a restaurant or hotel dining room, you may either put your party in the hands of the banquet manager and decide with him or her on your menu and then let the establishment do the rest, or you can keep a firm control over the party and put your own strong personal stamp on the proceedings. This personalization is achieved through a combination of some of the following actions:

- Working hard with the chef to make a very special menu
- Choosing special linens . . . or having them made . . . or bringing them from home, particularly your own beautiful lace-trimmed napkins
- Having your own florist do the table decorations
- Bringing some of your beautiful centerpiece decorations from home, such as your candelabra, silver pieces, porcelain candy dishes, porcelain birds, and the like
- Supplying chocolates or nuts on the table in pretty containers
- Having a favor at each place at the table

o Doing place cards with matching menu cards
o Arranging for a trio of musicians to serenade during the cocktail hour or during dinner

Things to Remember

o Get there early, so you can oversee the placement of your place cards and check on all the last-minute details that inevitably require correcting.
o Hopefully you already have solved the problem of how your guests will park, and have given instructions on your invitations (in the lower right-hand corner).
o How clean are the restrooms for your guests? Check them out in the planning stages, and insist that they be freshly cleaned on party day. Bring in your own guest soaps, paper guest towels, and room freshener from home to put there on the night of your party.
o Call the morning of the party and request that the linens, if being supplied by the hotel or restaurant, be freshly pressed for your party.
o Make certain there is a comfortable place for your guests to mingle during cocktails, preferably not in the room where you will have dinner. Have nuts and little things for guests to nibble on during the cocktail hour.
o Sit down to dinner right on time, when the food is at its height of preparedness—even if some guests have not yet arrived.
o Bring along some extra cash to tip the maître d' and the chef and the main waiters ($10 to $20 each), if you were very pleased with their performance the night of your party.
o Arrange to bring your beautiful, expensive flowers home after your party—or arrange to have them picked up and taken the next day to a hospital, hospice, or home for the elderly.

Restaurant Manners

It's very offputting to someone if you continually finish your conversations with "We *must* lunch sometime" or "I'll call you for lunch" but then you never get around to it. Based on the philosophy that one should "put up or shut up," you should either make a lunch date with that person or stop saying that you intend to.

Having lunch or dinner in a restaurant is a most pleasant way for friends to get together. But the restaurant is also the main place of business outside the office, and an executive's manners, or lack thereof, are under merciless public scrutiny here.

The following are a few etiquette tips to be observed by people eating in a restaurant for social or business purposes:

When You Are the Host

• *If you should have to cancel this date, call your guest yourself to apologize—don't have your secretary do it.* Reschedule the lunch right then and there, before you forget about it and lose a friend or potential customer.

• *If you have to cancel again, reschedule the date at once, and send a note of apology.* (If you have to cancel a third time—which does happen in this crazy business world—reschedule the lunch. Also send that person a gift (like a basket of fruit), with a note of apology, so your guest will really believe that you are as upset as you say you are over the inconvenience you have caused him or her.

• *Be very specific about date, time, and place* when you extend your invitation.

• *Select a restaurant close to your guest's office or home,* featuring food he or she likes. Ask about food preferences before booking a table at a place featuring fish or Oriental, Middle Eastern, African, Indian, or Tex-Mex food.

• *You, by virtue of having called the other person first and having reserved a table, are the one who pays.* There should be no confusion about that. In fact, don't ever go to a restaurant with anyone without the matter of who pays being clearly understood beforehand.

• *Reconfirm with your guest (or that person's secretary) on the morning of the lunch appointment.*

• *Reconfirm also with the restaurant,* and reiterate your desire for a good table. (My definition of a good table is one that is not in front of the kitchen's swinging door, does not face the restrooms or telephones, is not in front of the main door on a cold winter's day, and is not directly beneath the main air-conditioning duct on a hot summer's day.)

• *Arrive five minutes before the meeting time in the restaurant.* Go directly to your table, after checking your coat. It is most embarrassing—even infuriating—to the guest if the host is late. The host should be awaiting any guests at an untouched, pristine-looking table (which means that you don't touch your napkin, order a drink, use your bread and butter plate, or crumble breadsticks all over the table).

• *As host you should rise when the guest approaches the table,* or in very crowded conditions at least make half an attempt to do so.

• *The guest(s) should always be given the best seats* (against the wall on banquette seats, for example, or in the seats facing the main part of the room). If there is a chair facing a blank wall or the restroom, take it yourself instead of allowing a guest to sit there. If there is a seat in the direct path of the waiters rushing in and out of the kitchen, it should be occupied by the host, not a guest.

• *If you have several guests, know ahead of time where people will be seated around the table.* Make a penciled drawing of your table plan and put it in your pocket (or handbag) before going to the restaurant. Then your guests can take their proper seats quickly, without confusion and without clogging the aisles.

• *Allow your guests (eight or less) to choose their menu selections themselves.* Beyond that number, it is much easier on everyone concerned, and much less time-consuming, if you preorder the meal.

• *Even though you may not drink yourself, offer a premeal cocktail to the guest.* If your guest orders something—even club soda—you should follow suit, whether it's a glass of soda, club soda, fruit juice, or, in hot weather, iced tea or iced coffee.

• *Help your guests with their menu selections.* If the restaurant is noted for certain specialties, mention what they are. Be able to translate the foreign names for dishes (because you have briefed yourself on the menu beforehand). If your budget is limitless, mention to the guests, "The lobster here is fabulous." (If you're on a tight budget, you shouldn't be in an expensive restaurant in the first place.) If you suggest items in the low or middle price range to your guests, they will probably follow suit and order in that price range, too.

• *When a guest's order arrives, urge him or her to begin eating at once, while it's hot.* If your order arrives before your guests', however, wait until their food has arrived before you begin eating.

• *If you see your guest not touching the food on his plate, inquire once casually, "Is it all right?"* If it is not, you can take action with the waiter. (Your guest may wish his meat cooked more, or he may have ordered the main course without sauce and they brought it with sauce.)

If, however, your guest dismisses your question with a shrug, "No, I guess I'm just not hungry, that's all," don't press him further. Let it be. There is something he does not wish to say publicly, so don't make him. (He may think the fish is tainted, or he may be allergic to shellfish, or the meat may be too raw for him to eat but he doesn't wish to send it back, and the like.) Some people love to be conspicuous in restaurants, but some would prefer to eat nothing rather than have a fuss raised over them. So play it by ear.

• *As host it is your responsibility to cut the banter short, and get down to the business discussion.* Usually about ten minutes of small talk is sufficient.

• *Never give the waiter or captain a hard time in front of your guests.* Save the sermons and criticisms of the terrible service for after the departure of your guests. (Even go back to your office or home and write a letter to the management—they should know what went wrong.) To criticize the waiter in front of your guests will only upset them and make them worry over how you are feeling.

WHEN YOU ARE THE GUEST

• *If you must cancel the date, call your host yourself, don't have a secretary do it.* Ask your host if you can reschedule the lunch date right then and there, but with you as host this time.

• *Be absolutely punctual.* If you are going to be even ten minutes late, have someone call the restaurant to pass this message on to your host.

• *If you arrive before your host, go directly to the table, but don't order a drink or eat bread. Leave your napkin undisturbed.*

• *If you are late, don't slow up the meal service for the rest of the people at the table.* Simply order the next course being served, so that you eat in unison with the others and don't force them to wait for you.

• *If your host does not drink but offers you a drink and you want one, order one.* The polite thing to do is to say, "Look, I don't want to hold you up if you have a time problem today. Why don't we order lunch and then the waiter can bring me a cocktail?" or "I think I'd prefer a glass of wine with lunch, so let's order our meal and forget the cocktail."

• *Either one cocktail or two glasses of wine at a meal are enough.* If you order more, your host will surmise (probably justifiably) that you have a drinking problem.

• *If nothing is said by your host about ordering wine, don't bring up the subject.* You can always live through a meal without wine, and you really don't have a right to order it by yourself.

• *Don't order the most expensive items on the menu.* Take your lead from your host as to the price range in which to order. If he or she gives you no helpful suggestions, order in the middle price range, not in the lowest or the highest.

• *Anyone who wishes a separate menu from what the host has ordered for all his guests may ask for a substitute* (however, without demanding to see the menu and making a big fuss). For example, if you don't eat meat, you may say to your host upon the arrival of the mixed grill platters, "Would it be all right if I just ordered a salad?" Your host will, of course, answer in the affirmative, and you can then choose from among the salads the waiter tells you about. (In your host's home you would not do this, however; you would simply eat the foods you can and push around the rest on your plate.)

• *As a guest, never deal directly with the waiter; that's the host's job.* If you want something, softly mention it to your host, and he or she will call over the waiter.

• *If you are at a business lunch, don't try to force your host into discussing business before he or she is ready.* Continue to make small talk at the beginning of the meal. It is the host's perogative to give the signal when it's time to get down to business.

• *If you are someone's guest, don't even try to pay the check.* You can always reciprocate by treating your host to a return lunch.

• *Always write a thank-you note to your host right after your restaurant meal (or at least within three days' time).* It does not have to be longer than three sentences, taking five minutes in all to write, address, and stamp, as for example:

> Dear Joe,
> It was wonderful seeing you today, and to see you looking in good form, as always. And how I enjoyed those soft-shell crabs! Thank you for a memorable lunch . . .

When you write a thank-you note, even for something as pedestrian as a restaurant lunch, it gives pleasure to your host. It also signifies that you are a person of refinement and good manners—a reputation anyone should find desirable.

Behavior to Avoid in a Restaurant

○ Table hopping (an obvious attempt to draw attention to oneself; also a hazard for passing waiters)

○ Talking on a telephone brought to the table (again, a frenetic desire to draw attention to oneself)

○ Strewing the table with papers and documents, so the poor waiter can't even find a landing place for the plates for your meal

○ Putting a woman's handbag or anyone's tote bag or briefcase on the table

○ Talking loud and boisterously

○ Eating so slowly that you hold up everyone else and make them very fidgety

○ Remaining at the table when you have a long choking or sneezing fit, instead of quickly departing for the restroom

○ Using your napkin as a handkerchief (instead of quickly departing for the restroom)

○ Using a toothpick or a fork to dislodge food in your teeth (instead of rinsing your mouth out with water in the restroom)

○ A woman's putting on makeup (except for a quick, inconspicuous swipe of powder from her compact at the end of the meal)

Tipping at the End of a Meal

Because the subject of tipping gives rise to so many questions, I've discussed it at length in a separate chapter at the beginning of the book. This is an area in which manners—or the lack of manners—really show. Look back to chapter 6 for guidelines on how to show your appreciation for—or express your dissatisfaction with—service given in a restaurant.

MUSIC MAKES THE WORLD GO ROUND

Nothing gives more zip to a party than music. Talented hosts use it to create a mood, to "decorate the air of my party place," as one woman described it, and to make people feel relaxed and comfortable—or alternatively, to wake them up and get them going on the dance floor.

Background Music

Background music is strictly that—pleasant sounds in the background against which people greet each other, chat, stroll around, or sit conversing at the dinner table. Your guests are not supposed to be straining to listen to the lyrics in background music. Singers do not perform as background musicians, nor do featured solo instrumentalists. A cocktail party, for example, is not the moment to stop the action, grab everyone's attention, and have them listen attentively to someone give a solo performance.

Background music is very attractive during the cocktail hour. (If you're using tapes, have someone turn up the volume bit by bit as more people arrive, so that a snatch of music can be heard along with the babble of voices in the air.) This music is also welcome during dinner—soft, low, and unobtrusive, so no guest complains that it is difficult to talk or hear the dinner table conversation. After dinner, it makes sense to change your music, to introduce a new part of the evening. If you're using taped music, you could go from Cole Porter during the meal to a tape of a new Latin rhythm group after dinner.

If you are lucky enough to have live musicians, during the cocktail hour you might have a piano player, or even better, a combo (piano, guitar or sax, and drums, for example). Or you could introduce background classical music during the meal. You might have a harpist or chamber music quartet play throughout a large dinner. (Before the musicians leave the dining area at the conclusion of dinner, as host you should go up to the group, thank and praise them, turn to your dinner guests and give the players' names, so that your guests will applaud them.)

CLASSICAL MUSIC

There are good classical musicians in every region, and usually they are eager—and need—to make money by playing or singing at your parties. The lesser-known ones (we're not tal' ing about having Byron Janis come by to give a Chopin concert after dinner for you) might charge you anywhere from $100 to $500 per performer for playing at your party. (In smaller towns, the charge may be less.) Check into the music teachers in your community, as well as the faculty and advanced students in the music departments of the local schools and universities. Others will have heard them play, and you can go on their recommendations. But listen to them *yourself.*

- *If you are hiring musicians, be sure to*

  o Sign a contract with them or their agent.
  o Have them understand *exactly* what you want them to do. A friend of mine once hired a musician to play for her grandparents' anniversary party; he arrived without his accordion, thinking he was supposed to play the piano—but there was no piano!
  o Go over the content of their program with them.
  o Settle on when they should arrive.
  o Check on what they will be wearing. (To be on the safe side, tell the men to wear black dinner suits, the women long black dresses—they can't be conspicuous fashion disasters if they conform to that!)
  o Be firm about the exact length of time they are to perform.

An after-dinner concert of any kind of classical music should last no longer than twenty-five minutes to a half hour. People are relaxed, full of good food and wine, and want to have some time to talk before they go home. An interlude of concert music provides a perfect polish to a dinner party, but it should not drag on, no matter how excellent the musicians may be. A friend hired a chamber music orchestra and told them to play for thirty minutes after dinner. They wouldn't stop. They went on and on for an hour, while the host kept jumping up to applaud them after each "final" piece. Without giving him a chance to intervene, they segued into the next piece. The situation became comical. Finally the host told the leader of the quartet that the piece they were playing was absolutely the last one, and there were to be no encores!

Dance Music

How nice if you can afford an orchestra for your dance! In a big city, there are usually two or three musical organizations headed by well-known band leaders that supply orchestras, pianists, trios, quartets, and bands of any size for any kind of party. If you're holding to a tight budget, there might be a school or college dance band in your town that is terrific. Perhaps you can persuade a rock group in one of the local spots in your town to play for your party—provided you hold your party on the group's night off. You might have heard that someone in town had a great little dance band at their daughter's wedding reception. Call and find out who it was. Often the orchestra or group will have its own agent, so you would deal with that person, not the musical leader.

Hiring a Musician or Any Kind of Performer

Some performers have horror stories of how badly they have been treated when performing in a private home. One told me how a well-known woman kept him waiting to perform four hours after the agreed-upon hour. He was made to stay in the pantry and stood, leaning against the wall, because there wasn't a chair and he wasn't allowed to find one. He was not given anything to eat or drink; he was not given a hanger or a place to change his clothes—he had to do that in a utility closet. Fortunately, that kind of story is the exception.

- *You are a considerate host, as far as the performer is concerned if he or she*

  o Is given an opportunity to rehearse, try out the piano, or look over the sound system or whatever else needs checking.
  o Is given a bathroom to use to check makeup and appearance and a room in which to change and rest, with a comfortable chair and a closet or dress rack.
  o Is provided with an iron and ironing board, if that is needed for any costume.
  o Is given something to eat and drink, either before or after the performance, as requested.
  o Is properly introduced to the audience by the host before performing. (If a group is involved, the name of each person in the group should be stated.)
  o Is properly thanked for a good performance by the host—if it *was* a good performance!
  o Is sent a letter soon after the party, praising his or her or the group's performance. (It is very valuable for a performer to have written recommendations in order to obtain new bookings.)

TO TIP OR NOT TO TIP

You do not have to give a performer anything beyond the amount specified in the signed contract for the performance. However, if a fantastic performance was given—if your guests were immensely pleased, and you were, too—it is certainly nice to give the performer(s) a gift of money to show how pleased you were. You would never tip a Pavarotti who sang at your fancy New York benefit, but you could certainly give $10 or $20 to a singer-pianist in Toledo who absolutely made your party. Musicians like to be thanked, and since most have to scratch hard for a living, they enjoy seeing a host's appreciation back-stopped with a little cash.

Using Music Tapes

If you want to have a dance at home to the accompaniment of your own carefully selected tapes, hire a good disc jockey. It is worth the money. He or she supplies the sound system, knows when and how to change the tempo and kind of music—and when to adjust the volume. The perfect disc jockey for your party is a college or post-college friend of your children (preferably one who does this professionally) who loves all music, who is up on all the latest musical crazes of the young but appreciates the Frank Sinatra–George Gershwin appetite of the older generation, too. I remember asking one disc jockey how he handled the musical choices at his jam-packed nightclub, and he replied, "I look over the crowd and divide it into three categories: the 'blue rinse set,' who want the music of the forties and fifties; the 'yup-heads,' who want pop rock and music like the flamenco beat of the Gypsy Kings from Spain; and the 'kids in their twenties,' who want to hear anything from the Buckwheat Zydeco group [black accordionists from New Orleans] to the Sugar Cubes, a popular rock group from Iceland. I give 'em," he continued, "the kind of music that will move 'em, according to how many of each group are in the club at any one time."

People who want to buy the latest tapes of the "in" music have only to read a publication like *Rolling Stone* magazine to find out what groups everyone is talking about. When you educate yourself on who's new and "hot" and acquire their tapes to play at your party, you'll impress—and educate—your guests.

THE PROTOCOL ASPECT OF YOUR PARTIES

A knowledge of the basic tenets of protocol in entertaining helps you entertain both graciously and efficiently. It helps to know how to receive people, where to seat them at the table, and how to toast them as guests of honor.

How to Receive Your Guests

If you are a couple, one of you should be stationed with an eye on the front door, so you can immediately greet every person who steps through it and direct individuals to where they should put their coats. The other half of the couple should be in the living room or wherever cocktails are being served, to make sure the guests are meeting one another. If you are giving the party by yourself, you should station yourself between the cocktail serving area and the door, so that you can do both jobs at once.

SHOULD THERE BE A RECEIVING LINE?

If you are having a cocktail party for more than thirty people, you and/or your spouse and guest of honor should be in an informal receiving line as close to the entrance of the room as possible. ("Informal receiving line" means the hosts stand around talking to guests in a small group, keeping an eye on the door and able to regroup quickly to shake the hand of any new guest who arrives.)

If you are having a party of a hundred or more, you should have a receiving line of yourself or your spouse (who can cut in and out of the line), co-host if there is one, and guests of honor. The number one guest (either gender) should stand next to the number one host (either gender) of the party. At purely social parties, spouses always stand in line together. At business parties, the spouses may or may not have to stand in line—rarely at a large lunch, often at a large dinner. There are different formulas for receiving lines. For example:

- The company's chief executive officer is giving a party for a very important Japanese businessman. The formation of the line might be as follows:

1. The chairman and CEO of the host company
2. The Japanese guest
3. The president of the host company

- If the Japanese businessman's wife accompanies him, the receiving line would look like this:

1. Chairman and CEO
2. Japanese businessman
3. Chairman's wife
4. Japanese businessman's wife

- Mr. and Mrs. John Mowinckle are having a big wedding anniversary cocktail buffet for the parents of Mrs. Mowinckel. The receiving line would look like this:

1. Mrs. Mowinckel
2. Mrs. Mowinckel's father
3. Mr. Mowinckel
4. Mrs. Mowinckel's mother

ADVICE ON HANDLING YOUR RECEIVING LINE

- *Never have more than four people in the line at any one time, if you can help it.* It becomes ponderous and too much like a wedding reception to have so many people standing together. Also, the longer the line, the more interminably long it takes to get through.

- *Spouses can cut in and out of the line,* subbing for their mates. At a large corporate party, senior management can take turns standing in the receiving line with the guest of honor.
- *When the receiving line becomes a veritable logjam,* with people stretching out into the street, the following steps should be taken:
  - Someone representing the host should urge people to come inside, get a drink, and go back into the receiving line later.
  - The guests should decide for themselves to go get a drink—and pass through the line later when it isn't so congested.
- *On the subject of drinking in a receiving line:*
  - Hosts should not have drinks in their hands—there should be a small table behind them, to hold whatever it is they are drinking. They can turn around and take a discreet sip every now and then, without anyone really noticing they have a glass of water, champagne, or anything else behind them.
  - Guests should not go through the receiving line with drinks in their hands. They can sip their drinks until shortly before they pass through the line, then they should put down their drinks somewhere and retrieve them after meeting their hosts.
- *If almost everyone has arrived, the receiving line may be disbanded,* but sometimes guests continue to arrive virtually throughout a two-hour period. If your large cocktail party (for hundreds) is from five-thirty to seven-thirty, the host or hosts and guest of honor should stay in the receiving line from five-thirty to about six-forty-five.
- *Many times at large parties the guests and hosts do not know each other.* In the receiving line, either the guest introduces himself or herself to the host, or the host gives his or her name to the guest passing by; the host then turns to the person on the right and introduces the guest to that person, who then introduces the guest to the person standing next on his or her right. (At a really fancy party, an "introducer" brings each guest up to the head of the line and gives that person's name in a strong, firm voice.)
- *If a couple is giving a large party involving mainly the husband's business associates,* he stands first in line, so he can introduce people to his wife, who is standing next to him. If they are giving a party for *her* business associates, *she* stands first in line, so she can introduce them to her husband.

Name Badges

Don't use them unless you absolutely have to! They look terrible on anyone's suit or dress—particularly on a dress. They are much too commercial to look decent at a party in someone's home or club. If there is no name badge, people have to be more alert and do their own detective work to find the identity of the person to whom they're talking. That helps make the party go, rather than deterring it.

If you are required to have name badges at an evening party (no one really minds them at lunch or in a hotel ballroom or convention center), wear yours high up on your upper right shoulder. Your name is most easily read in that spot by right-handed people. (If you're at a convention of all left-handed people, wear your name badge on your upper left shoulder!)

A name badge should contain the person's first and last name, and company name, if it is pertinent. For a host corporation, if the company name is already part of the name badge, the person's title should be included under his or her name, if he or she is part of senior management. People like to know the positions of the people they are talking to.

Signing in the Guest Book

If you plan to have a guest book at your party (it should be a handsome leather or fabric-covered one), put it on a table away from the congestion created by arriving guests. In other words, don't make guests sign, check their coats, and wait in a receiving line all at the same time. Put the persons overseeing the guest book signing in a chair at a table in a corner of the cocktail area.

The best way of handling a guest book, in my opinion, is not to have one, because it creates one more traffic problem—and there is, after all, a guest list. The second best way to handle a guest book is to have someone carry it up and down the receiving line, letting people sign as they wait to go through the line.

One more caution: *Have a supply of good black pens for people to use for signing in the book.* The last guest book signing I did was not a pleasant experience. The pen leaked all over my fingers, and I spent my time at the party sipping champagne and wondering if the ink stains would ever come off the thumb and third finger of my right hand. My consolation: Everyone else had the same stains on their thumbs and third fingers.

Seating Arrangements

People have friends over for dinner all the time, and no one worries about who sits where. However, it's more efficient and more stimulating to seat any kind of table with a little thought.

Family Meals

Within your own family, it certainly does not matter who sits where at the table (unless you have to separate certain siblings who tend to fight all the time. Even so, it is helpful for young people to learn that father and mother—the figures of authority—sit opposite each other at the ends of the table or in the center of a rectangular table, and that grandparents are seated comfortably and in "places of honor." (If the family dining table is round, the two take seats opposite each other at some point in the circle, as in the illustration below.) It is all part of teaching children deference and respect for their elders, which includes passing the food to others older than they are before taking it themselves, and waiting to eat until their elders have begun.

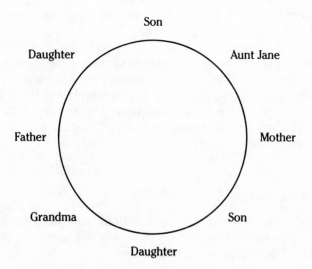

Son	Grandma	Father	Eldest Daughter	Son	Youngest Daughter

Daughter	Son	Mother	Grandpa	Oldest Son	Aunt Cynthia

WHO SITS IN THE HOSTS' SEATS?

There is always a host for every gathering. Often there is a co-host who sits opposite the host—such as a spouse or a business associate close in rank or importance to the host. In the case of a widowed person, a brother or sister, an in-law, or other adult family member may act as co-host, taking the seat opposite the host.

A word of caution here to someone who has recently lost a spouse: Do not put someone you have been dating in the co-host's seat soon after your spouse's death. Others feel a little squeamish seeing the late spouse's seat at the table occupied by a newcomer who unconsciously (or consciously) quickly assumes the role of a person only recently departed.

When there are several tables, such as at a large private party, a member of the family or a close friend acts as a host of each of the round tables. His or her place card should read "Host." There are duties attached to this honor—for example, making sure everyone is fully introduced and ensuring that the conversation flows around the table, without leaving anyone sitting with no one to talk to. This is why you should choose people who are competent, not just important (or rich!), as the hosts of your or your company's party tables.

At a corporate-sponsored affair in a hotel ballroom, for example, you might have the chairman, president, and senior vice-presidents hosting the tables. At your wedding anniversary dinner-dance, you might have your sister Anne, brother-in-law Bill, your Aunt Louise, and your college-aged son Harry hosting four of your tables. It does not matter whether the host is a man or a woman. What does matter is that it be a person who will represent you personally or your company in an attractive, well-mannered way.

GUEST SEATING AND RANK

• *It is a mark of graciousness to give any prominent guest in your home a seat of honor.* The number one seat for a man is at the hostess's right; the seat for the second most important man is on her left. The number one seat for a woman is at the right of the male host, the second most important woman sits to his left.

• *A person who has rank deserves a place of honor* (see also chapter 23, "Addressing People Properly.") If you have invited a person of rank to dinner at your house, or if that person will be your guest in a restaurant, seat him or her to the right of the host of the opposite sex.

  o *A present (or past) elected official*—governor, mayor, senator, congressman, police chief, alderman
  o *A present or past appointed official* (an ambassador, head of a commission)
  o *A high-ranking military officer*
  o *A White House appointee* (member of the president's cabinet or sub-cabinet, head of a government agency)

Even when your guest is no longer in office (or on active duty), unless you have a guest who presently holds office and would therefore outrank the one out of office, give the former official a place of honor.

• *A person holding a high religious office deserves a place of honor at your table.* However, a clergyman should not have to be as high as an archbishop to deserve a seat of honor. Your own rabbi, parish priest, or minister deserves a good seat at your table.

• *There are people of no rank who are given "top" seats nonetheless out of courtesy:*

  o An elderly person
  o A foreign guest
  o An adult houseguest
  o The honoree(s) of the party—someone with a birthday, wedding anniversary; someone who is retiring, being promoted, going away, has gotten engaged, had a baby, earned an honor, won a competition
  o A senior professor
  o A community leader
  o A respected, senior business leader

• *The spouse of a person of rank enjoys equal rank at the table.* In other words, if a man is the number one ranked person at the party, he is seated on the hostess's right and his wife is seated on the host's right as the number one ranked woman present. If he is the second ranked person, he sits on his hostess's left and his wife sits on her host's left. If

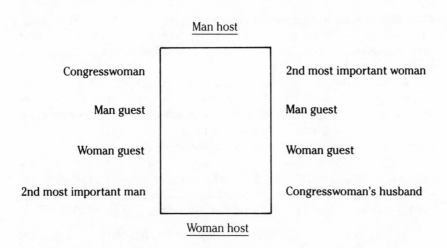

Man host

Congresswoman   2nd most important woman

Man guest   Man guest

Woman guest   Woman guest

2nd most important man   Congresswoman's husband

Woman host

a woman is the number one ranked person, the same seating arrangement applies, since the host and hostess would always have the first-ranked person of the opposite sex to their right. For example, at this dinner party at which a Congresswoman is present, she is seated on the host's right, and her spouse therefore sits on the hostess's right.

• *Anyone who entertains a lot and has guests with city, state, or national office rank, should know where to go for help in seating that meal.*

o For questions on the rank of *city officials,* call the mayor's secretary and ask who handles protocol matters for City Hall.
o For questions on the rank of *state officials,* call the governor's secretary and ask who handles protocol matters for the state capitol.
o For questions on the rank of *Congressional figures,* consult the *Congressional Directory* (Government Printing Office, Washington DC 20401).
o For questions on the rank of *White House staff, cabinet members, and Washington diplomatic corps officials,* consult *The Green Book,* which lists the entire precedence of these officials (The Social List of Washington, DC, 10335 Kensington Parkway, Kensington, MD 20895). For questions of *military rank,* any local military office will give you the order of rank of the officers of any of the branches of the military.

"GIVENS" IN SEATING ANY OF YOUR GUESTS

• *Seat people in alternating sexes around the table—man-woman*—unless you are short one or two of either gender, in which case, you would be obliged to seat two of the same sex next to each other (which is no great problem). You might put one of those same gender guests on your left, so he or she will feel honored instead of feeling that he or she is "extra."

• *Make sure that you don't seat two bores next to each other, two overly shy people next to each other, or two overly talkative people next to each other.* The success of a table conversation stems from variety and balance, not from the overkill of people competing next to each other in talking or in maintaining a painful silence.

• *When friends come to dinner, seat them next to people with whom they would most enjoy themselves.* There are logical reasons for who should sit next to whom at your parties. Think it out ahead of time, like this hostess, who in pondering her dinner party decided to

- o "Put saucy Abigail next to cranky old Mr. Hamilton, because he loves pretty young things. In recompense, Abigail will have an attractive young man on her other side, so she won't mind putting up with Mr. Hamilton half the time.
- o "Put Louise next to the exchange student from France, because Louise speaks French, and the exchange student is newly arrived and hasn't learned enough English yet.
- o "Seat George next to Jim Jones's wife, because George is job-hunting and has revealed that he has an appointment with Jim Jones next week to see about a job. George might be able to impress her and do himself some good.
- o "Put Alfonso and Jennifer next to each other, so they can talk about wildlife conservation all night. Both are hipped on the subject, they have never met each other, and it is a stroke of genius to seat them together.
- o "Seat Grace next to Bill. He has been so despondent since his wife's death, and if anyone can bring him out of his funk with sparkling, funny, wonderful conversation, it's Grace.
- o "Put Mark on my left, because he drinks too much and has become impossible lately, but he and his wife are dear old friends and I know I am the only one, other than his poor wife, who will take it." (The hostess then resolves to give herself a fascinating man on her left at her *next* dinner party.

You, as host, know better than anyone else how the synergism of talents of your party guests will work, according to how you seat them. People should enjoy or learn from the people they talk to at dinner. If they are brimming with personality, they achieve happiness in giving to the others, in leading the conversation, in making people laugh. If they are quiet and good listeners, they counterbalance the talkers while enjoying the flow of conversation around them. The host should put all of the guests on his or her chess board, figure out the moves, and do the best seating possible to aid the party chemistry.

PROBLEMS OF SEATING A TABLE OF A MULTIPLE OF FOUR

At tables of eight (or four couples), and all multiples of four thereafter, you should seat the co-host down one to the right, instead of opposite the host in his or her rightful place. To illustrate, at a dinner of twelve, with six men and six women, if you put the co-host opposite the host, there will be people of the same sex sitting next to each other around the table:

However, if you seat the woman co-host "down one," the sexes will be able to alternate around the table:

If you have one person too many of one sex at a table of a multiple of four (such as seven women and five men), there is no problem in having the co-host sit opposite the host. Two people of the same sex will be sitting next to each other on either side of the table, allowing the co-host to sit opposite the host, as illustrated in this luncheon for twelve:

Woman host

Man guest	Man guest
Woman guest	Woman guest
Woman guest	Woman guest
Man guest	Man guest
Woman guest	Woman guest

Man co-host

LOGISTICAL DETAILS OF SEATING A LARGE PARTY

If you're in charge of a large function, whether a business dinner or a social event like a wedding anniversary dinner dance, the procedures used to seat the dinner are the same. Here are steps to follow:

1. *Decide on what kind of round tables you will use—those that seat eight, ten, or twelve people.* (Tables for eight or ten are better for conversation.) Let's say you are giving a dinner for fifty and will use five round tables that seat ten each.

2. *Take five large sheets of plain paper. Draw a circle four inches in diameter on each. Number each table 1 to 5.* Put ten little nicks around the circumference of each table, to designate a guest's place.

3. *Make a seating chart name card for each guest on a piece of paper.* Do this by typing a separate list of male guests and female guests, leaving enough space around each name so that you can cut them out and use them to put around the table charts, as in the following examples:

Georgia Ames	Roderick Ames
Marianne Andrews	Joseph Andrews
Fabienne Arthur	Dr. Lee Arthur
Susan Barker	William Baskin
Georgia Berrigan	Charles Berrigan

4. *Decide who will be the host (and co-host, if there will be one)* for each of the five tables. Take their names (from the guest list you have just cut into name tabs) and attach them with tape to the designated table in the host's place.

5. *Put the guests of honor in their proper places to the right of the hosts of each table.*

6. *Seat all the other guests* by attaching their name tabs by tape to the various tables, making sure to seat husbands and wives at different tables and to alternate men and women guests—unless you have too many of one sex.

7. *When the seating has been decided for your party,* wait until just about two hours before the party starts to have the final flat list typed up of guests' names with their table numbers. The reason is that there are often last-minute drop-outs in large parties, necessitating changes in seating . . . and in the flat list numbers . . . and in the table card numbers . . . and in the placement of the place cards on the tables.

Once you feel there will be no more last-minute changes, have the list of names and numbers typed up in duplicate copies. Give one to everyone involved in running your party, so that there will be several people helping guests find their tables in the ballroom when the cocktail period is over and people come in to dinner.

8. *The table cards with each person's name and table number should be placed alphabetically on a table in the entrance area.* The guests can be directed to go to that table to find their cards after checking their coats and before greeting you, the host. (A man usually sticks his table card in his jacket pocket, a woman in her handbag.)

9. *Alternatively, guests can go to a table at which a party assistant (or assistants) sits with the list of guests and tells people what their table numbers are.*

10. *Inside the ballroom, there should be a stanchion on each table,* holding a large white card upon which the table number is printed. (The headwaiter should be instructed to have the stanchions removed once the guests have found their proper seats and have sat down, because they obstruct guests' view of the room.)

Points of Protocol for an Official Social Function

If you are running a large civic event—of historic, military, or philanthropic interest or in honor of some beloved person who held high office—there are some points of protocol to follow to start off the function. The sequence is as follows:

1. Dais guests march in (to optional drum roll). Guests at the ballroom tables listen quietly but remain seated.
2. Colors are posted by the military. Guests stand for this, at respectful attention.
3. Guests sing "The Star Spangled Banner" (optional), remaining standing.
4. A member of the clergy gives the invocation while guests remain standing.

PROPER HANDLING OF THE FLAG

• The flag of the United States of America is always accorded the place of honor, with flags of other countries positioned to its own right (to the left, from the perspective of people sitting in the audience and gazing at it on the stage).

• When there is a row of domestic flags on poles of equal heights, the United States flag should be in the center, raised on some sort of platform, so that it is slightly higher than all the other flags.

• When displaying the flag vertically or horizontally against the wall, the flag's stars should always be on the top, to the flag's own right (to the audience observer's left).

• The American flag always flies at the top of the pole when more than one flag is flying from the same pole.

- The flag may *not* be used:
  - To cover a car or any vehicle (except when firmly attached to a staff)
  - To cover a ceiling
  - To cover a lectern
  - To drape a platform. (Use striped red, white, and blue bunting instead, with a dark blue stripe at the top.)

(For more information on the display of the flag, contact the National Flag Foundation, Flag Plaza, Pittsburgh, PA 15219.)

THE ART OF TOASTING

The ancient ritual of toasting with wine is a special asset anyone should learn—that is, anyone who expects to have guests for a meal on occasion. Knowing how to toast is an act of kindness, because it makes people feel good; it is an art, because its success depends on timing, intuition, and a smooth articulation of a message. It is a skill replete with nuances. It doesn't matter what kind of drink you have in your hand—a glass of water will do if you are merely making a symbolic gesture. When you raise a toast to a person for some reason, suddenly the place where you are and the people present take on a special cachet. You might suddenly raise a glass of soda to the person standing next to you at the beach hot dog stand—"Geoff, the news you just told me is *great!* Congratulations! Here's to you!" Suddenly, your hot dog and soda lunch becomes a celebration, and you have made the object of your toast feel very happy.

It doesn't matter if a foursome is having lunch in a cafeteria or eating dinner at Maxim's in Paris, at least one toast is always appropriate. (As a friend of mine expressed it, "There's always something to celebrate—like being alive, for example.")

Short Toasts

It is a nice gesture, when you have ordered drinks in a restaurant or in a bar and the drinks arrive, to make a toast to the person or people in your group. You simply raise your glass to the person (or people) next to you and say,

- "Here's looking at you."
- "Here's to you."
- *"Kanpai"* (Japanese).
- *"Kanpei"* (Chinese).
- "Here's mud in your eye" (World War I vintage).

o "All the best."
o "Cheers."
o *"Skoal"* (the Scandinavian toast used throughout the meal).
o *"Salut"* (international).
o *"Cin-cin"* (Italian).
o *"A vôtre santé"* (French).

You immediately take a small sip from your glass, and the other person (or people) then repeat what you said and take a sip, too. It is the person buying the drinks who ordinarily makes this short toast, but it does not necessarily have to be that person.

What Prompts the Making of a Real Toast

• *Someone is starting a new venture:* "Gook luck with the new company."

• *Congratulations are in order* (for getting married, having a baby, being promoted, winning the lottery, losing the desired twenty-five pounds, and the like): "We're very proud of you, Giovanna. This is sensational news. Congratulations!"

• *Thanks are in order:* "We owe you a big vote of thanks, Jim. You really rallied around. Here's to a great friend of this family."

• *A foreign business colleague is your guest:* "Henri, it's good to have you here with us—and in such good form, even after having just made the long flight from Paris. I raise a toast to you, to your dear wife, Madeleine, back in France, and to the success of our project!"

• *A friend's good news deserves special mention:* "Hey, Pete, I just heard your daughter Melanie graduated from law school at the head of her class. She's a real credit to her old man. I raise my glass to Melanie!"

• *A guest decides to praise his or her host:* "I don't know about the rest of you, but I've just had the best dinner I've had in years. I suggest we toast the person responsible for this culinary splendor. Here's to Mary—thank you, and what night will you invite us again?"

• *A great friend raises a joking, teasing toast to the groom-to-be at an engagement party:* "Well, Harry, you've finally come into your own. At college you were always a hundred yards behind me. I was always making better grades ["Not true!" jovially interrupts the groom], and I was always much more adept at sports ["Not true!" laughs the groom again], and I was always better liked and much handsomer than you ["Not true!" shouts one of the ushers], but somehow," the toaster continues, "you captured the loveliest, smartest, sexiest, and most sought-after woman in this city. ["True! True!" interrupts the bride.] Harry," continues the toaster, "I would like to say, old buddy, that you are one lucky guy, but also a very smart one. I drink to my friend, and congratulate you on getting Sally before I did. A toast to the fortunate Harry!"

Helpful Points of Etiquette on Toasting

• *When you sit down at the table, don't grab your glass of wine and start drinking it right away*—because your host may be planning on making an immediate welcoming toast, and you wouldn't want to begin drinking before that. However, if none is forthcoming and you see your host or hostess drinking from his or her wineglass, follow suit, because they are obviously not planning on giving an opening salute to their guests.

• *In many European countries and often in this country, it is the custom at the beginning of the meal for the host to give a welcoming toast to the guests, usually from a standing position.* A formal kind of person might say, "My dear friends, welcome to our house. We are happy to have you around this table, and let us all enjoy each other and this food." An informal kind of person might say, "Georgia, Ruth, Sam, Aggie, and Walter, it's good to see your smiling faces around this table. Welcome, and let's enjoy our dinner!" The sequence is as follows:

   o Host toasts his guests, takes a sip, then sits down.
   o Guests mutter low-voice thanks for the welcome (a phrase such as "Nice to be here") and then raise their glasses in a return gesture of thanks to the host.
   o Guests may now drink from their glasses.
   o More toasts may be raised at dessert time, when the host toasts the guest(s) of honor.
   o The guest(s) of honor returns the toast.
   o Other guests now join in the toasting, if they wish.

Some people manage to live out their lives by attending many dinners at which there is toasting, and yet never have to give one themselves. Extremely shy people find toasting very painful; they should not worry about it, except on their wedding day, when tradition demands that they raise at least one toast—to their new spouse.

• *If you are on the receiving end of the toast, do not drink to yourself.* Just nod and smile your appreciation at the end of the remarks; don't pick up your glass to drink from it. If you wish to return the toast to the person who made it to you, or if you just wish to address the gathering in general, you can stand up and do it right then or later in the meal.

• *If you are the one toasting, say your little speech, look at the person being toasted,* and when you are done, raise your glass and then drink, still looking right into the other person's eyes. Then nod and put your glass down on the table (and sit down, if you are standing).

• *Practice your toast beforehand* if you're nervous about having to make one. Rehearse it in front of your bathroom mirror two or three times, so that your timing will be smooth and you won't forget the punch line.

• *Brevity is key.* I have seen more toasts absolutely ruined when the toaster, who knew he had a good thing going, went on and on and on. Two minutes is a perfect toast length. Five minutes is all right if you're witty and well prepared—a Johnny Carson or Dave Letterman type. Most of us can't hold people's attention for that long. When everyone is full of wine, they don't want to have to concentrate listening to someone's long toast; they just want to be entertained.

• *Don't give a toast when you've had too much to drink.* When someone has imbibed even a bit too much, the tendency is to rise to the feet and then deliver oneself of a rambling, senseless monologue. It's a great way to irritate everyone present!

• *Stand up if you're at a big table, even if your toast is only a minute or two in length.* People who are seated can't see you when you talk down the table from a sitting position. Besides, it does more honor to the person you're toasting if you stand for it.

• *If you're sitting at a table for six or eight, and your remarks are very informal,* you do not have to stand. Remain seated, but get everyone's attention by saying in a voice slightly louder than usual, "Ladies and gentlemen, I happen to have something to say!"

• *Don't tap your wineglass with a knife to get everyone's attention.* You might break it—hundreds are broken every year this way. Your rising at the table will draw enough attention to your impending toast.

• *Be careful of protocol—don't give a toast to the guest of honor before the host does!* If there is a champagne glass on the table along with a wineglass, it means that champagne will be served with dessert. It is most likely that the host will rise just after the last glass at the table has been poured and give a toast to the guest of honor or to the special occasion for which the meal has been organized. If you feel like giving a toast to your hosts and it is obvious as dessert draws to a close that your host is not going to raise a toast (nor is anyone else), rise and thank your host for the good dinner with a short toast. It will be appreciated, I assure you.

• *Leave bathroom humor out of your remarks.* It does not work in mixed company—and often does not work in company with just your own sex.

• *Always end on an up note, even if you've been teasing the honoree during your entire toast.* People want to be left with a nice feeling, not a possible joke at someone's expense.

• *Know when to stop the toasting at your party.* This is a responsibility of the host or whoever is in charge (like the master of ceremonies at a banquet or the best man at wedding festivities). This person should be intuitive enough to know when the evening should come to an end. At a certain moment, enough is enough. Long, awkward pauses between toasts is the signal, and instead of waiting for yet another person to jump to his or her feet, glass in hand, ready to make another toast, the person in charge should say, "All good things must come to an end, such as this dinner [or lunch]. Thank you all very much."

The two best toasters I know today are political columnist Rowland Evans of Washington and Paul Fay, Jr., of San Francisco, a great friend of John F. Kennedy and a member of his Washington administration. When either of these two are hosts (with their respective wifes, Kay and Anita), the guests wait expectantly all through dinner for the toasts. Each man starts with the guest of honor and then goes around the table, telling something funny and wonderful about each person. It's never the same, no matter how often you are their guest. By the time everyone has finished laughing and savoring the witty compliments thrown in their direction, the dinner is over, and the guests depart feeling that life is beautiful.

Toasting is an art—and a gift to some people, too.

ENTERTAINING WEEKEND HOUSEGUESTS

Whom to Invite

• Experienced hosts know this rule, usually learned through experience: *Invite the proper number of guests*—not just one person if that person is heavy going, and never too many people for the available space. Houseguests really want to be comfortable!

• *Invite only the people you really crave as guests.* If you are forced to entertain for business or some other reason, invite those people for lunch on Saturday or Sunday. You can always put up with someone for *one* meal or two hours. Business people you don't know well and close personal friends often won't mix well for a forty-eight-hour stretch.

• *Invite those you really want far ahead of the date.* The recipient of your invitation will be flattered and will probably have a free schedule, too. If you're inviting friends to ski in the mountains, invite them in October for February. If you're inviting them to visit you in Washington during the Cherry Blossom Festival in April, ask them in November.

• *Think kindness.* You might have a friend who has suffered a blow recently and needs cheering up. You might know someone who has recently moved into your town and really hasn't had the chance to meet people. Introducing that person to congenial company at a weekend house party could be the best thing that will ever happen to him or her (or them). You might be able to introduce an unmarried friend to another single person he or she has never met, and be responsible for the start of a new romance—or a lifetime friendship, which is even better.

• *Become a master at designing the perfect weekend group.* You don't have to have people all of the same ilk and interests. Insert a little spice into the group—perhaps a friend from another country, a stranger in town, a person of entirely different interests from those of your own friends. People are basically nice, want to meet new people, want to be nice to them, and want to get along with them.

On the other hand, if you invite a terrific tennis player, there should be another excellent player in the group; if you invite someone who loves to dance, there should be someone else in the group for him or her to dance with. If your guest of honor only likes to play bridge—constantly—you had better make sure there are three other adamant bridge players around somewhere!

In all my years of spending weekends in many countries, time and time again I have been part of a completely diversified group of strangers who shared no background or interests with one another. In a letter to my mother, written when I was a single woman in my early thirties, I raved over a house party I had attended outside Salzburg. The party consisted of our hosts and their guests: an Austrian ski instructor with the "brain of a pea," as I described him; a very leftish French journalist who kept baiting me with his anti-Americanism; an incredibly intellectual couple of music professors from the University of Geneva, who gave us all an inferiority complex (he played the cello, she the flute); a painfully shy Indian student from the University of Salzburg; and myself. Yet we had an absolutely splendid time and formed lasting friendships. It was all thanks to our host, the group designer, so to speak, who had assembled a very unlikely combination and *made it work.*

When Not to Invite Houseguests

If you are exhausted from the wear and tear of having houseguests every single weekend at your resort place in the past, resolve this year to save at least every other weekend for yourself or you and your family alone. Next year you might plan on having houseguests only once every three weeks. This will immeasurably reduce your exhaustion. A summer or weekend place should, after all, provide you with some rest and relaxation. To anyone who asks to visit you on one of your "private weekends," just say, "Unfortunately, we're busy that weekend." (They don't have to know that you'll be busy with yourselves that weekend!)

Getting Yourself Organized

To host people with great success—whether it's for a week, weekend, or just overnight—requires deft planning, executed with a talented manager's skill.

One couple who entertain every weekend during the summer months make two plans, one for themselves, to remind them what to do before the guests come, and a second schedule that is drawn up and sent to the guests to help them get organized.

- *The schedule you make for organizing yourself for the weekend might include*

  o Arrival and departure times for each guest, including arrival times for flights, trains, or car services
  o Location of bed and bath for each guest
  o List of guests' known food allergies (such as shellfish—important to know at a seaside place!)
  o Full menus for Friday, Saturday, and Sunday
  o Hours for food to be served in-house
  o Logistics on all party activities outside the house, including transportation arrangements
  o Golf course tee-off times and tennis court reservations
  o List of extra athletic equipment on hand to lend guests
  o Church service information for Sunday morning
  o Alternative activities planned in case of rain
  o Number of cars needed to borrow or rent

- *The schedule you send to the guests might include*

  o The approximate hour at which they are expected on Friday evening and the hour at which they are expected to leave
  o A map of how to get to your house
  o A list of—and a brief, amusing description of—the others who have been invited (even if it's just one person)
  o A list of the times and places for all athletic and social events, meals, and free-time periods for shopping and sightseeing opportunities
  o The athletic equipment required ("Better bring your own clubs"; "Bring some tennis balls"; "Don't forget your boat shoes.")
  o A list of the clothes they will need ("You'll need whites for our tennis club"; "Men will need sports jackets but no ties"; "Bring a raincoat or a light topcoat.")

Preparing the House

I once asked the late Gloria Guinness, renowned for her beauty and her considerable talents as a hostess, what she considered the rule of success for having houseguests. "Very simple," she replied. "Sleep in your guest room before any guest who is too polite to tell you what's wrong sleeps there."

I've always remembered that—and remembered all the times I've been someone's houseguest and there was no trashbasket anywhere, or the bedtable light didn't work, or there were holes in the screens and the mosquitoes sailed in at night to hold a regatta over my bed.

You will hear other houseguests complain—out of earshot of their hosts, of course—about there being no vestige of even a corner of a bureau drawer in which to put clothes, or a free hanger in the closet on which to hang a dress or suit. The litany of hosting mistakes includes forgetting to leave soap in the bathroom, insufficient towels and face cloths, lack of a warm blanket for the bed when it's cold, and a mattress so full of lumps it's guaranteed to make its occupant miss a night's sleep.

WELCOME ADDITIONS TO THE GUEST ROOM

A good host not only checks out the comfort of the bed and bedding, but he or she also makes sure there is

- A meticulously clean and sweet-smelling room
- An electric fan or air conditioning available in the guest room on an incredibly hot night, or an electric heater on an incredibly cold night
- Something interesting to read on the bedside table
- Something delicious to munch on in the room (cookies, candies, fresh fruit) in case the guest becomes hungry
- A good strong lightbulb in the reading lamp
- A clock that works
- A radio or television
- Pencil, pen, and a writing tablet—even stationery for a last-minute letter that needs to be written (plus a couple of stamps!)
- A thermos of water and a glass

• *The little touches matter.* Along with everything necessary being in place, it's nice to put a small bouquet of fresh flowers in the guest room. One of my favorite places to visit is the Charles H. G. Rees house on the sea in Watch Hill, Rhode Island. Filled with houseguests every weekend, it has been a tradition for years for one of the Rees daughters in residence to go around each evening removing the bedspreads, folding them neatly and turning down the beds. The little things matter in this life.

Welcome Additions to the Guest Bathroom

o A toothbrush glass for each guest
o An extra roll of toilet paper
o A box of paper tissue
o A shower cap
o A sponge and detergent so the thoughtful guest can clean the tub after use
o Insect repellent for summertime use
o Air freshener

These items are not necessary but will be gratefully acknowledged by guests:

o A fresh razor and blades, in case these were forgotten
o New toothbrush and toothpaste, in case either was forgotten
o Shampoo
o Clean comb and brush (often forgotten)
o Electric curlers
o Hairdryer
o Hairspray
o Deodorant
o Adhesive bandages
o Aspirin or analgesic
o Mouthwash
o Hand lotion
o Sun block

How to Organize the Sleeping Quarters

• Usually the oldest person in the group gets the best room or bed. (Or, if you have a guest who is frail, he or she merits the most comfortable quarters.)

• High school students or younger can make do with individual sleeping bags, if necessary, for a weekend.

• If you have parents or a parent with a young child, put them the farthest away from the other guests because of the inevitable noise. Borrow a cot for a young child who's out of a crib; don't make him or her sleep in a parent's bed. (If you have a baby accompanying a parent, borrow a crib and linens from a friend or neighbor.)

• Don't expect two tall or husky people to fit into a single bed, no matter how much passion the two may generate together. In fact, two large people can't even fit comfortably into a regular double bed. If you don't have enough single or queen-sized beds, invite fewer houseguests (or else invite all small people!).

• Don't expect to put two unmarried people automatically in the same room if you know they have been going out together. Ask each separately, "Do you wish to share a room or use separate rooms." You might hear one story from one of them and a totally different story from the other. So ask each of them.

If you feel it is morally wrong to have two unmarried people sharing the same room in your house, put them in separate rooms but tell them beforehand—"We are putting you in separate rooms." The unmarried couple should understand. Your house is your house, and guests should conform to *your* standards and rules, not theirs.

How to Plan the Food

Give your guests the kind of food you like yourself, and they'll be happy. As a host, you should not have to spend all your time preparing complicated dishes for your guests. In this world of takeout food and frozen gourmet meals, there is no need to spend long hours toiling over the kitchen stove.

If you have planned and prepared your menus and then a houseguest arrives with food and wine, expecting to see you serve it that very evening or at some point during the weekend, don't be ashamed to say no. Explain to the guest that you are absolutely delighted with such a delicious present, but, because all of the food (or wine) has been planned for this weekend, you will freeze (or save) his or her wonderful gift for a very special occasion in the future. If someone brings you a big ham, you don't have to serve it as a main course at a meal if all your meals are already planned. Have it around for people to snack on at a porch lunch or at the cocktail hour, and keep reminding your guest donor of "all the wonderful meals at which we'll serve it in the near future."

Here are the menus prepared by a talented cook for her six houseguests on a recent weekend on Cape Cod. She prepared most of the food before her guests walked in the door, so she was able to be with them, not in the kitchen, most of the time.

- *Friday night dinner:* boiled lobster, coleslaw, garlic brown bread, lemon sherbet and brownies, white wine and coffee
- *Saturday breakfast:* choice of three cereals, fresh fruit, bacon, eggs, English or bran muffins, coffee or milk
- *Saturday lunch:* hamburgers or hot dogs at the beach concession stand (or, in case of rain, sandwiches at home)
- *Saturday dinner:* Barbecued steaks, mixed green salad, a casserole of chopped spinach, artichoke hearts, and sour cream, fresh fruit compote, macaroons, red wine and coffee
- *Sunday breakfast:* Melon, fruit juices, the host's renowned waffles with strawberry jam or maple syrup, coffee or milk

o *Sunday lunch:* Beach picnic (or, if it rained, a living room floor picnic) of roast tarragon chicken, a cold pasta with vegetables, whole wheat rolls, fresh raspberries with *crème fraîche,* red and white wine, and coffee

This host always plans her food a week ahead and markets, cooks, and freezes in bits and snatches during the week before her guests arrive so that she does not have to spend long periods of time preparing the meals. No gourmet restaurant could do it better.

I know other hosts with weekend retreats who bring everything with them from the city in hampers and cold storage bags. They don't spend much time in the kitchen either. One such host remarked, "I have everything so organized ahead of time that my major job in getting a meal on the table is opening the bottle of salad dressing and pouring it on the prewashed, pre-prepared salad."

Necessary Attributes in an Accomplished Weekend Host

• *A love of one's fellow men and women.* Let's face it, you really have to love people to put up with them as houseguests. Seeing friends for lunch or an occasional dinner party is *nothing* like having them totally dependent upon you for room, board, and emotional sustenance hour in and hour out. This is when the mirror cracks. But if you love people—if you are a caring, wonderful host—this is your moment to shine. Nothing gives your friends greater pleasure and nothing relaxes them or cheers them up more than a wonderful weekend at your home. They will remember your many kindnesses forever, and you will go to the top of their list of "people we love."

• *An intuitive expertise in the science of group-mixing,* which includes dealing with infighting, as when one houseguest accuses another of cheating on the tennis court . . . another guest tries to bed someone else's spouse . . . or a guest drinks too much and becomes verbally abusive. Developments of this kind call for a weekend host sometimes to serve as a counselor, referee, discipliner, or grown-up nursery school teacher!

• *Patience.* The host needs an unlimited supply to deal with moments such as when a guest borrows his desperately needed car and disappears for hours . . . or uses up the whole household's supply of hot water with an endlessly long bath . . . or breaks the host's favorite $300 Steuben highball glass by letting it fall off the porch railing . . . or announces, as the group is leaving for the dinner dance, that he is so badly sunburned that he wants to go to the hospital's Emergency Room instead of the country club.

• *Creative talent,* so that when things go awry a substitute plan as good, if not better, than the original one can be put into execution. (For example, the snow's not good enough for skiing, so the host arranges a hike to a nearby aviary and wildlife center with a forest ranger scientist guide.)

• *A large supply of elbow grease.* Guests require a lot of work, if you count the number of sheets and towels you have to wash, the number of salad greens you have to buy, wash and chop, the cases of wine and soda you have to lug from the store to your kitchen, and the energy (and false smiles) you have to summon when your sixth houseguest gets up and wants breakfast at the sixth separate time that morning.

THE CONDUCT OF THE HOUSEGUEST DURING A SUCCESSFUL, HAPPY WEEKEND

H ere are some basic tips on how to be the kind of houseguest who receives repeat invitations:

• *Have a positive attitude from start to finish.* Be determined that nothing—the poor quality of the weather, the other houseguests, your host's children, the discomfort of the bed assigned you, or planned activities that go amiss—will affect your cheerfulness and enthusiastic participation. I have seen more than one "up" houseguest who laughed at everything that went wrong and buoyed everyone's spirits to save what otherwise would have been a disastrous situation.

• *If you're not feeling well, cancel out beforehand.* If you should arrive, for example, with a bad cold, half the household will be miserable worrying over you, and the other half will be worrying that they will catch your germs. If you come down with a bug during your stay, just don't say anything about it. Suffer through the weekend gamely and courageously. (Like everything there are exceptions. If you think you have come down with something very contagious, like chicken pox or measles, *do* say something about it.)

• *Don't ask to bring your children or your pet—and certainly don't show up with them as a surprise!* Children should be expressly invited by the host (not subtly suggested by the guest), and about the only kind of unannounced pet you can bring that won't upset your host is a goldfish in his own small bowl.

• *Arrive when you say you will—not before, not after—and leave when you're supposed to.* This rule of good conduct means that, even if your flight home is canceled or your car breaks down as you leave the driveway, you do not burden your hosts with it. You simply find a solution by yourself.

• *If you don't have presentable luggage, borrow some for the weekend.* It's a real downer for your hosts to see you arrive with all your possessions in plastic shopping bags.

• *Bring the proper clothing.* If you don't know what to bring, if you don't know what's scheduled, or if you're not familiar with the climate in the place where your host lives, ask some detailed questions before you pack. Don't expect your hosts to provide extra sweaters or raingear. Provide your own. Bring your own athletic gear, too, whether it's ice skates and skis or tennis racquet and balls. If there is a Saturday night party somewhere, find out how to dress for it. And if you have to share a bathroom "down the hall" with other guests, pack a bathrobe.

• *Have your own agenda,* in case your hosts are busy with chores and don't want you helping them. In other words, bring a good book!

• *Offer to pitch in and help with everything,* whether it's fetching someone at the station or picking up extra ice for the cocktail party, arranging flowers or making hors d'oeuvres, taking great-grandmother for a drive or watering the parched lawn. The dishwasher might need emptying and the table might require setting for the next meal. Your host's child might need an hour of baby-sitting so your host can run some errands. Just offer to do anything. But if told a firm "No," take your host at his or her word. Many host couples prefer to do all the chores themselves, so that things are done properly and on time. A guest offering to help is sometimes more of a hindrance than a help. However, a guest who offers to do nothing often has his or her name crossed off on the future invitations list.

• *Accept your host's schedule with a smile.* Be a joiner and a good team member for the weekend. At the same time, if your hosts are the kind who like their guests to organize their own activities, be a creative self-starter. Don't keep asking, "What should we do now?" Beat yourself at solitaire, or try your hand at a jigsaw or crossword puzzle. Bring some good books with you, or take long walks by yourself and commune with nature. (If it's a book-reading weekend, here's a tip: Bring along your own 100-watt lightbulb for your room!)

• *Be neat in your room.* Keep it tidy and picked up all the time, so that your hosts will enjoy walking past it instead of feeling the need to duck the mess in it. Make your bed first thing (yes, that includes the bedspread). Keep your towels on the bathroom racks, not on the floor, and your toothpaste in the tube instead of all over the basin. Keep your makeup or shaving paraphernalia in a neat pile, so that other guests or family members using the bathroom will have room to stow their things, too.

• *Be on time.* The entire group appreciates any member who is punctual and mindful of the schedule to be followed. It's important not to sabotage the logistics of moving people from one place to another, which is the task with which your house party hosts must cope.

• *Don't try to discipline your host's children, even if such action is warranted.* Grin and bear it. You will soon return home to a childless household again, or to your own home with its well-behaved children.

• *Don't complain, even when there's just cause.* If the ski lifts are so crowded that you can't get on them . . . if the motorboat has no gasoline, so you can't use it . . . if the tennis courts are so soggy that all tennis for the weekend is cancelled . . . if the ice never arrives for your host's cocktail party, speak not—just help out. Keep smiling and joking, and say it doesn't matter. You'll be able to talk yourself and everyone else around you into believing that it really doesn't.

Houseguest Presents

The better you know your host, the more sensitive you probably are to his or her desires and needs in relation to household presents. I know houseguests who

○ Brought an inexpensive camera and several rolls of film to grateful hosts who didn't have a camera but could really use one.
○ Brought home-made frozen casseroles to their grateful hosts, parents of children whose mouths were constantly open, like baby birds waiting for food.
○ Brought bottles of wine to grateful hosts who drink wine with every dinner. The wine was a better quality than their hosts could afford, and it was given with the admonition, "This is only to be enjoyed by you two, not consumed by your houseguests!"
○ Stock the lakeside cabin of their grateful hosts with a new set of family games every time they visit, because it inevitably rains and they know how often those new games will be used.
○ Always bring some new outdoor sports equipment—a badminton set, a croquet set, or a volleyball and volleyball net—enabling the family and guests to play games together all weekend.
○ Can be counted on each year to bring a bagful of movie cassettes (with accompanying boxes of popcorn) to keep everyone happy if it rains.
○ Bring all the latest magazines to leave behind for their hosts' enjoyment.
○ Inevitably stock their hosts' pantry with difficult-to-find gourmet goodies to enjoy in the future—a basket of fresh fruit, gourmet pâtés and crackers, ice-cream sauces in jars, and tins of special puddings, cookies, and cakes.

The host makes the weekend by having the kindness to invite and prepare for the guest—but the guest really makes the weekend by showing his enjoyment of it. It's a nice joint operation!

Not to Forget: The Thank-you Letter

As a houseguest, you may have brought a present with you, or you may have sent it afterward, but neither the generousness of your gift nor the enthusiasm of your thank-you telephone call lets you off the hook. A written thank-you is obligatory in the world of manners.

When you stop to think of all the trouble, caring, and expense your host went to, to go on record with your thanks seems a small enough recompense. A well-written letter of thanks brings a smile to your host's face, is passed around to his or her family, is read and reread, and if it's a really beautiful letter, it's saved. Who knows, it may turn up some day in a collection of twentieth-century letters published in the twenty-first century (if the publisher could ever find enough good letters from our era to fill a book).

The structure of a nice thank-you letter from a houseguest to his or her host is as follows:

• The guest writes on behalf of him- or herself and spouse (or accompanying children) and addresses it to the wife of the family but makes it clear the letter is meant for both husband and wife. ("Dear Joan, George and I had the most magical time with you and Allen this past weekend . . .")

• The first paragraph should state what a great time the visitors had. ("We were both work-weary and you managed to give us a wonderful rest, but also a tremendous amount of fun. It was the best kind of therapy for your bedraggled city friends . . .")

• The second paragraph should discuss how nice the house is—or the lake or mountain or farm vista, or whatever the place has to offer. ("Each morning I looked from my bed out across that luxurious rolling green lawn to the flower beds and concluded that my hosts are living in a paradise, not just the country . . .")

• The third paragraph should mention what fun you had doing the various activities. ("I will never forget our doubles game. Even though George and I almost got a divorce in the middle of the first set, we finally had to agree on something—that you two are far superior players, and that you were nice even to play with the likes of us . . . The Sunday picnic was memorable. You managed to feed us all a feast with such seeming effortlessness! We are in total admiration . . .")

• The fourth paragraph might comment on the other guests, if there were any, or on the host's children. ("We really enjoyed meeting the Abells—stimulating, amusing, and nice at the same time. And of course, the biggest treat was seeing how Jessie has grown into such a lovely young lady. You must be very proud of your daughter. She was so nice to us . . .")

• Then state your thanks again and sign off. Be sure to thank both hosts equally. (A friend of mine recently reminded me how often her new husband's friends visit them in Gulfstream, Florida, and write him a thank-you note without even mentioning her name—when she has done all the work!)

If it is a lot of work to have someone over—whether it's for a sixty-hour weekend, for a three-hour dinner party, or for a sixty-minute drink—it is also one of the most rewarding of activities. The amount of pleasure you give by extending the warmth of your hospitality to others is immeasurable. But it's also an investment. You get back all that pleasure you gave, with interest, by realizing what you have contributed to other people. Entertaining is the way to make friendships grow deeper, the route to newly acquired friendships, and the most effective way of adding to your own personal growth.

Have you ever noticed how a good host is basically a very happy person?

16

Gifts That Show
You Care

There's a little bit of the child in all of us that makes us love receiving presents all our lives. It's so nice to have someone put a gaily wrapped box into your hands. There's the anticipation of untying the bow, then removing the ribbon, and finally opening each end of the festive paper to take a peek. Even the very rich who claim to be blasé about gifts, who will yawn and say, "There's nothing, after all, I really need, and there's nothing I really want," confess to feeling at least a twinge of excitement when they see a box they know is for them lying on the table or under the tree.

In a way, it's too bad that gift-giving for holidays, special occasions, and joyful celebrations is also such big business throughout the world today, because things can get terribly materialistic. (For example, many of us feel our mothers are not properly honored just by money expended for a gift on Mother's Day.)

But if we step back and become children again, both in giving and receiving gifts, there's great happiness to be derived. We delight someone else because of the gift—either the one we gave or the one we received and for which we showed real appreciation.

The true spirit of gift-giving is very basic—uncontrived and noncommercial. It is simply a gesture to please someone else, particularly a person we love—or even just like.

WHEN YOU SEND FLOWERS

Flowers are a joy to receive at any time of the year. Some people prefer florists' arrangements already firmly anchored in a bowl, to which they need add only a little water. Others much prefer receiving a gift of cut flowers—even six will do—that they then arrange in their own container.

• You send flowers or a plant—preferably a plant—to someone who is ill in the hospital—unless he or she already has some in the room, in which case, send them later to the patient's home, when he or she has returned and is recuperating.

• Flowers or a plant are a nice way to say thank-you for a meal. It is preferable to send them the morning of the dinner, so they can be used for the festivities; otherwise, send them the day after. While it is an international custom to show up at the door the night of the dinner with cut flowers, this frequently throws the host into a panic of unwelcome extra work—trying to find a vase for them and to put them in just the right place while greeting guests and getting the dinner into shape.

• They are a great way to say congratulations—for graduating, getting engaged, having a baby, being promoted, winning a tournament, doing well in a TV game show, sticking to a diet, successfully stopping smoking, being elected to do a tough job for a nonprofit organization.

• They are a traditional way to recognize a pertinent holiday—such as Mother's Day, Valentine's Day, a birthday or wedding anniversary, and Christmas, Hanukkah, Easter, and Passover, of course.

• They say "Cheer up," when someone has been having a tough time and could use a little sunshine in his or her life.

• They are ideal when saying "I'm sorry" (don't forget the note) after you have offended someone, intentionally or not.

• They are a wonderful way to welcome someone into a new house or apartment.

• They say a warm "Welcome home" to someone who has been away on a trip or otherwise absent for a prolonged period of time.

WHEN A COUPLE GETS MARRIED

Wedding Shower Presents

It is important to remember that there may be more than one shower, and you still must give a wedding present, so be careful with your budget on shower gifts. Guests bring separate gifts or couples bring gifts—usually of the kitchen variety or for the bar. For ideas for kitchen gifts, see the suggestions in that category for wedding presents. Gifts in the bar category include

- o Wineglasses
- o Cocktail shaker
- o Bar knife
- o Can opener/bottle cap remover
- o Highball glasses
- o Martini pitcher
- o Small cutting board
- o Old-fashioned glasses
- o Long stirring spoon
- o Wine bottle opener
- o Ice bucket

LINGERIE SHOWERS FOR THE BRIDE

The most important thing to remember about this kind of shower, usually given in a home by one of the bride's woman friends, is that the host must know the exact size of the bride for the various kinds of lingerie and communicate that to the guests while organizing the shower. (After all, some women are bigger on the top than on the bottom, and vice versa, so knowing that the bride takes a "Medium" slip will not help you when you are buying bras or panties for her.)

Many of the items in the list of suggestions below are very expensive. It is logical for two or more friends to band together to give a joint gift if the item is expensive.

- o Nightgown and matching peignoir
- o Flannel nightgown
- o Bras
- o Pantyhose
- o Silk camisole top and pants set
- o Lacy garter belt
- o Winter bathrobe
- o Panties
- o Lingerie cases
- o Half slips
- o Matching bedroom slippers
- o "Racy" stockings
- o Summer bathrobe
- o Wooly winter slippers
- o Teddys
- o Full-length slips

At a lingerie shower, the groom often makes a surprise appearance at the end to take his fiancée on to another engagement. He is then shown all of the lingerie, which occasions merriment and laughter—a fitting finale to the shower.

Co-ed lingerie showers have become a fad recently, with guests giving lingerie for either of the couple or to both, as the gift-giver chooses. It can create a lot of fun. Naturally, both bride and groom are guests at these occasions.

Wedding Presents

The bride and groom are really fortunate if they

- o Have registered in the Bridal Registry at either a local store or one with branches all over the country. In this way, they will receive what they have selected.
- o Inherit wonderful antiques and bibelots from relatives (one-of-a-kind objects, either valuable or valued for their sentiment and family traditions).
- o Are given checks, if money is a major problem in their lives.

- • *Someone on a tight budget who is giving a wedding gift should*

- o Band together with two, three, or more people who are in the same bind, so that the joint present will be a nice one
- o Haunt everything from an auction house to a tag sale, to pick up some small memento that is attractive and unique

- • *A first-time bride and her groom need*

- o Furniture
- o Bedding—mattress pads, sheets and pillowcases, blankets, electric blanket or quilt, blanket covers, bedspread or quilt, dust ruffles, pillow shams
- o Bathroom paraphernalia—towels, washcloths, bath mats, wastebasket, towel racks, storage cabinets
- o China, glassware, and flatware
- o Table linens—place mats or cloths to fit the table and napkins (both sets of white and in a color or pattern)
- o Barware—highball glasses, old-fashioneds, all-purpose wineglasses
- o Lamps
- o Wastebaskets
- o Decorative accessories
- o Vases, cachepots, and other flower containers
- o Storage containers

○ Cleaning equipment—vacuum cleaner, carpet sweeper, mop, broom, pail, or whatever

• *For their kitchen* (to give as shower or wedding presents), almost anything you can think of—from a really substantial gift like a microwave oven or food processor to small accessories that every cook needs, and that you can find in profusion in the kitchenwares section of all good department stores. If you buy assorted small accessories, tie them together with ribbon, plunge them into a small pitcher or pot, shape wrapping paper or foil around the pitcher or pot, allowing the utensils to stick out of the top, and tie ribbon streamers around the container.

• *For their china, silver, and glass gifts*, you may follow their dictates on the Bridal Registry, or if they have not registered, review the china, silver, and glassware needed for an average meal and purchase what you can afford in any of the categories. It is always better to ask their parents—or the bridal couple themselves—what they really want and need. Today, young couples are not shy about letting you know!

• *Other things that newlyweds might need or appreciate include*

○ Delivery of the morning or evening newspaper for a year
○ Their choice of a magazine subscription, to start as of their wedding date
○ A monogram die at a stationer's for the bride to order her new stationery. (The gift of the monogram die *and* a box or two of stationery is *very* welcome.)
○ Gift certificates to their local supermarket
○ A wonderful clock for their mantel or bookshelf
○ A gift certificate to a good print shop (rather than a print itself, as your taste probably won't be theirs)
○ Gift certificate to a lamp store. (Newlyweds never have enough lamps.)
○ Money, of course—a nice check

GIFTS FOR A COUPLE WHO MARRY AFTER LIVING TOGETHER A LONG TIME

A couple who has lived together for a year or more will often already possess many of the basics, such as common cooking equipment. However, they often do *not* have a full complement of pretty, nonutilitarian possessions. Ask them what would please them most (if they are not already registered in a store). They may, for example, have all the frying pans they need but no beautiful sheets and pillowcases. They probably have a trash pail, but no good-looking wastebaskets. They probably have an odd assortment of wineglasses, but not one full set of good ones. If you've been in their home before the wedding date, all you have to do is look around to discover something that they need.

<small>GIFTS FOR THE SECOND-, THIRD-, OR FOURTH-TIME BRIDE OR GROOM</small>

It doesn't matter how many times a family member or a good friend marries. It doesn't matter how much money you figure you have expended on his or her wedding gifts over the years. It doesn't matter whether or not you are invited to the latest wedding. What does matter is that you show you are a friend and supporter and that you wish this person all the happiness in the world. Instead of being cynical, take a positive attitude. *This* marriage is going to work!

The oft-married bride is going to have the basics in her household, so you don't have to worry about buying her sheets or knives and forks. In all probability, she is well supplied. Therefore, give her a little bibelot or a small gift you find in your general wanderings through stores. For example, you might find

- o An attractive pair of bookends
- o A pretty telephone book slipcover
- o A pair of unique-looking salad servers
- o A picture frame (for their new wedding photo)
- o A set of bar glasses (as these items are always broken over the years and a new bride needs some matched sets)
- o A set of dessert plates (because the same applies as above)
- o An embroidered pillow with a relevant amusing saying
- o A pair of giant coffee mugs for their breakfasts
- o A new coffee maker (because her old one is probably battered)
- o A music box that plays "That's what friends are for"

The Bride's Dilemma: To Return or Not to Return Gifts

• *A bridal couple who receive an ugly eyesore of a gift from a family member or a very close friend should not return it.* A family antique must be received with enthusiasm and delight—even if you find it grotesque. It is far better to put up with a monstrosity than to hurt someone's feelings, especially when that someone means a lot to you. Put the monstrosity in the closet or garage, and take it out for display every time the donor comes for drinks or dinner. After a year, you won't have to even do that any more.

Also, remember that decorative objects go in and out of fashion. How I would love now to have so many of the things my grandmother tried to give me. I felt they were hideous and fended them off, but pieces of Victoriana and *la Belle Epoque* would now be considered so chic— and are worth so much! So save the inherited eyesore. It, too, might come back into vogue.

• *A bride who has received three identical presents* (water pitchers, for example) should return two of them and get something else she likes in return. She should also tell her friends what she has done. Her individual thank-you notes to all three friends would praise the "fantastic water pitcher and the terrific tray we received from the three of you." In this way, each person feels the bride kept *her* water pitcher, and everyone receives credit for two gifts, instead of one.

HOLIDAY GIFT-GIVING

Organizing Your Holiday Gift List

It is a very good idea to list all of the gifts you have given—and received—each year (on your computer, if you have one) so that you can review the record to remind you of how to organize this year's gift list. Purge the list of names and addresses of people to whom it is not necessary to give a gift this year. Update all the addresses, name changes, and marital status of your married or now divorced friends. Many people organize their holiday gift lists into these categories:

- Family
- Close friends
- Business associates (including secretary)
- Apartment building staff
- People who make life worth living (including any of these: housekeeper, baby sitter, hairdresser, masseur, gym instructor, building superintendent, newspaper delivery person, and the like)

Just because you gave a gift to someone last year does not mean that you must give him or her one this year. Gift-giving should never become a meaningless habit; it should be a sign of special remembrance or a way of saying thank-you for something done for you during the year. Perhaps you want to cheer up someone who has had a tough year. Next year, when things are better for that person, you won't have to send a gift.

Just because someone gives you a Christmas present does *not* mean that you must give one in return. Someone may give you a present to say thank you for any number of reasons, and you do not have to return that gesture. Simply write a warm thank-you note.

Baking and Making Your Own Christmas Gifts

If you don't have the money to buy Christmas gifts this year, don't borrow money or go into debt. Your family and friends will understand.

For years one of our favorite Christmas presents in New York came from a friend who was eternally broke and in financial difficulties. Each Christmas morning at eight she left outside our door one of her warm, freshly baked loaves of bread, wrapped in silver foil and tied with ribbon. It was a wonderful present, and now that we have moved from New York, our family will miss it very much at our Christmas morning breakfast table.

I know other people who are creative and have written poems or done original sketches on a blank card as their Christmas presents for their friends. One friend, an unpublished writer who is always without funds, walks the dogs of her friends who live in the neighborhood once a day during the busy two-week Christmas season as her gift to them.

Never be ashamed not to be able to buy someone a gift. Buy a Christmas card or write a letter to friends in which you say you wish you could give a gift, but this year you are unable to—but you send the gift of love and admiration and sincere wishes for their future good health and happiness. Isn't that what Christmas is all about anyway?

Organizing Your Own Family's Christmas Day

Here are some tips on bringing order out of chaos on Christmas Day (or on Christmas Eve), when the presents will be opened:

• If you were really forward looking, you would have bought a large quantity of Christmas wrap the preceding January, when stores dramatically slashed the prices of this normally expensive item.

• Gather the gifts you have bought, the gifts from family members to one another, and presents that have arrived from the outside, and place the items for each member of the family in a new, thirty-gallon garbage bag, with a name tag attached to the enclosure. Then the bag can be emptied out in a special spot for each person by the tree—or wherever the gift-opening will take place. As each person opens a present, the wrapping can be stashed back into the garbage bag. (Don't throw out these garbage bags for a couple of days, in case a gift card or an address is missing.)

• Give each person a little notebook and pencil, to write down who gave him or her what as each package is opened. This will facilitate written thank-you's later. (The lists of gifts for the little ones, or course, must be handled by an adult, or even better, by an older sibling who writes well; it's good practice for the latter.)

PRESENTS TO AND FROM ONE ANOTHER IN A VERY LARGE FAMILY

Large families (five children or more) have found that, as the children grow well into their teens, the business of buying gifts for one another becomes a giant logistical problem. The problem is compounded when the children of that family marry and have children of their own but still gather for the family Christmas.

One solution that many have found viable is having the children—in the summer, when they are all together for some occasion—draw the name of a sibling from a hat. That person is the only sibling who gets a present, but it is a handsome one. And if that sibling is married, with children, the donor takes care of those presents, too.

Thank-you's for Holiday Gifts

Yes, every gift definitely should be acknowledged in writing—not just a telephone call or thanks said in a chance meeting on the street, but a bona fide note, written in your own hand, or typed or done on a word processor. *Gifts should be acknowledged on the record.* It is only basic politeness! The thank-you note should be written no later than two weeks after receipt of the gift. If parents spent more time helping their young children write their thank-you notes to Grandma and Aunt Sally for their Christmas presents, the children would grow up into adulthood writing these letters automatically. There would also be many happier Grandmas and Aunt Sallys than there are today. (So many today become apoplectic with anger at nieces, nephews, and grandchildren who never say thank you for the Christmas and birthday presents their relatives labored long over in selecting and mailing!)

Here's a Christmas thank-you a friend of mine received from her wonderfully polite little grandson:

Dear Gramma,
You are rely nice to sen me the red truk. It goes fast and krashes rely wham. I lov you Gramma. You sur no yur truks.

That grandmother has shown that thank-you letter to everyone from the postman to the manicurist. It is dog-eared from being read and reread over this entire past year, and I could only agree with her when she showed it to me again recently and said, "Don't you think he'll be a great writer? I mean, with that power of expression already in evidence?"

You don't have to write a thank-you note to a member of your immediate family, but it's a sweet and lovely gesture if you do!

Business Holiday Gifts

Some heads of corporations and large professional firms don't care about the gifts they give—and it really shows! On the other hand, there are many chiefs of industry, finance, and the professions who care a great deal about showing their appreciation at the holidays to all their associates and hard-working employees.

The way in which a business gift is given is as important as the gift itself. When an executive has his or her secretary pick out a gift and mail it, with a business card inside to tell the recipient who sent it, the present is cold and impersonal. When the executive selects a gift he or she *knows* will hit the spot with the recipient, and then has it wrapped beautifully and writes a charming note to go with it, *that* is a nice holiday gift!

When an executive spends time on the selection of—and really researches—his or her gifts, they have tremendous impact. An executive who realized that the head of his ad agency was crazier about his dog than anything else in life gave the man a new doggy food bowl and a mat to put under it, both inscribed with the dog's name on it, as his Christmas present. (It cost very little, but it was a major success.) An executive who realized that the president of his company was an ardent bird watcher gave her a really fine new pair of binoculars. An executive who knew that his doctor, who had spent a lot of time helping him back to health, lived in a Japanese-style home gave him an antique Japanese *shoji* screen.

Business Holiday Gifts from a Senior Executive

The executive first establishes his or her budget for that year. Then he or she chooses any of the following people to be the "gift manager" and to handle all the gift chores:

- A very smart executive secretary
- A very smart spouse who has plenty of extra time
- A personnel office or other administrative executive
- A paid gift consultant

This gift manager should have the following talents:

- Good taste (right down to the wrapping on the gift).
- An ability to bargain for the best prices.
- A thorough knowledge of the market—what's new and great, what's "in" and "out" in consumer tastes.
- A knowledge of certain businesses' rules of ethics. (For example, some media people are allowed to accept gifts only up to $25 in value, others only up to $10; others may accept "only what they can eat.")
- A talent for selecting an item that reinforces the company's desired image.

Something extravagant, gaudy, or tasteless should never be chosen as a gift, because it would hurt the way in which the public thinks of the company. A gift that has absolutely nothing to do with what the company makes, would also do nothing to help the corporate image. For example, a paper products company would send customers a great box of fine stationery, not a silk umbrella; a steel manufacturer would send customers a handsome stainless steel picture frame, not one made of wood or velvet.

- *The gift manager works through the following avenues:*

  o By buying from the leading mail order catalogs in the country
  o By working with the personal shoppers or the corporate gift departments of the leading stores in that city
  o By dealing with the outside gift consultant's resources for custom-ordered items

In almost all cases, a person buying a large number of items or making a costly order can get a "corporate discount" to make the total bill a little less onerous.

- *The people who receive the senior executive's gifts are*

  o *Close friends and peers in the business community.* This gift might be anything from a $250 case of good wine to a $2,000 new stereo for the friend's boat.
  o *The board of directors.* Often these people stand by the CEO in times of great travail, spending long hours coping with crises. The CEO might send a handsome clock to each director, with just his card enclosed. But then again, he might pen a handwritten note that says, "This clock will never be able to mark all the supportive, helpful hours of your time that you have given me this past year. I appreciate your help more than I could ever express in words."
  o *Senior staff members.* If bonuses are given, then a small gift—a personal touch—is all that is necessary. A new recording from the city symphony or an art book from a city museum would be appropriate ($30 to $50). If it is the kind of business where bonuses are not given, then each individual might receive something nice for his or her home, such as a new television, a set of fine crystal water and wineglasses, a piece of equipment for his or her favorite sport, or some excellent additions to the wine cellar of a wine connoisseur ($100 to $300).
  o *Customers or clients.* The customer's gift, if it bears the company logo, should bear it modestly. Only someone who works for the company wants to wear a necktie with the corporate logo or use a keychain with the logo emblazoned on it. Smart executives manage to downplay the logo in their holiday gifts, so that the recipients will really use them. For example:

An icebucket will have the logo incised on the inside of its lid.

A set of four bar glasses will have the logo etched in a minuscule fashion, so that you would have to look hard to see what it is.

A wine bottle opener would have the logo incised on one of the arms.

A leather diary for the coming year would have the logo stamped on the inside back page.

o *A senior executive's personal secretary:*

If she has been with him a year, something not too personal, like a scarf ($50).

If she has been with him five years, a $100 gift certificate to her favorite store.

If she has been with him ten years, a $200 handbag that the boss picks out. (It will probably be returned, but no matter—it's knowing the boss went to a store to pick it out that counts!)

If she has been with him twenty years or more, she should be on the company bonus list, or she should receive a gift of stock in that corporation or a check to take her and her spouse, mother, or child to Europe for two weeks.

What Employees Give to Superiors and One Another for the Holidays

• *You do not give your boss a gift.* It would embarrass him or her, and think how expensive it would be if every boss felt that he had to give a present back to every employee who gave one! Besides, to give the boss a gift (other than a nice holiday greeting card, something you have baked at home, or a small plant or something else that is just a gesture) looks like apple-polishing.

• *A secretary is the exception to this rule.* A secretary usually enjoys a very close relationship with his or her boss—perhaps even with the boss's family. Therefore, a gift for the family, such as food, a Christmas plant, or Christmas cookies she bakes herself, is appropriate. What is not appropriate is to give a gift that is expensive, because that would be embarrassing to the boss.

• *Employees should not make a big thing out of exchanging presents in the office.* An office that is awash in gift wrapping all over the desks and cabinets is a nonproductive office. Give your gifts to friends in tote bags that they can take home, rather than open gifts in the office. Better yet, send each gift to the person's home, so he or she won't have to lug it home on public transportation. (If your friend has a car, then there is no problem.) Exchanging gifts in the office is also very tough on those who don't receive gifts. Of course, if you are the kind person who brings into the office a Christmas tree ornament or a chocolate Santa for everyone in the office (not exceeding $5), that is really nice. (Find a non-Christmas chocolate gift item for Jewish or Muslim friends who do not celebrate Christmas.)

GIFTS FOR OFFICE MESSENGERS AND OTHER SERVICE PERSONNEL

There is a whole category of employees who serve the corporation who might be remembered either by the boss, by the boss and all the executives, or by everyone in the office. When a gigantic box of cookies goes into the mailroom for the mail people and messengers, with a box of small plastic bags and ties (so that each person can take home his or her fair share) it is *really* appreciated. So is an enormous basket of fruit, or a box of individually wrapped cheeses. This kind of gift is also appreciated by

- Employees in the nurse's office
- The company garage staff
- The men and women in the mailroom or photocopying area
- The maintenance people, including the night cleaners
- The elevator starters in the office building lobby

All of these people do their share to make it a very pleasant place to work. Often some of the office workers give them individual gifts of cookies and candy if management does nothing for them.

- *Give thought to the appropriateness of a gift* for a co-worker, especially a co-worker of the opposite sex.

  - *Nice gifts for women to give other women:*

    A frame with the recipient's child's picture in it
    Gloves
    Handbag
    Nightgown (be sure of the proper size, of course)
    Hosiery (in the right size)
    Fragrance
    Lipstick (in the color the recipient wears)
    Potpourri or sachets for bureau drawers
    Lingerie or stocking case for traveling
    Bureau drawer organizers

  - *Nice gifts for men to give other men:*

    Tennis or golf sweater
    Colored socks for a natty dresser
    Silk tie (bow tie if the recipient favors them)

Men's fragrance
Large bar of shower soap

o *Gifts (not overly personal) for either sex to give either sex, married or unmarried:*

Items for a desk—inkstand, family picture frame, letter opener, clock, leather-covered dictionary, bookends
Books relating to the person's business or interests
Music tapes for the car
Golf balls or tennis balls (whatever the preferred sport)
A beautiful plant for the office or home
A gourmet food basket
Chocolates
Wine or the person's liquor preference
Membership in a local museum
Fruit or Pastry of the Month subscription
Clever new calculator, pocket radio, or gadget of the year
A pen and pencil set, or just a good new pen
Leather agenda for the upcoming year
Subscription to a new art magazine (if the recipient is interested in art)
Chef's apron and cooking tools
The newest-style sunglasses
Two theater, ballet, concert, or opera tickets
Set of bar glasses
Set of wineglasses

Hanukkah Presents

Hanukkah (also spelled "Chanukkah") is an eight-day celebration of an ancient Jewish military victory in 165 B.C., revered in Jewish history. The menorah, an eight-branched candelabrum, is often seen in the window of Jewish households during this time, and also shares the lobby space of office and public buildings along with the Christian Christmas tree. Hanukkah, the dates of which change on the calendar each year, is usually close to Christmas week.

A candle of the menorah is lit each day during the celebration, until all eight are lit.

Jewish people give their family members and friends gifts at this time. Gentiles and members of other religions should also give their Jewish friends their gifts during this period rather than on Christmas. There are special Hanukkah cards that a person who is not Jewish may appropriately send to Jewish friends in place of Christmas cards.

GIFT SUGGESTIONS FOR OTHER PEOPLE AND OCCASIONS

Baby Presents and Christening Presents

Many of the presents you might give a baby will be suitable only when he or she is older—the first book for his or her library, for example, or a gift of stock, or a silver porringer to be used as a bowl for nuts or chips in his first apartment.

When you're buying an article of clothing, buy something for an infant a year old or two years old, because the parents and grandparents will have outfitted the baby for the first months of his life. Also, babies grow very fast. Look at the baby's parents. Are they big people? Buy way ahead in this case. (My husband and I are both big people, and our children were already in six months size clothes when they came home from the hospital, and were wearing two-year size when they were eleven months old! I have now reached the point where I buy a sweater, dress, or boy's pants suit for a three-year-old, so that it can be put away for future use. (The parents are always grateful.)

SUGGESTIONS FOR BABY

A parent or godparent (or a group of office associates who know that money is tight for this couple) might buy the nursery furniture and the "wheels" for the infant. Other possibilities:

- o Bureau
- o Changing table
- o Child's wardrobe (armoire)
- o Nursery lamps
- o Crib and bedding (blanket, sheets, baby pillow and pillowcase)
- o Carriage or stroller (with blanket for carriage)
- o Playpen (for the future)

OTHER GIFTS FROM RELATIVES AND FRIENDS

Find out from the parents if they already have a practical item listed below that you might wish to give; ask if they need a particular item right now:

- o Set of practical terrycloth bibs (for feeding)
- o Nightgowns
- o Cotton carrying blankets

- o Crib mobile
- o Decorative box for diaper pins
- o Two-part electric feeding tray
- o Electric bottle warmer
- o Nursery wall clock
- o Music box
- o Clothing (or even better, a gift certificate to a good store)
- o Nursery night light
- o Picture frame
- o Nursery hangers
- o Baby book
- o Baby's first books to start a library
- o A check
- o Gift of 100 shares of stock
- o Money market fund opened in child's name

WELCOME GIFTS IN SILVER

- o Rattle
- o Teething ring
- o Mug (engraved with baby's initials and birth date)
- o Pusher
- o Long feeding spoon
- o Short-handled fork and spoon (engraved with baby's initials)
- o Frame (with birth date engraved)
- o Silver or pewter porringer (with engraved initials and birth date)

JEWELRY FOR A BABY GIRL

- o Gold bangle bracelet (adult size, to save)
- o Tiny gold circle or heart pin to wear now
- o Tiny pearl bead circle or heart pin to wear now
- o Small pearl necklace to wear when she is four (or an old-fashioned gold chain, add-a-pearl necklace)
- o Small gold chain with Virgin Mary or her saint's gold medal (for Catholics) to wear now and put on an adult charm bracelet or keychain later
- o Diamond earrings (a small single stone set in platinum or gold for pierced ears) to give her when she is sweet sixteen (a wonderful godparent's gift)

Suggestions for Gifts to Give Young People on Any Occasion

The occasion could be Hanukkah, eighth grade graduation, confirmation, Bar or Bat Mitzvah, birthday, or whatever. These gifts run the gamut from $10 to $1,000.

o Pet of one's own—if the parents agree
o Private telephone line
o Stereo equipment
o A book (ask a good librarian what to get, according to the age and sophistication of the teen)
o The best new dictionary on the market (again, ask a librarian)
o A globe of the world (since geography is so dismally taught!)
o Something for his or her bicycle, if that is the mode of transport
o Physical fitness and exercise aids (for boys anxious to develop their muscles or girls anxious to be slim)
o Gift certificates to a video rental shop, music store, electronics store, clothing store, or costume jewelry store (for girls)
o Camera and related equipment
o Items related to the sport of choice (whether a new volleyball, tennis racquet, skis, baseball bat, golf clubs, tennis or golf balls, or ice skates)
o Clothing related to the sport of choice
o Heavy sports sweaters
o Newest kind of skateboard (for the expert in the art)
o Goggles and snorkeling equipment
o Diary (with an excellent lock on it)
o Suitcase or backpack (whichever is needed more)
o Latest calculator
o Shortwave radio
o Sewing machine
o Pair of tickets (for teenager and friend) to a much-prized sporting event, rock concert, horror show preview, or classical music event (if the teenager is musical)
o Series of lessons of choice in computers, piano or guitar or other instrument of choice, a foreign language, karate, any sport, ballroom dancing
o Trips (for teenager and friend) to

A place like Washington (with visits to the White House, Mount Vernon, the FBI building, the National Gallery, the Air and Space Museum, for starters)
Europe (with a parent or teacher along on this one)
The city where tickets to a major event are waiting (such as the last game of the World Series, the Rose Bowl, or a great historic celebration)

New York for a great concert or opera (for a musical teen)
Disneyland or Disney World

o Money (a check)
o Bond
o Money market fund opened in his or her name
o Gift of stock

Gifts for the Elderly

The elderly deserve special thought in the gift you present at holiday time, on their birthday, or when you go to visit them in a retirement or nursing home.

Do some research before you buy that gift. Don't waste your money buying something you think will be appropriate. Do some homework on the project. Talk to the person who either lives with them or sees them regularly (a relative, nurse, or home care specialist).

o In a cold climate, there might be a need for flannel pajamas, a warm robe, bed socks, a wool scarf, gloves, or a throw
o What kind of reading material do they most enjoy *now*? Would a magazine subscription be more appropriate?
o If he or she uses a cane, how about a stunning new cane in a special color or design? (Have someone measure the person's cane, so that you buy one of the proper height.)
o If the elderly person's quarters are gloomy-looking, how about something to cheer it up? Maybe a new lamp with a white transparent shade to give maximum light, a pretty plant in a porcelain container (requiring little care but with a long life), a saucy new pillow to put at the person's back when he or she is sitting, some room fragrance to make the area smell wonderful.
o The newest photographs of the grandchildren, attractively framed.
o Books in large print for people who have trouble with their eyes; books on tape for the visually handicapped.
o Food to please the palate—perhaps a mailing from Fruit of the Month or Pastry of the Month.
o A lively new hobby to espouse—for example, an aquarium, complete with gravel, decorative rocks, and plastic plants for the bottom, air filter, heater, lots of tropical fish, fish food, and a booklet that teaches their owner how to care for these lively creatures!

For Someone Who Is Ill or Injured

There are many creative possibilities that will be much appreciated. Here are just a few ideas:

o Bring your camera into the office, and take a group photo of your sick or injured friend's office colleagues, all grinning and holding a big sign that says "Get Well!" Then bring it framed, to put by the patient's bed.

o Construct a free-standing "tree" on a table in the ill person's room, on which the patient can hang all the get-well cards received.

o See that he or she has one light, delightful book to read.

o When the person is feeling much better and the doctor permits it, see that he or she has plenty of allowable edible treats and plenty of friends who come for short, non-noisy visits.

o Bring the patient (whether in a hospital or at home) something that smells delicious, like bath soap, body lotion, or room fragrance.

o Arrive with a box of notepaper, and the patient will love you, because there are always thank-you notes and "I'm okay" letters to write. If you have a stamp already affixed to each envelope, the patient will love you even more.

o Remember, for a child, no matter how many stuffed animals he or she might have, there is always room to love one more.

A Houseguest's Present for the Host

• *A first-time houseguest would bring something like*

o A baked ham, for everyone's enjoyment (and the gourmet mustard and rye bread slices to go with it)

o Fresh berries the host may not be able to buy in that town

o A large cheese, like Bel Paese, Brie, or Edam (with wonderful assorted crackers, too)

o The newest, hottest book that everyone is talking about (complete with a bookbag mailer, addressed to the bookstore, to allow for the exchange of the book for another choice, if the host has already read this one)

o Paper cocktail and dinner napkins, printed with the hosts' initials or the name of the house

• *An old-hand houseguest, knowing the foibles of the house, would bring something like*

o A new blue shower curtain to replace the ratty old blue one in the guest bath

o A new set of badly needed towels—or beach towels—for the household

o A new ice bucket to replace the one with the broken handle

- A matching set of bar glasses, because none of the host's glasses match any more
- An oversized tin of the hostess's secret, unmitigated passion: a special kind of butterbrickle
- New set of mugs, since none of the hosts' mugs match any more

Gifts for a Housewarming

When you attend a party in someone's new house (or newly decorated house), it is customary to bring some small gift to mark the event. You are, in effect, congratulating your hosts on their lovely house or apartment.

There are certain gifts that are always useful. (If your hosts have one of these, it may be old and dilapidated and they would enjoy a fresh new one.)

- Telephone book cover
- Wastebasket
- Bedside lamp
- Decorated tissue box cover and matching toothbrush caddy
- Hanging board to hold a host of keys
- Bulletin board for family telephone messages
- Message pads with the family name printed on them
- Marvelous framed photograph of the exterior of the new house
- Year's subscription to a leading decorating magazine
- Monogrammed doormat

A LITTLE ADVICE

- *Perishable gifts* (flowers and certain foods) should only be delivered when the recipient is home. This requires someone calling ahead to find out when the family or person will be in residence.
- *Put your full name and address on the card or on the enclosure envelope.* Make it easy for the recipient to identify who sent the gift (a card scrawled "Pat," "Betty," or "Joe" might be any one of five people). The address makes it easy for him or her to send you a thank-you note.
- *Don't put your gift in a box from a fancy store like Tiffany's,* hoping the recipient will think it came from there. (The recipient may try to exchange it and discover the deception.)
- *Take care in the presentation of the gift.* If you have beautifully wrapped it, drop it off in a handsome tote or shopping bag, so that excitement and anticipation is immediately created by the outside wrapping.

People love to receive a gift with something tied to the ribbon. At the holiday season, you can find everything from little snowmen and miniature Christmas tree balls to small angels, miniature ice skates, and little skis. You can tuck fresh holly into the ribbon at Christmas, tie on a sprig of violets in February. One young man I know, in pursuit of a young lady, sent her a gift beautifully wrapped with many ribbons, and from the bow dangled a shiny new key (the key to his apartment).

The Japanese, the greatest gift wrappers in the world, wrap very special gifts in kimono fabric as the outer wrap. Leftover remnants of fabrics used in making clothes can be used for gift wrap; so can leftover unused wallpaper. One young impecunious artist friend of mine wraps up his home-baked cookies each year in brown butcher paper, and then paints an enchanting Christmas scene for each person.

Taking a few pains with the presentation of your gifts means simply that you care—a lot, rather than a little.

• *People love imaginative gifts* that include an element of personalization or a surprise. Here are some examples of "thoroughly merchandised gifts" that really please the recipients:

  o Anything engraved, incised, stamped, or embossed with their name or initials
  o A stamp box filled with stamps from the Post Office
  o A camera with a roll of film ready to go inside
  o A picture frame with the recipient's spouse or child or house or boat inside
  o A tie-case for him for traveling, with three new ties inside it
  o A hosiery case for her for traveling, with three pairs of pantyhose inside
  o A suitcase with the person's name printed on the attached luggage tag
  o A gym bag containing a towel and two pairs of athletic socks
  o A pretty plant in a pretty porcelain *cachepot*
  o A lovely tin box filled with cookies or chocolates
  o A book on fishing, with two new flies attached to its cover
  o A charcoal grill with a bag of briquets and a can of starter fluid inside beneath the lid
  o A French dictionary that, when opened, reveals two round-trip air tickets to Paris

• *The gift you give as a surprise—when there is no reason for it— is the best kind of all*. For example, it is a real act of love:

  o When you bring home from a trip abroad an item that a friend collects, indicating that you really thought about that friend
  o When you surprise a friend who married recently with a tape

cassette you had secretly recorded of all of the toasts made to the bridal couple
o When you chop down a tree that fell in your yard and deliver a neatly tied bundle of wood to your friends who have fireplaces
o When you deliver vegetables or flowers from your garden with a note saying, "Hope you will enjoy these!"
o When, after your friend tells you she is giving a big party and doesn't know how to cope, you leave a list under her front door the next day of all the equipment you will lend her for the party (such as card tables, trays, glasses, and tablecloths)

*   *   *

Next in value to the gift of life—the one gift we all have but rarely appreciate sufficiently—are gifts from the heart. They have absolutely nothing to do with money and everything to do with timing, presentation, and what is written on the gift enclosure.

The successful gift is an act of love. It makes the recipient feel pampered and loved or admired. The price or the purpose of the object do not matter—whether it's a vacuum cleaner, a gold ring, a fishing rod, or a thermos jug. It's the way in which it is given that matters. Many of us would rather receive a little sketch a friend made of our little house in the woods than an emerald necklace, simply because the sketch would come from the heart. When you show someone that he or she is worthy of your thought and research, you have made that someone feel very special.

PART V

DIFFICULT TIMES: HEALING YOURSELF AND OTHERS WHEN TROUBLE STRIKES

The resilience of the human soul and body is truly incredible. People can have bad things happen to them repeatedly and yet overcome every disastrous development with courage, determination, and even humor.

Of course, there are always those who take something like the advent of a hangnail as a disaster and spend most of their time griping about one thing or other, however minor, all day long.

This chapter is not for those other people and their hangnails. This chapter is about serious difficulties, and hopefully it will offer at least a few ideas for helping and healing to those wrestling with real problems. There is a solution to almost everything in life if you look hard enough, if you have people around to help, and if you have a little thing called faith—faith in God, country, or just yourself.

When you have been dealt a blow in life, it's a call to arms in defense of yourself. If you call up the determination and adrenaline needed in striving to overcome—and mix it well with the energy derived from others who care about you—you'll possess a very powerful strength. And as you learn to cope with the little things that go wrong, you will find yourself able to face bigger challenges with aplomb.

You may rightfully say to yourself that there's a large chasm between recovering from the loss of your spouse and recovering from making a social gaffe, but the act of recovery is the same. It means you are in charge, you are in command, you are going to settle accounts—do what you have to do (always with others' feelings in mind) and get on with life. Healing yourself, apologizing, making amends—each requires drawing on that precious energy we all have but sometimes deny having. When faced with a spill, it means looking at that glass of water and telling ourselves it's still three-quarters full, not one-quarter empty!

17

The New Manners and the Loss of a Spouse

It is shattering to lose a spouse, whatever the circumstances. I remember what a friend said who had gone through a terrible divorce. "Everyone always feels so sorry for someone whose loved one has died. I don't want to sound self-pitying, but I'm bitter about the public perception of a widowed versus a divorced person. At least the widowed person may have had a happy married life—at least he or she had that. And everyone gives a widowed person so much sympathy, love, and support. Not divorced people. When a husband or wife cheats and walks out the door to marry someone else, no one feels noble sorrow for the one left behind. Patronizing sympathy, perhaps. Real sorrow, no. The general attitude is, 'Well, he or she obviously did something to deserve that kind of treatment!' "

DEALING WITH A DIVORCE

The best action for a good friend to take in regard to a divorced person is to rebuild his or her pride and sense of self. It is, of course, much tougher to be the person who was left behind in a divorce. Not only is there the sense of personal loss, but there is also the gossip in the community to confront. There is the pitying that begins for the jilted person, and the constant irritant of the former spouse who has found a new lover and now circulates among old friends wearing a happy face.

How Should You Behave When You Have Divorced?

• *It's wise not to divulge every gory detail of the marriage breakup to whoever will listen.* "Less is better" at a time like this. Let it all out to a couple of close friends, ask them to remain discreet, and keep the personal details out of your general conversation. If you wear a Mona Lisa smile and remain aloof from the gossip, everyone will know you are going to be fine and recover quickly. (People like to be around winners, not eternal losers.)

• *Leave out of your conversation any financial details or legal matters*, including custody rights pending in the court.

• *It's better not to date someone or even be seen in public with a single person of the opposite sex until after the decree is signed.* Not only is circumspect behavior important in regard to your reputation in the community, but it is an important factor in the legal proceedings.

• *The people who matter the most are, of course, your children.* Make a conscious effort to spend much more time with them than usual. They are suffering as much as you, perhaps more.

• *Refrain from criticizing your former mate to your children at any time*—now or in the future. No matter how responsible your former mate was for the breakup of the marriage, making recriminations against him or her through your children is wrong.

• *If your former mate has a new love, avoid spreading gossip about the relationship.* You will only look jealous and spiteful to others. Attempting to sully the reputation of your former spouse in your community will have the worst possible effect on your children.

• *Don't imitate those who mail printed "divorce announcements" to their friends*, as though there were some happy news to impart. (Some people even send out engraved divorce announcements, which cost the same as wedding announcements!) Call your family and friends in the city with the news, and notify your out-of-town relatives and friends with short personal notes, giving your new address and telephone number if they are to change. A sample note:

Dear Denise and Bob,

I thought you should know that Greg and I have decided to begin divorce proceedings. It is really very sad, but it has been a long time in coming. Greg is living temporarily at his mother's (telephone: 000-0000). The children are holding up well, and they and I will be staying in this house for now.

There should be happier news the next time we communicate. Love to you both.

How Should People Behave When Their Friends Divorce?

• *If you love both people, don't take sides.* Don't criticize one to the other, even if one person has obviously wronged the other. Your job, as a friend, is to try to get each member of the couple into an affirmative, cheerful mood once again—to turn away from the hatred, disappointment, and embarrassment he or she may be feeling. It takes time, but a friend with a positive attitude who keeps talking about interesting things to do and see, great books to read, wonderful trips to take, will probably gradually get through to the emotionally upset friend.

• *Don't keep probing for the reasons.* If your divorced friends want you to know the reasons, you'll be told. When a friend tells you he or she is being divorced don't ask, "Is there someone else?"

• If there *is* someone else, don't serve as a gossip conduit, supplying information to the one left behind regarding all the activities of the other spouse and his or her newfound love.

• If one spouse quickly remarries, don't take out your spite on the newlyweds out of loyalty to the divorced former mate. The seemingly precipitate remarriage eventually will be old news, and you can't keep a feud that really doesn't concern you going from the sidelines forever.

• If you are friends of both, extend an equal number of invitations to them the first year of their separation, so that one won't suffer the added crisis of feeling that the other has taken away his or her good friends. If you invite one to dinner, invite the other to dinner a couple of weeks later, and let each know that's the way you're playing it. If you give a party with eighty or more people—like a Christmas open house— you can successfully invite them both. Make sure they know that they are both invited, however, so there will be no unpleasant surprises. They can operate at different ends of the room.

After that first year, if you are much more friendly with one than the other, you can forget about inviting them an equal number of times. Hopefully, by then the other person will be able to fend for himself or herself socially.

Of course, if one member of the divorced couple behaved badly in the marriage, there is no reason to keep your friendship flourishing with that person.

• A divorce is a time to really help out your friends—by doing things for their children. These victims of divorce need all the attention they can get at this point. If you get them out of the house, take them to amusing events, help them laugh and enjoy themselves, you are performing a generous act of kindness for everyone involved. Don't forget them in the months to come. They will need your continuing kindness.

WHEN YOU ARE WIDOWED

In today's world we observe far fewer rigid symbols of mourning than in years past. It is not necessary for a widow to wear black and a heavy veil at a spouse's funeral, nor are guests any longer required to wear black; any nongarish color is acceptable. The obliteration of starchy rules about mourning attire is one more step toward trying to help the bereaved get on with a normal life.

In the weeks following a funeral, others may feel uncomfortable around you. Most people don't know what to say to someone who has lost a spouse. They don't know whether to ask how you feel, wordlessly hug you and pat you on the back, inquire about how they may help, or else ignore the entire unpleasant subject and talk about happy things.

Many of your friends and acquaintances simply can't handle seeing you, someone they love, immersed in grief or depression. Everyone wants you to snap back to your usual good self; they feel helpless when confronted by your display of grief. Even if it doesn't matter how many times in private you open that door of grief, after time goes by you should close it in public and put a lock on it.

A sense of humor, of course, is the greatest saving grace of all. A widowed friend of mine, who had had a great marriage and lost his wife to cancer, was complimented by a group of his friends on his incredible spirit and snap-back ability. He laughed and said, "It's all of you who helped me put her death behind me. You were impossible—so embarrassed, unnatural, and ill at ease when trying to comfort me. I finally couldn't stand it any longer. I had to return to my old self in self-defense!"

Having young children, of course, is a real blessing. They need your attention and you need theirs; suddenly you'll notice there is a marvelous in-house support group already in place and functioning. The dependence of the young upon you is the best therapy in the world. Again, willing a positive attitude is key. If you conclude that your spouse certainly would have wanted you to get on with your life, you *will*.

• *Seek the help of bereavement support groups and/or therapists.* (See the next section of this chapter, "Making the Adjustment to Being on Your Own Again," for more detailed advice.)

• *Use your closest friends or relatives as volunteer punching bags for your emotional outbursts.*

Sometimes you really need to let it all hang out, particularly during those early, terrible sinking spells. There are times when it's a good idea to express in words how bad you feel, so *talk*—to the right person. An occasional emotional explosion in front of one or two really close friends allows you to hold your emotions in check in public. This is a period in life through which you should not delay your passage or procrastinate. Rather, see yourself passing through it quickly. Since we're all different, some manage faster than others. But remember that your "punching bag" friends cannot serve you endlessly in this capacity. It is not fair to them, nor productive for you. Look upon your passage through a state of grief as a learning experience from which you will graduate and go on to other, much happier kinds of learning experiences.

When you reach the point where you can talk about your loss in a normal way with friends and business associates, and when you can once again discuss other subjects with enthusiasm, you will have attained a major victory. When others look at you without immediately thinking of a crippling sadness in your life, you really are on the road to recovery. People who recover from a terrible sadness are stronger, better people.

- *It's very normal to have mementos and framed photographs of your late husband or wife around the house.* Hopefully, you won't try to paper the walls with them. That can make others feel very uncomfortable. One widowed friend reported that her suitor told her one night that when she reduced the number of framed photographs of her late husband from twenty to three in her house, he would ask her to marry him. The next morning she wrapped up nineteen of the photographs and put them away to distribute later among her grown children. That night, when there was only one photograph of her late husband left on display, her suitor put an engagement ring on her finger, and they were married a month later.

Another friend, a divorced man, had two photographs of his very beautiful ex-wife in his rather active bedroom. When he told me he wasn't having any real, lasting success with women, I suggested that he get rid of those photographs. He did, and now the only photographs of females in his house are those of his new wife and baby girl.

Resuming a Social Life

Advice on when a widowed person should resume a social life should be tailored to each person—because some are ready sooner than others. A widowed person who starts dating within a week of the funeral is asking for public disapproval. (Some don't care if there is public disapproval; my remarks are targeted at those who do.) It is appropriate for a widowed person to have dinner quietly with a person of the opposite sex within a month's time, particularly if the dinner takes place in the widowed person's home. It is also appropriate for a widowed person to go out for dinner in a group as soon as he or she feels like it, but it's wise to wait from three to six months before regularly dating another person alone in public. Even if it is the most harmless of get-togethers, your dating may be perceived as a courtship.

It is just better taste to wait a while before anyone can float the rumor of your having an affair or even looking for another marriage partner. I remember one friend's description of how she felt when she learned her daughter-in-law was seen dining and dancing with a man ten days after the woman's husband, my friend's son, was buried following a plane crash. "It was exactly as though she had whacked my face with an ice-cold washcloth," she described it, "and then whacked my heart with several more."

• *The parents of your late spouse are very important.* After all, they are suffering from an intense grief, too, and your sensitivity will help them. Spend time with them following the funeral. Don't shut them out in your own grief. Talk about their child—your spouse. Share funny, wonderful anecdotes and memories of the great times with them. Give them photographs and mementos of their child that will give them great pleasure in the years to come.

• *If you remarry, tell the family of your late spouse before anyone else.* Bring your fiancé(e) to meet them, and try to make the transition of your new marriage smooth for them. Make them understand that you and their son or daughter had a special relationship and love that should not be compared to your love for someone else. You are only embarking on a new and different life.

• *The most important responsibility in your remarriage is to keep the relationship strong between your children and those grandparents.* Some of the ways in which you can do this:

- o Invite them to all the children's birthdays and special days like Christmas and Valentine's Day.
- o Allow the grandparents to take them out for an occasional Saturday lunch and the rest of the afternoon.
- o Invite the grandparents for special observances, like Mother's Day and Father's Day.
- o Make sure your children remember their birthdays with a card and a telephone call, and the holidays with a small gift—perhaps something they make at school.
- o Invite the grandparents to those special times when the children are performing (such as a ballet recital, the class play, a team sports game, and the like), and of course, to activities like school graduations.

It is quite normal for your ex-in-laws to fear your new mate will keep their grandchildren from them, or that you will lose interest in keeping their emotional bonds strong with your children. Quickly address those fears.

MAKING THE ADJUSTMENT TO BEING ON YOUR OWN AGAIN

The Task of Healing Yourself

Regardless of the circumstances surrounding the loss of your mate, there's some very good advice contained in an old Chinese symbol for crisis: Half of it signifies danger, the other half signifies opportunity. A newly single person should fixate on the *opportunity* half. If you have lost your husband or wife, your life is undergoing great changes. Look upon those changes as a positive force for the future, when the healing is done.

Utilize the energy of the forces that catapulted you against your will into a newly single life. Channel that energy into shaping a frame of mind that will help you automatically to respond to opportunities as they arise. Use that energy for sharpening your senses, expanding your horizons, making new friends, and becoming open to fresh ideas. If you have children, look upon your crisis as an opportunity to grow much closer to them and to help them become much happier, even stronger human beings as a result.

Remember, too, that *the more energy you will yourself to have, the more you will have, the more you will get done, and the happier you will become*. There is always a reservoir of energy inside you waiting to be tapped. Don't waste it. Harness it to get you through this period of hostility against a divorced mate or departed lover—or grief, guilt, and perhaps even anger against a loved one who died. There's a new life to be led!

Some of this assistance is available right under your nose—perhaps in a caring, imaginative friend or in a clergyman at your house of worship. You usually receive this encouragement passively; it's almost handed to you. But much of the most effective assistance available to you must be actively sought, not passively received. It needs to be researched and discovered through your own ingenuity.

• For those with the right mind-set, help equals opportunity. The first step in the process of self-evaluation is *not to be ashamed to seek all the help you can get*. Many widowed and divorced people or people who have lost their longtime lovers are walking a very rocky path because they feel it is weak and embarrassing to seek psychological counseling or to enter a support group. If you are one such person, tell yourself that those experts and those services are there to help *you*, not just everyone else in the world.

   o Find out about the free counseling services offered by your local social service agencies.

o Ask your doctor about counseling services he or she recommends.
o Seek out other newly single people who have sought—and found—effective assistance.
o Check the activities of single, divorced, and widowed groups listed in the newspapers, particularly the various church and temple groups. Attend their self-help meetings. If you don't like one group, try another.
o Through your children's school faculty or parents' group you may hear of a counselor who will have answers you seek.
o The head of Human Resources at your office might have some leads.
o Volunteer service in a field you feel passionate about will be fulfilling because *it feels good* to know you are helping others who need you.
o There might be a new hobby that will consume you with enthusiasm and fill your hours with a really enjoyable activity. Anything that gets you going again is good in itself.

One young widow I know, two weeks after her husband's death, forced herself to attend her suburban church altar guild meeting for the first time. When she was introduced by the chairman to the forty-odd women present as someone who "is new in town and who has just lost her husband," she burst into sobs and the entire group rallied to comfort her. A women's network went into action. Within two weeks, the young widow was enrolled in a computer school run by the sister of one of the guild members, and she had a new, reliable baby-sitter—found by one of the other members. She also went to see a counselor suggested by another member. A year after that first altar guild meeting, she had a job she loved at an important nonprofit foundation; she later married a man introduced to her by another guild member.

I'm not suggesting you are going to have that kind of incredible luck because of one meeting, but usually you get something out of anything you try honestly to do. As you gain experience in trying out new solutions, you will find you become a first-class survivor, not a third-class one. It's the person who stays imprisoned at home endlessly wallowing in self-pity who faces a life of depression and never-ending grief.

The task of healing is really your own, and the time it takes is totally individual. After all, who knows you better than yourself? What is going to get you out of the grieving period and back into the mainstream other than your own will? And who can really evaluate the best road for you to walk down more intelligently than yourself?

We all need help at one time or another in our lives. If you investigate the many services and options open to you, you will probably find at least one that takes you out of a sad, despairing frame of mind and into a high-energy resolve to begin anew. If the first one you try is a dismal failure, try again. And again.

Getting Strong Again on Your Own

If you are newly single, it's important to concentrate on the positive side of being by yourself. An affirmative attitude makes it easier to find a mate and get married again—if that's your hope. You're more attractive when you're a happy, positive person. People want to have you around, and invitations follow. And if you don't wish to remarry, concentrating on the up side of life will make you even more content with being alone and determined to get the best out of life. I've noticed that the happiest divorced and widowed people are those who appreciate the gift of life. Everyone reading these words is alive; the alternative is not a happy solution to problems.

It's a good idea every once in a while to stop and think, "I have a will and control over my life."

There are many emoluments to living alone. Just ask some of the people who as adults have always lived by themselves and lead active, involved lives with plenty of fun attached. Forget any selfish hermit you may know. He or she is not typical of those who live alone. Remember instead all of the singles of your acquaintance who lead productive, happy lives, and remember that there is a great difference between *being alone* and *being lonely*. For example, you might:

• *Realize that you have the choice of either sinking into a self-pitying lethargy or of springing into action.* You can willfully summon your own supply of adrenaline to provide increased energy. Now is the time to establish new goals. Now is the time to get your life, your home, your children's lives organized. Start by writing down on paper (or making a file in your computer of)

- o Your financial assets and how you will exploit them to the fullest
- o Your liabilities and what steps you are taking to cope with them
- o Desired travel plans and what's out there available to you (charter groups, cruises, museum-sponsored tours, and more)
- o Educational and artistic goals you would like to seek—to play the piano, learn French, take a course in philosophy, join a bridge group, take a music appreciation or art history course, learn how to sew, garden, cook Chinese food
- o Volunteer work you will undertake—to help feed the homeless, become a docent at the museum, visit the elderly, read to the blind, help your church, temple, or hospital, train to become a literacy volunteer
- o Physical self-improvement activities (after getting your doctor's

okay)—start to jog, join an exercise class, work with a trainer, undertake a supervised diet, have a makeover and change your hair, cosmetics, and fashion look

• *Read*—voraciously, with joy. Not just the junk stuff, but good literature. Discover it for the first time, or rediscover it from your college days. Reading is a great soother and a leveler. It fuels your conversational abilities, makes you more interesting to be around.

• *Write letters.* Reach out to all your old pals. Write them catch-up letters to tell them what has happened to you, about all your new plans, and about how you are not going to waste time on tears. There's too much to do in life. You'll probably hear back from every one of them. Your upbeat letter will cause them to reach out to you again, and you will find all kinds of nice things happening because of renewed friendships—the very best kind.

• *Realize you now have a new independence*, enabling you to schedule yourself as and when you please. (Now you can go to *all* the ballgames instead of having to alternate with the concert series.)

• *Make the interior of your home more attractive*, even if you don't spend any money on it. You have more room for your possessions. Consider simply rearranging the space to be more comfortable and efficient. Try a more cheerful coat of paint on the walls, and a couple of new lampshades.

All of the above takes time—and sometimes money. You now probably have more time on your hands (unless you're someone with small children). As for the money it costs to try new things, you can become creative in saving or making the necessary money.

I know a widow, for example, who went on a month's expedition to Egypt, first-class, fulfilling a lifetime ambition to see the Nile. She paid for the entire trip by spending several hours every week for a year, typing corporate reports on her word processor at home. (She had a reputation for being faster and more accurate than any of the in-house typists, and the company, for whom her late husband had worked, kept her busier than she even wished to be.)

The key to a quick recovery for the newly alone is establishing new personal goals for yourself, so that you become the best person it is possible to become—the most attractive and the most giving. A person like that is never lonely—just alone on occasion, and usually very happy to be alone on occasion!

The Newly Single Woman's Name—and Stationery

THE WIDOW

Traditionally a widow lived out her life using her husband's name— for example, "Mrs. John Brown" on her checks and printed stationery. However, many women today, after remaining widowed for many years, have begun to use their given names. Mrs. John Brown, for example, after five or ten years begins to use "Cynthia Brown" on everything from her stationery to her charge accounts. It is a natural evolution.

Today's nontraditional widow resumes her given name immediately on all correspondence. Instead of Mrs. Anthony Garrett, she becomes Jane Jensen Garrett (her maiden name was Jensen) as soon as her "Mrs. Anthony Garrett" stationery runs out. When she orders new mono- grammed towels, for example, she uses "JJG" (Jane Jensen Garrett) instead of "aGj" (her and her husband's joint monogram).

THE DIVORCED WOMAN

A divorced woman may no longer call herself by her husband's name. She is no longer "Mrs. Martin Boucher." She is "Mrs. Mary Louise Boucher." Her old stationery printed or engraved with "Mrs. Martin Boucher" at the top is no longer usable, and she can't really cross out "Martin" and insert her given name with a pen. She can always cut off and throw away the top part of the letterhead (printed with the incorrect name) and then use the rest of the paper for scratch paper!

Many women take back their maiden names after divorce, which I think is an excellent idea if there are no young children and if the ex- husband has remarried.

If the divorced woman has custody of the children, it is less confusing when they are growing up if she has the same family name as they. But if there are no children or if they are out of the nest, she should feel at liberty to resume her own name. For example, Gretchen Campbell Marsden marries and becomes Mrs. David O'Connor. When she di- vorces, she can be either Mrs. Gretchen O'Connor or Ms. Gretchen Campbell Marsden again.

In the "old days," a woman who divorced was known socially by her family name combined with her ex-husband's family name. Thus twenty years ago Gretchen O'Connor after her divorce would have been known only as Mrs. Marsden O'Connor. Fortunately, since that is clumsy—and since it does not impart the woman's first name—it is not used much in the new society. She is much more efficiently known as Mrs. Gretchen O'Connor (or by her maiden name, Gretchen Marsden.)

* * *

When one of your friends goes through a divorce and is left behind because the former spouse is involved with a new love, it's time to rally around. And that's doubly true when a friend loses a mate through death. You don't have to start racking your brains for a date to pair with your newly single friend. Keep in mind that he or she may need some time to adjust to life without the former partner and won't be open to a new involvement immediately. Have him or her over for dinner with your family, or take your friend out to a restaurant and a movie. Help your friend fight loneliness and the feeling of failure or loss by conjuring up interesting or amusing things to do, particularly in the evening or on a weekend. You don't have to serve as a supply source for potential new mates. Of course, if you should be responsible for introducing a new love into your friend's life once he or she is open to that again, that's the height of successful friendship!

18

How to Help Someone Who's Ill or Has Suffered a Loss

When a friend has been or is still seriously ill, a large dose of depression usually goes with it. That's why it's important to make a nice gesture not just when you first hear the person is ill, but to keep at it. At least once a week, check in by telephone or letter. No matter how busy you are, you can always spare five minutes to do something for that family member or friend who has had tough luck.

There are people who simply can't talk to someone who is ill. They go to pieces, don't know what to say, get depressed if they see someone laid up. Then there are the others—thank God for them—who are always calling up with a cheery voice to ask how the patient is feeling, always sending a little something to make the patient feel good (like his favorite ice cream or her favorite flower), always ready to take a person out shopping, run helpful errands, go the lending library—always showing that they care. That kind of support is good manners; it also is an openness of heart.

HOSPITAL ETIQUETTE

When a good friend or relative is hospitalized, there are things you can do to show you care—and things not to do, too.

• *Don't telephone the patient.* If the person is feeling very ill, you won't be able to speak to him or her anyway. If the person is on the mend, constant incoming telephone calls will be so exhausting that they could set back the recovery. Also, when from two to four people are sharing a hospital room, the constant ringing of a telephone is very unfair to the others in the room. With a shortage of nurses, even the sickest person sometimes has to pick up the telephone to answer a persistent ring, either because he or she hasn't had telephone service cut off or doesn't know what to do about it. If the call answered under duress is from you, trying to find out how things are going, he or she will put your call in the same category as a kiss of death, rather than regard it as an affectionate gesture of greeting.

• *Do call the patient's family or office to find out the latest news and to transmit your message.* A few days later, ask a family member when it will be all right to call the patient. Some patients instruct their families to have all calls held until they are home from the hospital.

• *Check with the patient's family to see if there is already a supply of fresh flowers in the room.* If there is, don't add to the lack of oxygen in the usually overheated hospital room by sending more. (The nurses are too busy to take care of them anyway, and there is nothing worse than a hospital room full of dying or dead flowers!) Instead, have flowers sent to the patient when he or she has returned home. Nothing cheers up a person more when he or she is feeling better and is back home recuperating in familiar surroundings than to see them embellished with lovely fresh flowers or a plant that he or she can take care of personally.

• *Even though hospital food is notoriously bad, your patient friend might not be able to eat certain things.* Therefore, watch what kind of gift of food you send. Ask a relative of the patient if you can bring a dish of hot pasta or if you can put some ice cream with your friend's name on it in the fridge at the nurses' station. The doctor has to give the okay. If the patient is not nauseated, a large box of chocolates is a great idea— to steal from personally on occasion, if the doctor permits it, but basically to offer to visitors, doctors, and nurses when they come into the room. Having a treat to serve visitors warms the atmosphere in the hospital room.

I will never forget one friend who, while lying in traction in her private hospital room, kept a constant supply of ice in a plastic bucket, in which sat one bottle of champagne after another. She wasn't allowed any herself, but decided to serve each of the ten bottles she had received as gifts. (She had suffered a bad accident at the end of a downhill ski race—which she won.) Everyone who came to see her (hospital staff excepted) was offered champagne, which made her hospital room one of the most popular visiting spots in town.

• *Do send reading material that is light, easy to read, and upbeat.* A hospital stay is no time to launch into *War and Peace*, but it is a time to read a collection of popular magazines that were presented as a gift, all tied up with a festive satin ribbon. One or two paperbacks to appeal to the patient's reading tastes are also nice to bring or send, but remember, someone who is hospitalized probably won't feel like reading too much. When he or she is recuperating at home, that's when the patient will start to read, enjoy food, and take pleasure in talking on the telephone with friends again.

• *Amusing or attractive get-well cards are always welcome in the hospital.* You should personalize such a card with two or three sentences, not just sign it. (Example: "The office is like a morgue without you. Everyone keeps asking how you are, and we all command you to get well quickly, so that the company becomes productive again.") If you don't have access to a studio card, send a note. Mail is always a treat for someone who is hospitalized.

• Of course, the classic present for someone who is in the hospital for a very lengthy stay is a cassette player with a recorded cassette of the voices of everyone in the family or in the office, sending special messages to the patient. I know one patient who was hospitalized for three months, during which he received a weekly cassette from his family. He always knew when he had come to the end of the recording, because the sign-off signal was always the barking of the family dog— the dog barked on command.

• *Visitors in a hospital room should keep their voices low, not only for the patient's sake, but the sake of any other patient in the room or in neighboring rooms.* It is not a time for boisterous, raucous humor, just gentle jokes and calm conversation. A patient loves to be cut in on the office gossip, to hear people tell about amusing parties they attended, good games or plays they saw, and amusing or upbeat things that are going on in the world. Sitting by a hospital bed is not the time to go into detail about the latest oil spill and how many animals and fish it will kill. Sitting by a hospital bed *is* the time to recount the story of the elephant that got loose at the circus and sauntered up a main thoroughfare of town before being captured.

• *Don't tell someone who looks terrible, that he or she looks "just great."* Instead talk about "how much better you're going to feel soon," and how "next week you'll have the roses back in your cheeks and be flirting with all the really good-looking doctors or nurses." (Since there are male and female doctors and nurses, either will do.)

• *If you're the one who's the patient, on your departure morning it's nice to leave a big box of candy or basket of fresh fruit at the nursing station to say "thank you" to all the staff who helped take care of you.* This includes doctors, nurses, nursing aides, orderlies, and volunteers. If you forget to leave a present behind, you can always drop a note to the head nurse of your floor, expressing your thanks to them all. Hospital staff work so hard, are so short-handed, and bear so much grief these days that any show of appreciation on the part of a patient brings a tremendous ray of sunshine into their lives.

WHEN A GOOD FRIEND DEVELOPS A LIFE-THREATENING DISEASE

You cannot act too quickly to show your concern when a good friend develops a life-threatening disease, such as cancer. When you hear a bad piece of news like this, speak first with someone close to the person and knowledgeable about the case, to determine how serious the condition is and whether or not the person involved wishes the nature of the illness known. In this way, you will be able to help dispel rumors, and you will become either an accurate source of information or the instrument of embargo on information concerning the patient—all based on your friend's wishes in the matter.

• When you hear bad news about a person's health and then happen to see that person in public, you certainly don't want to rush up and pour out your sympathy to someone who's valiantly trying to keep his or her condition secret.

• *Your quiet, unpublicized assistance to the family in coping with your friend's serious disease* is a gift that is simply not measurable. The friend or colleague who works silently and efficiently behind the scenes to help with anything that requires attending to becomes a beloved hero in the eyes of the sick person and his or her family. This help may consist of fetching special equipment, coping with legal matters, answering mail, making telephone calls, doing the banking and bill-paying, filling out medical insurance forms, sending over casserole meals, helping with nursing chores or whatever.

• After sympathizing with how "bloody awful" your friend who has cancer, heart, or lung disease must feel, take an upbeat approach with that person—"Of course, you're going to beat it! Of course, you're going to get well."

• If you know of others who have had the same disease and are now—long afterward—on top of their physical problems and leading productive lives, use them in conversations with your friend as illustrations of successful victories over the disease.

• Do research for your friend, seeking out current major articles on the strides being made in the fight against whatever it is he or she is suffering from. If a woman friend has had a mastectomy, and you run across articles on exercise tips or on fashions like swimsuits adapted for women with mastectomies, save them for her. It could help make a difference in her life.

• When someone undergoing chemotherapy suffers temporary hair loss and must wear a wig, the polite thing to do is ignore it. I have seen people thrown for a loop by the sight of their friend in a wig then make a joke of it (inappropriate) or go into phony raptures over how great the wig looks (also inappropriate). It is best to ignore the entire subject unless your friend brings it up.

• If he or she looks seriously ill, don't gush, "Gee, you look great today!" because your friend will know you are being insincere. But if a cancer patient really does look good in his or her new wig and has obviously made an effort with his or her appearance, a compliment is very much in order. "You look terrific today!" Just don't mention the wig. (Some people, of course, have a great sense of humor about their wigs, but it is best to let them initiate the jokes on the subject—not you.)

• As the months go by, don't keep confronting your friend with the past illness every time you see him or her. People get cured, or if not cured, so stabilized that they lead normal lives. In other words, just stop inquiring about the person's health or mentioning the "recent" sickness, which may not be so recent any more. After I passed through and out of colon cancer, I began to resent the people who for the next ten years clutched my arm anxiously every time they saw me, saying, "How *are* you, *really?*"—as though they expected me to keel over and die right in front of them. It made me uncomfortable that they still perceived of me as being sick, when in actual fact I was much healthier than many of them. When you beat something like cancer or a heart attack or a lung operation, you expect others to forget you ever had it.

• *When someone is actually dying, of course, any peppy, upbeat approach is inappropriate.* Just be there by his or her side, quietly talking when the person feels like it, and remaining silent when the person is tired or is dozing off. Hold the patient's hand, don't be afraid to touch or kiss him or her. And if you can offer religious comfort and discuss the joys of the "life hereafter," *do it*. It will be one of the last real favors you can perform for that person. I have a friend who is a proud atheist, who vehemently proclaims there is no God. Yet I will never forget the description of his actions one night when he sat beside the bed of a sick mutual friend. The nurse had just gone out of the house on a short errand. The patient suddenly sat bolt upright and said, "I need to see someone about God." Without hesitation the agnostic picked up the telephone by the bed and called the rectory of the Episcopalian church across the street. A priest was there in ten minutes—just in time to ease our friend's passage to death.

The fact that you are a constant visitor when someone is dying— even if you are not permitted in the room for more than a minute or two at a time—is a great comfort to the person who is sick, and also to the person's family. A grave illness is no time for abandonment, but rather a time for patience and solid support. Your friend's family may send you away because there is nothing you can do, but if you have left your name and telephone number and the message, "I'll be waiting; I'll always be there when you need me," you have no idea how much comfort that gives the grieving family. You also have no idea when someone in that house will pick up the telephone and dial your number because you *are* needed.

When You Have a Good Friend with AIDS

• Don't ask him or her about it. Let the person tell you first. He or she may not want you to know at first.

• Stop others from broadcasting the news about the illness prematurely, because there is sometimes severe discrimination against a person with AIDS. Ask the rumor-spreader, "Did he tell you himself he has AIDS? Do you know it for a fact? Well, then I think you shouldn't be telling me—or anyone else—that you 'think' he has become infected."

• When the person's condition becomes public knowledge, rally around him or her (or around the family, in the case of a child who has contracted it). If you are a caring colleague at work of a person with Acquired Immune Deficiency Syndrome, find out if he or she has seen an AIDS counselor. (There is an AIDS Clinical Specialist already on staff in many major hospitals.) Make sure he or she knows the number of the very helpful National AIDS Hotline (telephone: 1-800-342-AIDS). The GMHC (Gay Men's Health Crisis, Box 274, 132 West 24th Street, New York, NY 10011) is another source for help and information. Find out the name, address, and telephone number of the doctor in charge of your friend's case (and if he or she doesn't have one, make sure that he gets one).

• As a friend, make sure that as he or she weakens, someone is coordinating on necessary care—a relative or someone close to him. If a lover is nursing the ill person, give that person a much-needed break, and take over for a couple of hours. If he or she is alone (having been abandoned by family or a lover), when conditions worsen and the person becomes weaker, make sure that someone is preparing his or her meals, bathing him or her, and keeping his or her place clean.

• Urge everyone in your office or among your mutual friends to visit your friend regularly, to call up to see how he or she is, to send treats (a special flavor ice cream or a favorite casserole, for example), and to make certain he or she is receiving the proper care—such as taking medication regularly, seeing the doctor when necessary, being given regular baths, getting clean sheets put on the bed regularly, and so forth.

Some people totally reject an AIDS victim, and some families have been known to be downright cruel when confronting a relative with the disease. I will never forget a friend who suffered from AIDS whose lover had abandoned him and whose family had not spoken to him from the time they learned he was gay. When the parents learned their son was dying of AIDS, they took action only once, and that was to take every stick of furniture out of his apartment, except the bed on which he was lying in a weakened condition. His apartment had been furnished with family antiques, and his parents were afraid these would go to his lover, so left him to perish in a bare apartment.

We should do everything we can to help anyone die with dignity—whether that person is male or female, homosexual, or heterosexual. We are all human beings, after all.

There are many fine publications to give the family and friends of an AIDS victim to read. These include

o "Answers About AIDS"—a report by the American Council on Science and Health, 47 Maple Street, Summit, NJ 07901; telephone: 201/277-0024
o "Coping with AIDS—Psychological and Social Considerations in Helping People with HTLV-III Infection"—U.S. Department of Health and Human Services, DHHS Pub. No. (ADM) 85-1432, printed 1986
o "Medical Answers About AIDS" prepared by Lawrence Maas, M.D., published by Gay Men's Health Crisis, New York, 1987

HOW TO TALK WITH THOSE
WHO HAVE SUFFERED A LOSS

I remember talking to a very recent young widow when she was trying to tell how she felt. There was a need for her to put her feelings in words at that particular time. A third friend present, a man, was convinced that our widow friend should not even be allowed to discuss the tragedy. As she tried to eject from herself bits of grief, one at a time, he interrupted constantly, chattering on about what was happening in the Super Bowl contest. She finally turned to him and said in the nicest possible way, "Henry, I know you're trying to cheer me up. And I love you for it. Normally I am incredibly interested in the Super Bowl. Next year I will be again, but not this year. Would you mind?"

• *Be sensitive in your comments.* A friend should never say, "You're young, you'll be married again right away." That is not the comfort the survivor needs. When a person says to a widow, "Well, thank heavens you don't have any children, for it will be much easier for you to remarry," the insensitivity of the remark cuts right through her. It is also wrong to take away from the seriousness of a widowed person's grief by claiming that the children of the marriage will make everything instantly all right—"Oh, well, you have Jennifer and Bobby to think about now. You won't have time to think about yourself any more." Widowed people like their friends to acknowledge the seriousness of their loss, even if there is the comforting presence of their children.

When Someone Loses a Lover

If a relative or good friend of yours loses a lover—someone with whom there has been a long-standing relationship—that person feels the same grief as a married person feels who loses a spouse. Don't put down the person by thinking, "It's not as if they were married . . ." Whether the lover died or left your friend, the emotional devastation is the same as if the two had been married. *Even if you have disapproved of their relationship*, remember that the person left behind is suffering and deserves your support and sympathy. It's a time for you to

○ Check in on your friend or relative often, to see how he or she is doing. A friendly voice on the telephone just asking, "How are you coming along?" can mean so much to someone in distress.
○ Invite that person to dinner or for activities over the weekend— the toughest time of all to be alone.

Real friendship means support—in good times and in bad.

When a Parent Loses a Child

There is nothing that bears down so grievously on the lives and hearts of parents than to lose a child. Friends are desperately needed to stand by at the time of the death, and to be there in the future when a parent wishes to discuss that death. Understanding friends are needed for years to come, too, if a parent refuses to discuss that death and keeps bottling up the grief inside tightly. Some day all those emotions just might explode.

Be there for your grieving friend at the time of the funeral, but also in future years. Don't be afraid to bring up the child's name in a natural way in your conversation as the years go by. ("How Joey would have loved watching this game with us. I remember how he'd always sit absolutely spellbound in this very chair, with his feet up on the hassock, shouting and cheering in front of the TV during the whole Final Four games of the NCAA.")

Most parents become bitter if they feel their child has been forgotten by the world around them—either because the child's life is a subject that is past and not relative to the present, or because the subject is considered too painful to bring up by friends.

It's important to remember the special pain the family feels at times like holidays. Write down the child's birthday in your diary, and remember it in some little way every year. (Don't observe the anniversary of the child's death. Most parents prefer you to remember happy living memories, like birthdays.)

I know someone who has contributed ten children's books to the library of his small town on his friends' little girl's birthday every year since her death in a tricycle accident. The books are in a special section of the library, marked with her name "In Memoriam." There are now 150 books there, each one reminding its young reader of the girl in memory of whom the books were given. It's nice to do something special like that in memory of a child.

When Your Friend Has a Miscarriage

Be very careful and sensitive in talking to someone who has suffered a miscarriage. If there is one thing she does *not* want to hear, it's, "Oh, it's nothing. You'll have another one right away again. Cheer up!" That kind of "comfort" downgrades her grief.

We pour out our love and consolation when a friend loses a child. Yet when a woman suffers a miscarriage, we are often insensitive. Let your friend know that you are aware of the terrible shock she and her husband have suffered. Let her know that you know—"This is a very tough time for you. It's a tragedy. I'm here to help in any way."

19

Making Things Right: How to Get It All Together Again When You've Messed Up

To me, one of the worst feelings in the world is when I'm utterly embarrassed—either because I've done something to make myself look like a fool or, worse, because I've done something to offend someone else in a major way. Everyone has his or her own way of reacting to such a negative situation. When I find myself in one, my pulse quickens, I sense my heartbeat accelerating, there's a feeling of panic, and the bottom of my stomach feels as though a boulder rolling down the Grand Canyon had just hit it. Obviously, relief must be found in a situation like this. In my case, relief comes only when I feel the people I've wronged have forgiven me.

After years of practice in surviving such disastrous events, I have become an expert on what to do. Just to give you a look at a few experiences:

At age nine, I was a "portal page" along with Patsy Garrett at the Ak-Sar-Ben Ball in Omaha, Nebraska. This was the biggest social and civic event of the year, magnificently staged, with the crowning of a prominent king and queen, whose identity was kept secret until that night, and a procession of beautiful debutante "princesses and countesses of the Royal Realm of Quivera" in magnificent designer ballgowns.

Patsy and I were beside ourselves with the honor, prestige, and excitement of being the door-openers. Twenty-five thousand people had jammed into the Coliseum to witness the pageant, and we, the portal pages, were to initiate the entire proceedings. Clad in white satin, rhinestone-studded knicker suits, with white plumed satin berets, we were to open the great ceremonial doors when we were given the signal and the pageant would begin. Our signal finally came: the blaring of what seemed a thousand trumpets (but were probably only fifteen). Patsy and I moved across the stage in perfect unison (how often we had rehearsed) and in one graceful motion pulled on the great gold knobs of the doors. Nothing happened. Twenty-five thousand pairs of eyes were on us. The trumpets kept blaring. Some workman for some insane reason—most likely revenge against the ball officials—had nailed the portals shut right before the performance. We could hear the pageant director swearing at us from behind the scenes. Finally backstage they realized our problem, and we heard the director's voice through the doors: "Be calm. While the carpenter is summoned, stand together, you two, straight as arrows, your arms akimbo as though you are guarding the gates, and smile. Smile like you have never smiled in your life!" (Those were words of tremendous wisdom. I don't know about Patsy Garrett, but I've used that advice about smiling when in great adversity in public many times in my life.)

The trumpets continued trumpeting, we stood there smiling as though this entire humiliation were all part of the show. Finally the hammers arrived, the nails came off, and we could open the big doors. This was a worse embarrassment to me than the night I played a Rachmaninoff solo on the piano at a Convent of the Sacred Heart recital in eighth grade and the top of the grand piano came smashing down because of an improperly placed stick prop. The piano strings resonated with loud dissonance through my entire piece, and I could see my mother with her face buried in her hands (whether in grief or in laughter, I could never decipher), but my father's face read, "Continue—you have to go on." I smiled at the audience as I asked God why He let this happen to me, but I finished.

It's very intimidating when you embarrass and merit the wrath of the President of the United States as I have. I made President Kennedy furious his first Monday in office, because of the party I'd produced the night before in the White House. Applying my many years of embassy experience, I had bars strategically placed around the main floor to make a smooth flow for the party guests. The morning papers the next day screamed headlines about the Kennedys shattering several sacred traditions—serving liquor with the press present, having bars for the first time in the White House, and having a party on a sacred day—Sunday. I had broken every rule in one easy sweep, and a delegation of Congressional leaders immediately called on the President to express their horror and disgust. The President summoned me to the Oval Office and gave me a dressing-down for getting him into a well-publicized mess his first day in the office.

I was mortified for having caused him such embarrassment. I told him I felt like doing myself in. I told him I'd hire a skywriter to write in the sky that it was all my fault, and none of the Kennedys'. I told him I would march into the muskets of a firing squad, if it would help expiate for my crime. He laughed, put a consoling hand on my shoulder, and congratulated me on a really effective apology. "Never forget how to apologize like that, Tish," he said. "You're very effective, even if you did rob me of the chance to really give you hell." (By the way, there never again have been bars in the White House; drinks are always passed now at official functions.)

Not only did I have to apologize many times in my embassy and White House lives, but also in my business career. I have survived some real disasters. One was in connection with Burlington Industries' national interior design project, the Burlington House Awards. These were important annual awards given to people who had tastefully and creatively designed their home interiors. One year, as usual, I gave our mailing house a list of the thirty-two winners and another list of the several hundred losers in the competition. I wrote a sympathetic prototype letter to be sent to the losers over my facsimile signature, thanking them for entering, praising them for their lovely homes, but regretfully informing them they were not winners.

I wrote another prototype letter for the winners, congratulating them, telling them of the awards ceremony to come and all of the glory of the publicity they would receive. Unfortunately, there was a small error in the actions of the mailing house: They inadvertently switched the lists of names and mailed the "Congratulations, you have won a Burlington House Award" letter to the enormous list of losers, and to the small list of winners, they mailed the "Sorry, you lost" letter.

After meditating a few minutes on why God had let this happen to me, I concluded that the combination of AT&T's telephone lines around the country plus some acting prowess on the part of my staff could pull us through this impossible situation. I called the staff together and called in some of my friends with acting ability as volunteers. We took over several of Burlington's telephone lines for the next two days. I gave everyone a detailed rehearsal—an acting lesson, in fact—on what to say and how to sound as if performing in a Greek tragedy. We called hundreds of people, moving from one time zone to the next, calling back repeatedly if necessary until there was an answer. Finally, after two days, we had reached every single family of losers who thought they were winners. We used drama and pathos to explain our "unpardonable mistake." We threw our emotions full force into our voices, sounding truly upset and sincere about our apology. (*"Please* forgive us, Mrs. Snodgrass. How could we have done such a thing to you? Will you ever forgive us, Mrs. Snodgrass?") With the exception of one person, who was downright nasty about the mistake, the people we called were understanding and nice, and we were forgiven. They kept saying to the caller, "Look, it's all right. I'm not upset. Please don't worry about it!"

I told the management of Burlington about the mailing errors *after* everyone had been informed and the psychological damage was already healing. The power of an abject apology is unlimited!

MAKING AMENDS

If you forgot a lunch date with a friend who stood miserably on the corner in the rain and wind for forty-five minutes waiting for you, that friend is going to be justifiably angry—to put it mildly. Your feelings of anxiety and embarrassment for having done that to your friend probably will be even stronger than his or her resentment toward you. When you stand up someone—whether a customer or a friend—you never quite heal from embarrassment over what you put the other person through. You should not only make quick amends, but artful ones as well. An out-of-town business colleague of mine who left me waiting for him in an airport for over an hour did the following when he realized his error: (1) sent me a long Mailgram of apology, (2) sent me a dozen long-stemmed roses, (3) took me to lunch at the 21 Club the next time he came back into town, and (4) ordered a car to pick me up at my office and take me back again after the lunch. (I call that expiation in style.)

A friend of mine who had been stood up on a date was equally impressed when the blind date who had done this terrible deed baked two batches of Toll House cookies for her to prove his sincerity. Another friend who inadvertently forgot an engagement with an acquaintance she hadn't seen for two years, sent him an imported Italian prosciutto, which she knew was his favorite food. Her note read, "With every stroke of the knife as you slice this prosciutto, think of it as a punishment of me for having forgotten our date." He told her later he had only romantic thoughts of her when he cut off paper-thin slices of prosciutto, and since they were subsequently married, it all goes to prove two concepts: that not all missed appointments bring disastrous results, and that there is a little ham in us all.

I have forgotten more than my proper share of accepted dinner invitations because of being overextended, but also through sheer carelessness in how dates are entered in my agendas. (Keeping two books, one at the office and one at home, is often responsible for the mistakes.) My husband and I have also arrived more than once at a dinner party on the wrong night, thanks to my error. (It's a great feeling to arrive at someone's house all dressed up and to have your hosts answer the door in their pajamas and robes.) I have also put down engagements on the wrong date in my diary. Not to excuse myself, but these are all good reasons why a host should send reminder cards, containing all of the salient facts, to any guest who accepts his or her invitation on the telephone.

I have even invited people for an informal Sunday night supper at our house and then forgotten about it, forgetting even to mention it to my husband. When this happens, you have options. You can play upon your guests' sympathies, apologize with pathos and drama and immediately invite them to a later, much better dinner party than you had originally planned for them. Or you can bluff right then and there, pretend you were expecting them, and feed them pot luck that evening. (If you take the latter approach, keep an outward calm when you are in the living room with your guests, even if you must improvise frantically when you're coping in the kitchen.)

The more absent-minded you are, the more creatively apologetic you must be in order to heal the wounds. I have taken all of the steps listed below after being an unintentional no-show at a party given by friends—and I have been forgiven, so the same responses will probably work for you:

• *Telephone your hosts and make a dramatic, really sincere apology*. Admit that they have the right to be furious, and tell them you know how humiliated they must have felt with that empty place (or places) at the table. Ask your host if it would be a good idea if you casually called some of the other guests whom you know well to explain the mix-up— why you weren't there when you were supposed to be. (Often there is a legitimate excuse—a secretary may have written down the wrong date on the boss's calendar—and when the other guests know this, they are relieved.) The main problem to alleviate may be the social anxieties you have caused your host, particularly if it is someone you do not know very well.

• *Go to your host's house or office to offer an in-person apology*. This always makes a big impression.

• *Send or leave a note* (your apology thus goes on the record), accompanied by flowers or a gift.

Or follow through with with a combination of all three of the above.

When You Mis-introduce Someone or Forget a Name

Having spent many years in diplomatic circles, where I was required to introduce people properly, I have pulled some giant boners. At the American embassy in Rome, when the border wars between India and Pakistan were at their height, I introduced the new ambassador from Pakistan to the entire diplomatic corps as the new ambassador from India. (He did not immediately understand what I was doing, since I was making the introductions in Italian, a language he was not proficient in, but when apprised of what I had done, he left the embassy in a huff.) I wrote him a long letter of apology, delivered it to his embassy myself the next morning, and was admitted into his presence in order to make my apology more compelling. After looking sternly at me and telling me he would not have minded being introduced as the ambassador from any country in the world other than India, he put his head back and laughed, "This will have been the most amusing moment of my entire career. Thank you, Miss Baldrige, for having given it to me." As long as everyone maintains a sense of humor, all mistakes are forgiven and forgotten.

Most of us make mistakes in introductions all through our lives, although of lesser gravity than my India-Pakistan debacle. If you, for example, introduce an old friend by her former husband's name (knowing full well that she remarried years ago), just apologize and explain that you are "so bad at names, so careless with past and present names. *Please* forgive me for doing that." It's when you don't say anything and leave your mistake hanging in the air that the person you have mis-introduced becomes embarrassed, perhaps even irritated.

I remember Clare Boothe Luce, my boss at the embassy in Rome, telling me how often throughout her life she was publicly mis-introduced. As a speaker, she was constantly presented to large audiences as "the celebrated actress, Miss Claire Luce" (a woman with a similar name with whom she detested being confused). The author of *The Women*, a famous play about bitchy women all in the act of getting divorces, she once doubled over with laughter on the lecture platform in front of two thousand people upon being introduced as "that famous author of *Little Women*," Louisa May Alcott's syrupy book about a nineteenth-century family. Clare Luce told the audience she was delighted to have her book confused with Louisa May Alcott's incredibly successful classic, but added that she doubted Louisa May would feel equally delighted.

When my father, a well-known Republican, was running for Congress from the state of Nebraska, he was introduced to a national radio audience as "that famous leader of the Democratic Party from the state of Nebraska." He laughed and said that although his party was Republican, he would be very happy to annex the Democratic party into his own and give it the leadership it had been lacking all those years.

I remember how embarrassed a business friend was when he introduced a military officer above his proper rank. The officer spoke to the large throng and thanked his introducer for introducing him two ranks higher instead of two ranks lower. "You're going the right way," he said. "Just remember that anyone in the military will be delighted to be introduced at a higher rank any time—just any time!"

A flash of humor—and not a solemn correction—is what is needed when someone mis-introduces you. If you forget a good friend's name, or someone forgets yours, make light of it. Don't let the other person suffer. "Andy, I, too, forget names all the time. Don't think a thing about it. I'll forget yours next week. There, will that make you feel better?"

In other words, if you embarrass yourself by making a mistake in regard to someone else, you can contain the mistake by the speed and the creativity with which you offer your apology. And if someone else is embarrassed because you have been the victim of his or her error, keep your sense of humor and show everyone that you are a good sport.

When you make a minor social gaffe and apologize promptly and sincerely, instead of losing a growing friendship you often can cement it by showing that you are concerned and really care about the other person's feelings.

WHEN YOU ARE ANGRY

One way to make sure that others won't like us is to be unable to control our anger, whether that anger is justified or not. All of us become angry at one time or another; it is almost impossible not to, but there are ways of dealing with it. Some people deal with it by becoming unacceptably hostile. But most of us do not become antisocial. Instead, we kick the desk, put our head in our arms and cry, pound the table with a fist, or look around for a voodoo doll into which to stick a pin or two.

I believe that yanking your sense of humor from your subconscious and sending it up to do battle in the front lines with your temper is the very best way to handle the situation. For example:

• Have a private chat with your dog, pouring out your emotions and reciting all the injustices done to you. There is no being more supportive, no pair of eyes more sympathetic and understanding. Perhaps your cat or your bird would also be a good listener, but a dog—even a borrowed one—is probably your biggest eye-contact sympathizer.

• Write an absolutely furious letter to the person who wronged you. State everything that should be said, and castigate the recipient in the richest prose you can summon. Then read the letter aloud—with great dramatic embellishments—at least five times. Then tear it into shreds and destroy it. (*Under no circumstances*, mail it!)

- Try some yoga. Get a book on yoga if you are not familiar with any of its techniques. You either will relax from the breathing exercises and forget why it is you're so angry, or you will become tired and relaxed from trying to understand how to do the yoga. Either result will be beneficial to anger control.

- Practice any sport in which you have any glimmer of interest. Smash tennis balls against the backboard, bounce the basketball as hard as you can in the driveway, and drive your golf ball as though it were the devil incarnate. You should become spent from all that physical effort—enough to make you stand back from your anger and get a proper perspective on it.

- Clean house like you've never cleaned it before. Pretend you're vacuuming up your enemy into the dust bag or wiping him away with your polishing cloth.

- Do a physically demanding, much-hated chore—like raking all the leaves in the yard or taking everything off the kitchen shelves, washing them and the shelves, and putting everything back. You will be so proud of yourself afterward that the edge will be off your anger.

- Follow any great physical effort with a nice warm bath, including bath oil or bubbles or a special fragrance. (I'm addressing men as well as women!) How can you retain negative feelings lying in such a relaxed, sweet-smelling state?

- Go see a movie, and crunch hard on your popcorn. That munching action is very therapeutic.

- Better yet, go to a museum. There are so many anguished- or angry-looking people in the famous Old Masters paintings hanging on the walls; you'll conclude that they're far worse off than you are. You will begin to feel calm by comparison.

- Play music—your soothing, beautiful tapes, whether they're Madonna, Schubert, Chopin, or Sting recordings. Music is a wonderful way to calm down.

In other words, defuse your anger with deliberate countermeasures. Then the next day you won't have done or said anything you have to be sorry for. You'll be *in charge of yourself.*

PART VI
KEEPING IN TOUCH

The ability to use language, to communicate with people in times of joy and sorrow, and to persuade, soothe, enchant, or calm another person, is a great gift. It's called the *art of communication*. We all can be accomplished in this art, if we just make ourselves aware of how important it is to both our success and happiness.

We have a lot of difficulty keeping in touch with one another in today's busy world. Nevertheless, we need the support of our friends, we need the affection of our relatives, and we need to tell people we still think about them, that we hope they are well and happy. It does not take very much time. Whether you are making your second telephone call of the week to your shut-in grandmother, writing an old college friend who has been ill, or telling someone you see at dinner that their children are wonderful, *you are performing a human service, an act of kindness.*

20

Being an Interesting Conversationalist

It's no secret that our society is not doing too well these days conversationally. Many of us spend all day in front of a monitor, staring at a new kind of Esperanto computerese on a screen. Then we spend our evenings sitting in front of a TV or VCR screen, or we wear our Walkman earphones like wallpaper over our ears to shut out the sounds of the world. Where is the human element, the sparkle of the spoken word, the harmonious music of the human voice in all of this?

In our stressful times, more than ever it's people, not computers, we need and want near us. But no one needs people who are inherently boring. It's the good conversationalists who make us feel good, season our days, and serve as insurance that others will enjoy themselves. Stimulating people are magnets around whom we cluster quite happily.

The affirmative aspect of conversation is that anyone of average intelligence can become quite good at it. To be a good conversationalist is to be unselfish—as well as constantly learning. It requires a process of continuous self-education and an attitude of caring about other people—getting away from oneself and thinking of others. A good conversationalist thinks outside and beyond himself; he is neither limited to what is inside him nor constricted by an obsession with self.

541

THE TWO V'S: VOICE AND VOCABULARY

Your conversation is enlivened by a good vocabulary, but it is also transmitted through the voice. These are two important components in how you communicate and in how the public perceives you—in your business or social life.

Cultivating a Voice That Is Pleasing

When you hear that someone has a "great voice," that person probably

- o Is easy to understand, with good enunciation
- o Speaks without strain, at a low, comfortable pitch
- o Projects enthusiasm with the voice, rather than fatigue or depression
- o Has an unaccented voice—or, if there is an accent, it is light and pleasing, rather than exaggerated and unintelligible
- o Speaks at a controlled volume, neither too soft nor too loud
- o Has good pacing, neither too fast nor too slow, and even changes the pacing to suit the meaning of the words

Most of us don't have a clue what we sound like. When we happen to hear our voice on a tape, we are usually surprised: "Whose voice is that? I don't sound like that!" The sounds that resonate inside our head as we speak are different from those others hear—and from those you hear when you listen to yourself taped.

If you have an unattractive voice, you are very possibly unaware of it. Your family and friends are used to your voice, so they don't think about it or discuss it with you. A well-modulated voice is a tremendous asset, but a poor one can hold you back in your career, and most certainly in your social life. Since improving the voice is one of the easier tasks of self-improvement, and since there is help all around, it's worthwhile to consider taking action.

With the help of a good tape recorder, record your voice at length, reading something, conversing, and talking on the telephone. Those tapes will act like a magnifying glass held up to your voice. Carry the recorder around with you and make a few hours of tapes. You'll find that after a while you won't even notice the existence of the recorder, and you'll sound natural on it. Then sit down quietly and listen to all the tapes by yourself. Ask family members or a couple of good friends to listen to a few minutes of it (five minutes are sufficient). Ask them to be frank about what they hear regarding the quality of your voice.

If the general consensus (yourself included) is that your voice could stand improvement, find professional help. You will find free-lance speech therapists in most cities. There are drama coaches who work with local repertory groups, and professors in public speaking or drama departments at most colleges and universities. A voice coach will show you how to breathe properly, from the diaphragm, to enhance your voice. You will be given simple exercises to improve your diction and the tone, quality, and pacing of your voice. When you master your own voice and make it as attractive as it can be, you will be a more confident, persuasive public speaker. And it will also enhance your personal life!

The Force of a Dynamic Vocabulary

There is nothing more exciting to listen to than a person with an imaginative vocabulary. Our English language is so superb, so full of nuances (ask someone from another country about its level of difficulty), that we should be proud to use it well. Today, it seems there is more abuse than proper use of our language, but if more of us consciously try to be role models in such an effort, those around us may begin to follow. "Good language is contagious," I remember hearing the late writer and ambassador Clare Boothe Luce say one day. The trouble with her statement is that bad language is contagious, too. Street talk with its obscenities and foul language is creeping into our everyday vocabulary like weeds choking up fields of lovely flowers. Foul language is becoming so commonplace that it no longer shocks. Television does not help, with the writers of some shows consistently using bad grammar and one network star saying at least two or three times a day to many millions of people, "That's real nice," or "It's real good."

A good vocabulary is fostered in a child within a nurturing family life. One family I know always devoted five minutes at their dinner table each night to word games. A new word was learned, and each child subsequently made up a sentence that used it properly during the meal. Occasionally the thesaurus would come to the table, and one child would quiz his siblings and parents on the variety of existing synonyms for a word. Those parents instilled a love of the English language into their children that they have carried into very successful adult lives.

When a wordsmith like Bill Buckley is on the air on a television show, listeners often keep a dictionary handy and write down the new words he throws out so effortlessly. If you or I were to try to talk like Bill Buckley, it would sound very stilted and artificial, but perhaps we all can try a little harder.

Teaching children to enlarge their vocabularies becomes a game that is fun. Teaching adults to enlarge their vocabularies becomes a challenge. But again, just as parents are the role models for their children in using good English, so senior managers in the workplace have a great opportunity to inspire those they supervise with a love of the English language. If they use good English and develop rich vocabularies, even in their written memoranda, the younger ones coming up just might try to follow suit. Who knows, we might be able to beat street talk back into the streets!

SMALL TALK

One dictionary defines small talk as "casual or trivial conversation." I prefer to call it "amiable, unhurried communication." When you're making small talk, you're passing time, exchanging thoughts and opinions, perhaps acquiring a knowledge and amassing information you never had before (and perhaps will never need again). You make small talk while you're waiting with other party guests for your cars or with an acquaintance while you sit waiting in an airport. You make small talk on the station platform waiting for your commuter train or riding in an elevator. You make small talk waiting for the meeting to begin or the concert to start or all during any cocktail party you happen to attend.

In spite of its diminutive aspects, small talk is important. Knowing how to make it effortlessly is a gift as well as a social tool. It often becomes a combined business and social plus. It is an instrument of communication that renders a person attractive and makes him or her pleasant to sit next to at a dinner party, or across from at a lunch where business is being conducted. It's important to remember that:

At a business lunch	*At a social function:*
If you're the guest, make small talk until your host signals that it's time for the business discussions to begin.	Give equal time to everyone around you, particularly both dinner partners, even if one person is much more attractive and amusing than the other.
If you know the other person is married and has a family, ask him (or her) a very general question about it. If he drops the subject fast, follow suit. If he continues on the subject, it signals he is flattered by your interest.	If conversation bogs down, get the other person talking about him- or herself, a guarantee that the conversational ball will keep rolling during the meal.
Bring up light business subjects such as new companies starting up, stories of human interest, funny happenings. The other	Launch light topics of conversation, not depressing ones. Your partner is not going to want to hear about the auto accident that befell the man who lives down the street; he or she

person wants to enjoy his or her meal, not be depressed with your latest statistics of business failures.

If you know a good joke, the best time to tell it is during the soup course, before the serious business discussion begins—or quote an apt proverb, such as business advice from Lincoln: "When you can't remove an obstacle, plow around it."

would rather hear about the beautification project on your city's waterfront.

If you can quote an appropriate proverb, dazzle your dinner partner with your sense of timing. For example, if he expresses agreement with you, tell him you now feel like the great Disraeli, who said, "My idea of an agreeable person is someone who agrees with me."

The main thing to remember about small talk is to keep it light and upbeat. If you remember to smile while you talk, you'll make the person listening to you smile, too.

When Not to Make Small Talk

Of course, there are times when it is best to remain silent. When someone is concentrating—working, reading, intensely involved in the work at hand—leave him or her alone. At a dinner party, people are supposed to make chit-chat during the service of a meal. On an airplane, on a bus, a train, in the doctor's waiting room—wherever—a person concentrating should be left alone. *This includes one's boss when you are accompanying him or her in a car or waiting to see a client.* If your boss is studying papers in her briefcase, let her open up the conversation if she chooses to. And if she does, but then you see her start to go back to her papers with her eyes, return to your papers and let her work again.

If you are talking to someone sitting beside you on an airplane and he or she is working, leave that person alone. If you are the one being bothered by a "talker" (I seem to get one of these on almost every long trip), be very pleasant but firm: "I wish I could talk to you. I can see you are a very interesting person. But unfortunately I'm on a deadline and have a great deal of work to do before we land. I hope you don't mind."

SO WHAT *ARE* YOU GOING TO TALK ABOUT?

A good conversationalist is very aware of the kind of subjects that please most people, so he or she, in an act of leadership, pulls out just the right topic for the occasion. Then the give and take among the people present seems to ignite.

The good conversationalist also knows that a successful "conversational launch" depends not only on the subject, but on the occasion and on the kind of group.

If only one person in the group plays golf, a good conversationalist does not go on about that sport, because he knows only one pair of ears will really be listening.

If he is at a funeral, he does not discuss the latest gossip he has heard, because it's simply not an appropriate time to discuss such frivolous (albeit fascinating) things.

One of his funny and only slightly off-color stories may break up a group of men in the locker room, but that same story could fall with the thud of a sack of bricks in mixed company at his office.

A good conversationalist takes the temperature of the group and the occasion before leading the discussion. He is successful when he is sensitive to others and wants to please them—an unselfish point of view.

In general, there are some topics that please more than others.

Good Conversational Moves	*Bad Conversational Moves*
• Taking an item from that day's newspaper that's fun to talk about or introduces an unusual topic of interest	• Taking a grim, depressing item from that day's newspaper, guaranteed to make everyone feel discouraged
• Asking parents about their new baby	• Asking someone if his or her marriage is breaking up
• Congratulating someone for having recovered from an operation or illness	• Asking someone to relate the gory details about an illness or operation
• Proposing new ways of raising funds for an illness like AIDS	• Asking a couple if it's true their son has AIDS
• Providing news on sports of major national interest, such as the Olympics or World Series	• Giving a discourse on a sport known to few if any of those present
• Discussing heartening news of the economy	• Giving seriously depressing news of the economy
• Starting an informed discussion on local civic problems	• Becoming enraged and emotional about a community issue
• Describing fascinating new educational experiments you have heard about	• Damning the entire local school system as being outdated and hopeless
• Providing happy news of mutual friends	• Providing information on everyone's miseries
• Talking about the latest cultural performances of excellence	• Criticizing every new artistic event in town
• Divulging good news on the health and nutrition fronts	• Telling everyone how they now "can't eat this and can't eat that"

- Telling people to be sure to watch an upcoming TV program that is purported to be excellent
- Discussing how the local real estate market is doing
- Talking about ways to help a mutual friend who has lost his job

- Warning everyone that the upcoming program is reportedly inferior, not worth watching
- Asking anyone what they paid for their house or apartment
- Wondering aloud about what a mutual friend did to get fired

A good conversationalist is upbeat, and searches for the provocative topics that most people present care about.

If You Don't Want to Be a Bore

You can test to see if you are a bore by becoming aware of how people are responding to you at any given moment while you hold the floor and are talking. If they are looking around the room at other people or things . . . if their eyes are slightly glazed over . . . if they have sunk deep into their chairs so that they are practically lying down instead of sitting up . . . if they have given up trying to interrupt you . . . if, out of the corner of your eye, you see them glancing at their watches, beware—you are boring them.

It's the conversationalist who overdoes it, who won't get off the subject, who sticks to his or her topic like a gummed label that is the bore. The three topics most likely to bore are your health, your job, your children.

If you have had a serious illness and you run into your friend Gregg in the street, he will ask with genuine concern, "How *are* you, Jennifer?" Jennifer, give him a simple ten-second answer. He knows you are in the land of the living, and he is really not interested in your medications, the changes in the doctors handling your case, the status of your X rays, and the quality of your digestive system at present. You can answer, "I've been out of the hospital a month now and am doing just fine, thank you. I'm really lucky." Enough!

If on the bus you sit next to someone you haven't seen in a while and, to be polite, that person asks you about your children, mention each child's name (he or she will probably have forgotten their names) and give a report of only a few seconds' length on each. "Jim graduates from junior high this year, Harvey made the tennis team at Lehigh, and Mary Alice is finishing college this June and is going to Europe with some of her friends. They are all in fine form." Enough!

If you mingle after church in the courtyard with some friends you haven't seen for a while and someone asks you about your job, give a quick report. "I left Eagleton and have a new job in computer programming with Steers and Company. It's a great company and I really like my new job." Enough! The intelligent thing to do after someone has asked you about your children, health, or job and you have politely answered them, is to turn quickly to a new subject—one that veers in their direction, away from yours. "Enough about me. How is Hal? And your mother? Are you going to the lake this summer?"

EXTRICATING YOURSELF FROM A CONVERSATIONAL DILEMMA

It's a good idea to bring up an entirely new subject of conversation when:
- *A nasty argument has erupted.* (That's the time for a hero in the group to say something like, "Enough about that subject. What I want to know is who here is willing to make a wager on the outcome of the upcoming elections? Who's savvy enough even to know who all the candidates are?")
- *The stories are getting dirty in mixed company*, which leaves everyone feeling uncomfortable. ("Would anybody mind if I asked George a question? I'd really like to hear the good news about his promotion.")
- *Someone or several people are making mincemeat out of a friend of the group* who is not present to defend him- or herself. ("Let's stop attacking Suzanne and go into dinner and attack the shrimp cocktail instead.")
- *The conversation is way over the head of most of those present.* Even though two computer hacks may be enjoying their rapid dialogue on computer technology, a few minutes is long enough for them to hold the floor while cutting out the others in the group who do not understand the jargon. (It is appropriate for someone to then interrupt, "You're too smart for the rest of us—it's time to come down to our planet again or to go into the other room to continue your private discussion.")
- *Someone has just committed a gross gaffe* (such as making an uncalled-for ethnic joke, in response to which one of the people present says that it impugns his wife, and he does not appreciate the humor). What follows is usually a terrible stillness. It really helps if one person has the courage to break the chilling quiet. ("Well, I'm sure there will be apologies later. For now, I'd like to ask Terry, who has just returned from the USSR, and who has been trying to tell us about her trip all night, to take the floor and tell us all.")

It also helps if the person who picks up the conversational ball as a good soldier starts to talk and talk, in order to dissipate the tension. Hopefully, too, the person who made the error will take his or her offended friend outside and make the most earnest of apologies. (Such an offense also calls for a carefully written letter of apology, not just a verbal one.)

I don't know about you, but it happens to me all the time—I become trapped in a conversational booby trap by remarks I initiate to get a conversation going. As Clare Boothe Luce used to say, "No good deed goes unpunished."

Here is an example:

> *Me:* "I noticed your handsome wedding ring. Do point out your wife to me."
> *Dinner partner:* "She died six months ago."
> *Me:* "Oh, I'm so very sorry."
> *He:* Silence

If you find yourself in a situation like this and there is a long meal ahead yet to be served and eaten, you might face up to the challenge. To the man who lost his wife, real sympathy is in order: "I imagine these last months have been very hard for you. Do you have people—children perhaps—who are helping you cope?" (The usual reaction on his part will be to talk gratefully about the children, the in-laws, the friends who are giving him assistance; this conversation can last throughout an entire meal.)

The safest way to extricate yourself from an awkward situation is to direct the conversation toward the other person. Almost everyone likes to talk about him- or herself—even someone who seems loath to do so. Just keep floating different topics in his or her direction until that person reaches up to grab one of those colorful balloons.

The Conversational Hero

A conversational hero is the person everyone wants to sit beside. I remember sitting near a young man at a Sunday barbecue lunch who had been asked by his hostess to talk to her tongue-tied, painfully shy young niece. He asked her question after question, with one-word answers coming back. He told her about himself—his job, what he did in his leisure time—with practically no reaction. Finally, he put his elbow on the table, rested his cheek in his hand, looked her gravely in the eyes, and said, "I've told you everything about myself. I've asked you everything about yourself. Would you like to hear about my dog?"

With that she burst out in laughter; the ice was broken. He was and always will be a conversational hero, because he's basically kind and he uses his sense of humor to open up others.

A conversational hero will inevitably

• *Listen.* The primary asset of any good conversationalist is the ability to listen attentively to others.

- *Not interrupt.* No matter how hackneyed or boring, every speaker deserves to be allowed to finish what he or she is saying.
- *Show a great sense of humor.* To laugh at oneself—without putting oneself down too much or too far—creates the most charming kind of ambience.
- *Work tirelessly to charm a bored or boring, even bellicose guest*, someone who may have been important for the host to invite for some reason, but who, left alone to his or her own devices, is a real party destroyer.
- *Be able to talk on any subject.* This means that the person is well read and knowledgeable. It also means the person knows how to participate, even when the subject being discussed is not in the realm of his or her information.
- *Know how to defuse someone else's lugubrious conversation.*

Before dinner one evening, I overheard the following discussion between two tired women from Wall Street:

> "I feel terrible tonight."
> "I don't feel so hot either."
> "I got bad news about a friend today."
> "Join the club. My best friend died last week."
> "Well, I bet you don't have the mess at your office that we have. Another ten percent fired this month."
> "The very same thing's about to happen to us, only higher than ten percent."

The host, who heard part of this dialogue, moved in with lightning speed, like John Wayne in a fast gallop, to save the conversation. "From the sound of the two of you, you'll never make it into dinner, you're both so depressed! Cheer up. Come over here to this group. They're discussing just what you need—the incredible, hilarious pet tricks last night on Dave Letterman's TV show."

- *Know how to take a topic of conversation into new, interesting depths.* For example, people might be discussing all the historical pageantry of various national bicentennial anniversary celebrations of George Washington's presidency, which causes one person in the group to talk about the thrill of bringing his kids to see Mount Vernon, George Washington's home. This causes another person to announce that Mount Vernon has just published a little book of our first president's amusing "Rules of Civility" (in essence, an etiquette book for young people, written when he was fifteen). Someone else then discusses the new American history book that challenges the entire relationship between the American and French revolutions, which prompts someone else to bring the discussion to Hollywood—and a movie being made on an aspect of the two revolutions.

Good conversation is a pleasant—and kind—give and take on a

subject of mutual interest. People weave in and out of it, Virginia reel-style, as spectators, listeners, and participants. There are some people you always love to talk to—because they're upbeat, amusing, or inform-ative. These are the people who make you feel relaxed and part of their orbit. These are the people who, when you run into them or join them in a business or social situation, cause a reflex reaction in your facial muscles—a nice big smile.

Handling Prying Personal Relationship Questions

People may not have the right to ask prying questions about relationships between people, but they do anyway. When impertinent, even infuriating questions are asked of you, remember to

• *Keep your cool.* Control your quite justifiable anger, because if you become upset, it will only make you look guilt-ridden. You can teach others a lesson only when you are in absolute control of your emo-tions—and your vocabulary.

• *Embarrass the interrogator with a deflecting, non-answer.* Never answer directly an impertinent, uncalled-for question. This is a time for sarcasm—almost to shock the person who asked this question into realizing how out of line he or she was in asking it. For example, whether there's truth to the rumor or not, if someone asks you if your marriage is over because your husband is leaving you for another woman, reply with something like "Divorcing my husband? Wherever did you hear that?" That will put your interrogator on the spot.

Or if someone asks you, a bachelor, if you are going to be, or are, living secretly with a certain woman, as rumored, answer something like, "Why? Are you hunting for a roommate?"

Or if a friend asks you how far you have gone in your relations with a man you've been seeing, answer something like, "Why not ask George?"

• *It's all right to challenge your interrogator.* For example, "I can't believe that *you*, of all people, would ask me a question like that," or "I can't imagine a real friend delving so far into something so private." Or, "How would you feel if I asked *you* a question like that?"

THE ART OF GIVING AND RECEIVING COMPLIMENTS

When a compliment comes your way, doesn't it sound nice, and doesn't it feel good? Unfortunately, our society is so uptight and sometimes so overly frank that compliments don't exactly flow around us every day. Many people are afraid to give them, because they don't want to let anyone know what they're feeling inside. Others are afraid to receive them, because they're cynical and suspicious of the motives of any person praising them.

What a nicer, happier world it would be if more of us told each other nice things more often! If there was ever a true statement made, it's that as humans we *need* to be complimented. Children learn to be complimenters from their parents. If, for example, a little boy sees his father watch his wife come downstairs dressed to go out for the evening, and his father exclaims, "Don't you look *beautiful!*" that little boy has a good chance of growing up to say the same kind of thing to please his wife when he is a grown, married man, too. Too many wives never bother to tell their husbands how handsome they look, and too many husbands neglect even the most basic compliments, such as when a wife asks her husband, "Well, what did you think of my dinner tonight?" and he answers, "I ate it, didn't I?"

- *You don't have to lie if asked if you like something and you don't.* Some people are against paying social compliments just to please someone, unless the statement is totally accurate. I don't believe a person should lie, but a compliment that is said just to make someone feel good is, to me, a good end in itself. Today, many years after my four-year stay in Rome in my youth, I remember fondly all those Italian men whispering in my ear that I was "the most beautiful woman in the world." I knew they were saying the same thing to almost every woman they talked to, but it made me feel happy and wonderful; I couldn't have cared less about the insincerity of the remarks. It's a kind of game of pleasant teasing, but it bubbles inside you like good champagne.

For those who must be 100 percent honest all the time, someone might ask you if you like her new dress when you think it's most unbecoming. You would be truthful if you said "No, I don't like it, it's not becoming." But telling her the truth could really hurt her feelings. *Something* must be a positive about her appearance, so find it and mention it. Her dress might have one redeeming feature—its color, a pretty collar, or even nice buttons. Mention that detail, without saying whether or not you like the dress as a whole. "It's a very nice blue color," or, "That's a good neckline on you."

Compliments as Ice-Breakers When Conversation Has Bogged Down

A compliment is the nicest kind of ice-breaker when you are having a tough time getting a conversation going with another person. Even if the other person is as shy as you are, when you pay that person a compliment, he or she will usually react positively, and the compliment just might cause the recipient to start rowing her end of the boat.

I was seated in an airport gate area one weekend, waiting for my plane to depart. On the seats next to me were two people, obviously employees of the same company, who were trying to make conversation and not succeeding very well. There were many awkward pauses. Although I was reading a newspaper, I was aware of the shyness of both men, particularly the younger one.

His colleague finally said, "Sharp, I noticed how you looked when you got here tonight. That's a good-looking suit." Immediately, his companion smiled. "Thanks," he said, "I just bought it last week," and unconsciously straightened up in his chair and began to speak in a much more animated tone. From then on, their conversation flowed with ease.

• *When you're shy about speaking to someone of the opposite sex, remember the power of a compliment.* It really helps your conversational flow. It's as though you turned on a heater in a cold room. Even if the other person is too shy to give you a snappy reply, your saying something nice gets the words started. Think ahead about complimenting an acquaintance you would like to get to know better. Rehearse your compliment-paying before going out on a date—open a new file of compliments in that computer brain of yours. Then, when you're seated speechless next to him or her, go into that file, select an appropriate compliment, and come out with it. It doesn't matter whether it pertains to the other person's good looks, personality, ability, or intelligence— say whatever seems appropriate at the moment. For example, it might be difficult for a shy young man to say to his date, "You are so beautiful," but he might be able to say, "You look really good tonight" . . . or, "I watched you at the meeting the other day. You were terrific" . . . or, "You know something, you have very pretty eyes" . . . or, "I like dancing with you. You really know how to dance" . . . or, "I like the way you laugh. It's a nice laugh" . . . "That's a really neat dress you're wearing" . . . or, "You have a great sense of humor!"

• Here are some standard occasions in which a compliment should be paid:

  o When you know someone is wearing a new dress or suit. ("Hey, George, you look really special" . . . "Mamie, that's a great new coat!")
  o After your hosts have served you a delicious meal. ("Joan, that was the best lasagna I've had in years. You're a master pasta chef!")
  o After someone has made a public appearance. ("Your speech was *very* effective. If anyone can get that fund drive launched, it's you. Well done!")
  o After there has been recognition or an honor bestowed, either on your friend or colleague or on a member of that person's family. ("What wonderful news about Henry! He's a chip off the old block. He's headed for the top.")

- When someone has expended great effort on a project. ("Mary, your entry in the show was sensational. Your plantings were just so perfectly designed and installed; the whole Garden Club must be proud of you.")
- After a person has successfully and intentionally altered his physical appearance. ("You look so slim and elegant. The weight loss is very becoming" . . . "Your makeover course was a great success. You look terrific.")
- When a person has done something courageous. ("The way you stuck up for Roger and defended him was wonderful. You are the kind of friend everyone should have.")
- When a friend did a good job in competitive sports, whether he or she won or lost. ("Mark, you played well today. It's a shame you lost, but you were brilliant out there and next time you'll win.")

Know How to Accept a Compliment

If we Americans are not good compliment-payers, I think it's safe to say that we're worse compliment-receivers! How often do you tell someone how great he or she looks and instead of receiving a thank-you, you're given a protest? For example:

> "Mary, you look so pretty today."
> "Oh, no I don't! I have this awful pimple on the end of my nose, and the hem is coming out of my dress. I look terrible."
> "Albert, you gave an excellent presentation in the Board Room this morning."
> "Oh, no, it was awful. I choked up several times. I had a feeling no one could hear me, and I forgot the punch line to the entire thing. It was a disaster!"

When someone says something nice to you, say "Why, thank you!" or, "Aren't you nice to say that!" or, "I really appreciate those warm words." Whatever you do, don't deny the compliment or try to refute it. It puts the other person down who was only trying to please you. The perceptible lack of ability to accept compliments must be part of our national uptightness. Instead of feeling embarrassed and compelled to belittle yourself, be grateful and thank the other person for the nice things said to you. Relish them. Write them down and tuck them in a desk drawer. You can take out that note later and read it when you're feeling down.

When You Notice a Friend's Physical Change for the Better— or If You Notice a Friend Looks Ill

If a person has done something to greatly enhance his or her appearance, compliment that person without referring to a specific improvement. For example, to say, "You look absolutely wonderful!" may elicit a response such as, "Oh, so you noticed my weight loss," or "Do you really like my new hair color?" Then there will be further conversation. Or, your compliment may elicit only a curt "Thanks," in which case you should pursue the subject no further, because that person is obviously sensitive about people noticing the changes.

If a good friend looks ill to you, don't comment. Just continue talking about pleasant, upbeat subjects. If he or she brings up the subject, then, of course, you can come forth with all your sympathetic, loving support.

* * *

To have the reputation of being a great conversationalist brings magic into your life. You will be wanted as a guest at everyone's party; people will lean in your direction to hear what you have to say; people will quote you—the sincerest form of flattery. It's well worth acquiring the self-discipline and the knowledge it takes to become a good conversationalist. And when you become one, think of this: You will even amuse yourself!

21

Great Connections: Telephone Manners

HOW YOU SOUND AFFECTS HOW PEOPLE SEE YOU

You undoubtedly know people whose voices on the telephone are so attractive that talking to them is always a pleasurable experience. Theirs are happy voices that give a psychological lift, for the cheeriness in their voices is contagious.

It's a good idea to listen to your own telephone manners and voice and to make an effort to sound pleasing to whoever is calling. That means consciously putting a smile into your voice when the telephone rings, and saying "Hello" as though you're glad it rang (although the effort is much greater if the call forced you out of the bathtub, and the person on the telephone is trying to sell you a magazine subscription!).

When you answer the telephone,

- o Your voice can sound warm, cheerful, upbeat, happy to be talking to the other voice—"Joe, it's *great* to talk to you! I haven't heard your voice in such a long time, and we've been thinking about you. In fact, we were talking about you just the other evening, wondering how you were."

556

o Or your voice can sound cold, detached, and uninterested—
"Hello, Joe. What's up?"

o Your voice can imply that you are a caring person who thinks
about others, not just about yourself.

o Or it can communicate that you are an uncaring, self-centered
person who is simply not interested in anyone else.

• *In addition to the factor of warmth, a good telephone voice has*

o Clear diction. (Every sound is easily understandable.)

o A normal tempo. (The words do not tumble out too quickly or
drag interminably.)

o A pleasant volume. (The caller does not speak too close to or too
far from the mouthpiece, so the other person never has to ask,
"What was that? Sorry, what did you say?")

o A good pitch (not too high and shrill or funereally low). A speech
teacher who works for a telephone company said she likes
helping people change from "sounding either like a hog-caller or
a baritone singing after ten beers."

BASIC GOOD TELEPHONE MANNERS

*M*ake good telephone answering a priority at home and at the office.
The manner in which you answer your telephone—or your child or
your secretary answers for you—says a lot about your concern for how you
are perceived. In other words, *your* telephone manners will be judged by the
way anyone else answers who picks up the instrument in your office or
home.

At the office, write down for your secretary exactly how you want your
telephone answered. Don't expect her (or him) to have extrasensory powers
to know how you want things handled. As for your children, write down and
post on the wall by the telephone a simple list of how the telephone is to
be answered in your household, beginning with a bright, enthusiastic
"Hello!"—and not a loud "Yeah?" Be sure to keep a notepad and sharpened
pencil near every telephone in the house, so that lack of writing materials
can never be an excuse for not taking a good message. (Store a large supply
of pads and pencils. In the average house they last about two days by the
telephone, after which one finds them under sofas, beds, and in bureau
drawers.)

• *Your home telephone should be answered within four rings.* If
the caller has to wait for ten rings, for example, he or she may think you
are loath to answer the call at all. If you move around a large area and
always seem to be far from the telephone when it rings, have an extra-

long cord put on your telephone, add extensions, or buy a cordless phone to carry around with you. *An office telephone should be answered by the second ring.*

• *Always return your calls—within the same day, preferably, but if not, certainly within forty-eight hours.* If you can't return your own calls, have someone do it on your behalf, rather than just not calling.

For example, a husband returns a call on behalf of his wife:

> "Georgie left a message that you called for Lisa. She won't be back until next Monday. Is there anything I should tell her when she calls me tonight?"

A secretary should notify the caller when her boss cannot return an important call. For example:

> "I know how anxious you are to reach Mr. Walton. It now looks like that meeting he's in will last much longer than originally planned—perhaps well into the night. He left firm instructions not to be disturbed. Is there anything I can do in the interim? May I transfer you to Ms. Jennifer Hamilton, who is also involved in the project you called about?"

• *Call when it's convenient for the other person, not just for you.* Start off the conversation with: "Is this a good time for you to talk?" Some people prefer to handle personal matters in the evening at home, others early in the morning before going to work. Still others don't wish to be bothered at home with personal calls, and want to be called only at their offices. If you call someone at home, that person may be taking a soufflé from the oven, feeding the baby, or arguing with a spouse over their quarterly income tax filing. A caller should always be sensitive to the time pressures on the one he or she is trying to reach. I find that by asking an important person's secretary when the best time is to call, I receive invaluable information.

• *The caller should also be sensitive to the other person's ability to stay on the line for a lengthy period.* There are people who live alone and are lonely; there are those who are bored; there are others who like nothing better than to while away the hours talking. Then there are those who always seem to be frantic, overscheduled, and suspended in a continuous state of crisis and emergency. (I know this latter group well, since I am one of them.)

• *It is an act of human kindness to remember to call regularly those who are lonely* and who need the human contact of another person's voice. It is also, however, an act of human kindness to call those who are overly busy (even if it is because they are inefficient in their time management) only when necessary, and always with a minimum of time expended.

• *Show concern for the elderly when telephoning.* Since many elderly people have difficulty getting to the telephone, allow it to ring much longer than usual when you call them. And since many elderly people are hard of hearing, raise the volume of your voice to accommodate that problem when you speak with them; you can ask them frankly what sound level is best for them.

• *Always sincerely apologize to the person whom you have inconvenienced by dialing a wrong number.* When you erroneously dial someone, it is just plain nasty to slam the telephone down in that person's ear—as if it were his or her fault that you misdialed. (This usually happens to me when I'm awakened in the middle of the night. I only wish a fairy's wicked spell would attach the rude caller's ear to the receiver, so that he or she would have to listen to what I have to say to them!)

• *If someone has an appointment with you—at home or in the office—don't interrupt your conversation by taking the call of anyone who rings.* If you have no one answering the telephone for you, tell the caller you will get back to him or her when your visitor leaves. (Then write down the person's name and number so you don't forget to do so.)

• *But when you are with someone in his or her office and he or she must take an urgent call,* don't sit there, staring. Offer to leave the room. If he or she motions, "Not necessary," read something on your lap, go get a magazine, or stare out the window at the scenery.

• *Watch the background noises when you are on the telephone.* The sound of your television or stereo is magnified into the earpiece; the sound of your chewing your food is like a storm; if you're cracking your gum, it can sound like a machine gun firing!

• *Whenever there's a disconnect, the person who originally placed the call should place it again,* even if the problem obviously came from the other person's line.

• *When you're calling someone long distance to ask a favor,* and that person is not there, don't ask him or her to return a call that is potentially expensive. After all, it's you who are asking for the favor, so tell whoever answers the phone that you will call back when the other person returns. If you say to the person answering, "Please have Mr. Smith call me collect," the chances are Mr. Smith will call you back at his own expense—unless he is a student!

In other words, don't make the call asking for a favor at the expense of the person of whom you are asking the favor.

• *Cut a call short if you have to,* but with diplomacy and tact. A white lie is even warranted at this point, so as not to hurt the other person's feelings. "Janet, I'm sorry, but I have to go. My secretary informs me there's another call that has been waiting for some time." "Doug, forgive me, but I must leave right now for another appointment." You can always finish the discussion at another hour, week, or month. If, however, there was some urgent business you interrupted when you cut the call, you should call back within the same day.

• *Remember that people prefer good news to bad.* We are usually quick to spread bad news by telephone (someone has cancer, is getting a divorce, was fired, and the like), but we should be even quicker to spread good news by telephone (a marriage, birth, promotion, tournament win, someone's child awarded a college scholarship, and the like).

The Home Telephone

- Your home telephone is answered nicely with

  ○ A cheery "Hello," or
  ○ "The Jackson residence," or
  ○ A recitation of your telephone number, or
  ○ If you work out of your house, with the name of your company, such as "Jackson Residential Properties"

Again, more important than the words is the tone of voice—hopefully pleasant, warm, welcoming.

• *Family members should refrain from being line hogs.* A line hog is someone who ties up the line with frequent overlong conversations. As a single father of three children explained to me, "At home, *no one* could get through to me, nor could I ever make an outgoing call in the evening when I returned from work. I refuse to spoil the kids by giving them their own lines; if I gave them a new line to be shared, the three would be fighting over it the entire time, and there would be no peace in the house. We now have a rule whereby no one can make an outgoing call after six-thirty in the evening except me, unless it is an emergency. For all other calls they want to make outside, I keep a jar full of quarters on the hall table, and they may use them for the pay telephone right on our corner! They hardly ever avail themselves of that privilege. There is now peace in the house, and the kids are getting their homework done."

Security When Children Are Home Alone

If a stranger asks a child on the telephone, "Is your mother home?" the child, not recognizing the voice as that of a relative or a good family friend, should answer, "I'm sorry, but she is unable to come to the telephone right now. I'll have her call you back as soon as she is free."

If the stranger presses further—"Well, is she having a meeting there?" or "Does she have company?"—the child should respond, "She can't be disturbed."

Your child is not telling a lie; he or she is simply stating that mother cannot come to the telephone right now. You can make your child be at ease with this if you practice calling, acting as a stranger would, playing the devil's advocate, and rehearsing your child to react in such a way so as not to give a stranger any information. As you practice, there will be a lot of giggling and horsing around at first, but eventually, it will stick in the child's mind. (Your children, of course, should not be left home alone.)

Some mothers, forced by economic circumstances to leave their junior high children home alone while they are at work, have a system whereby no one answers the phone while the children are alone. If a parent wants to get through to a child, he or she dials twice in rapid succession—a kind of code—and the child knows then to pick up. ("Usually, however," a mother told me laughing, "I can never talk to them anyway, because they are on the phone with their outgoing calls in alternating turns, so there is no chance for any bad person—or good person—to get through to my house.")

The Office Telephone

Your office telephone is properly answered informatively. In the case of a woman who works for a large real estate firm, for example, her company policy might have her answer her telephone in this manner:

- o "Newstead Properties, Joan Jackson speaking," or
- o "Joan Jackson, Sales," or
- o "Joan Jackson, Commercial Sales"

If her secretary answers for her, it might be

- o "Joan Jackson's office"
- o "Miss (or Ms.) Jackson's office," or
- o "Miss Jackson's office, Ms. Farnham speaking"

- *A secretary should never answer with just her first name.*

She loses dignity for her position and herself if she uses a first name only. It is much too informal—and also not informative enough. If, for example, you have to go through an entire organization, trying to track down a "Betty Sue" instead of "Betty Sue Brown," you will have one tough time finding her.

An editorial aside: Some of the information systems businesses have a rule—part of their corporate culture—that only first names are to be used. That may work well inside the company, but it can't work all that well in relationships with the outside world. Many people are upset when on the telephone people they do not know call them by their first names. We need some dignity and a modicum of formality in order to make life more graceful and efficient.

- *Another cold and information-poor way to answer a telephone is with an extension number only.* One man I know automatically responds with a question every time he hears a voice answer his call with just an extension number: "Is this the computer speaking?"

• *Work with the secretary of the person you're calling.* Some people are ego-driven to speak only with the boss of the office they have called; they are incapable of dealing with the secretary. Well, the smartest way to deal with an executive who has an intelligent secretary is to go through her, leaving substantive messages, impressing upon her the importance of certain actions you hope will be taken, imbuing her with enthusiasm for an idea that you want to sell to her boss, and making her aware of your timetable. Many times in my business life I have realized that the secretary understands what I am calling about more than does the boss. Therefore, I always explain carefully the purpose of my call. She inevitably responds with good advice for me ("Call back tomorrow morning"; "Write it in a short letter"; "Send it Federal Express to his vacation address"; or whatever).

EDUCATE YOUR SECRETARY IN GOOD PHONE MANNERS

• *Instill in her the priority you place on courtesy* in handling incoming calls

• *Train her not to over-screen your calls* and make you inaccessible to people. No one should be put through the third degree when they try to reach you, such as:

"What is the business of your company?"
"And your position within the company is?"
"And when did you last speak to Mr. Thatcher?"
"Will he know what this is about?"

As her boss, you should furnish her with

o A list of everyone—family, friends, doctors, teachers—who should be put through to you immediately. ("Just one minute, Mrs. Ellsworth, I know Mr. Henry will wish to speak to you.")
o A list of secondarily important people whom you would like to speak to if you have the time. ("I know that Mr. Henry wants to take your call. He is on long distance right now, and there are two calls waiting, but when he finishes these three, we'll call you right back.")
o A list of people you never wish to speak to. ("I'm sorry, Ms. Rogers, but Mr. Henry is really tied up on several important projects at the present. He simply does not have the time to take any calls, so the only advice I can give you is to put whatever you wanted to say to Mr. Henry in a letter, and to send it to this office.")

• *Teach her not to put someone on hold for longer than fifteen seconds.* If you have to remain longer than that on the other line, have her tell the person on hold that you will call him or her back within minutes. (And then do it!)

• *A young executive should place all of his or her own calls to upper management.* A junior person should never have a secretary call a senior person. When the senior person gets on the line, the junior person should already be on the line, not his secretary!

• *When you are not in the office,* your secretary should automatically say, *before* she asks the caller's name, "No, I'm sorry, Ms. Gates is not here. Who is calling, please?"

If the secretary answers, "Who's calling, please?" and then says, "Oh, I'm sorry, Mr. Jones, Ms. Gates is out of town," Mr. Jones may very well think that Ms. Gates is giving him the runaround.

• *Teach her to be a deft transferrer of calls.* In other words, teach her about the company and who does what, so that when you are not available, she will know to whom she can intelligently transfer a call—to a person who will be able to get action or solve the problem.

Taking Good Messages

People should take efficient, legible messages for each other. Otherwise, they should not answer someone else's telephone.

• *The caller should not "overload" when leaving a message.*
A message should not be more complicated than this:

o The person's name leaving the message, plus telephone number (with area code and extension number, when pertinent)
o The time the person called
o The name of the person to whom the message is going
o One simple piece of information or instructions

If you leave a message with *if*'s, *and*'s, and *but*'s, you can almost be certain that it will not be transmitted with perfect accuracy. (The exception, of course, is a competent secretary, who can take the most complicated of messages perfectly. In fact, if I want something done right away, I ask the executive's secretary to do it!)

DEALING WITH A WELL-MANNERED ANSWERING MACHINE

When answering machines first began to worm their way into our lives, I swore I would never use them. I found them infuriating, inhuman, tacky, and without redeeming features. Now, because really great answering service organizations using real people are fewer in number, I have a different machine attached to each line—at home and at the office. They may still be infuriating, but they're a lot better than a telephone that rings unattended in a void. An answering machine allows you to communicate with someone without endless redialings when you're in a jam, such as when trying to catch a plane, with five angry people in line behind you, all waiting for the pay phone!

Good Manners for the Answering Machine Owner

- In your recorded outgoing message, do not inflict your latest flight of humor on the ears of those who call you. If someone is trying to reach you from a department store to arrange delivery on your new mattress, he or she should not be forced to go through a long recorded joke (which you thought screamingly funny, but which really is not) before being able to tell you what day your mattress will be delivered.
- Do not assault your caller's eardrum with a high-volume rendition of your favorite new, rather weird music before the beep sounds to take a message. A cool refreshing silence is what most people want—between the answering machine owner's recorded voice and the beep signal.
- Keep your message brief and to-the-point. Feeling rotten one day with a fever and a cold, I called a friend on an urgent matter, only to have to listen to an endless dissertation on problems between the Kurds and the Turks before finally I could leave a message. Even though I was impressed with her knowledge, my temperature rose an entire degree because of being held hostage to that spiel. (If you have hopes your answering machine will make you into a professional performer or lecturer, please control the impulse to buy one!)

Advice to the Person Leaving a Message

- Talk distinctly. Don't mumble. Speak slowly when you come to numbers, difficult names, or addresses. Repeat a telephone number you must supply, so there can be no mistake about it.
- Give your name, the date, and the hour of your message, which, hopefully, the machine's owner already asked you for on his or her outgoing message tape.
- Come to the point of your message quickly.
- Say "good-bye" in an up voice. If you sign off without one word, the other person may think you were cut off.
- Say something nice, too, before you sign off—such as "Hope all goes well with you, Johnnie. Good-bye."

A Caution About Answering Machines

The first piece of advice: Be sure to put your answering machine up high, so no small child can reach it. Often we rely too heavily on these machines. They can be inoperable, for example, without our being aware of it. The outgoing message may have been erased, or the machine may have run out of tape, or someone may have accidentally erased your entire message. Any number of little glitches may occur. Therefore, don't be angry at someone who "has never called back." That person may have called back and your machine was not working. It's up to you to get in touch again with anyone who does not get back to you. Don't implicitly trust a delicate machine when several pairs of hands may be manipulating it. (One of my friends bought herself an answering machine and found that six people in her house now use it for their messages.)

THE INTRUSIVE BEEPER

B eepers were invented for doctors on call and people involved in public safety, such as those in the police and fire departments. When an executive's beeper goes off in a restaurant, in a movie theater, or at a concert, because his or her secretary has a message to relay, the public is understandably irritated at the interruption and distraction caused by the piercing sound.

People not involved in saving lives should not use their beepers indiscriminately, as they often do, because it looks to others like a blatant cry for attention—undeserved attention.

*   *   *

The telephone can be a wonderful human extension of you. It really is a wonderful instrument. There's nothing wrong with the telephone—it's the people who abuse it who are wrong.

If you use a telephone with care and express your personality through its mouthpiece, the person on the other end of the line will *always welcome your calls.*

The telephone is an instrument to be respected, whether utilized for business, cementing relationships, or even as an antidote to loneliness. Respect for it means that you, the user, understand the rights of others in your house to use it, as well as the rights of those who are trying to call into your house—not to mention the rights of the person who has to pay the monthly bills!

22

Contemporary Correspondence: Writing Good Letters and Notes

A good letter not only relays feelings and emotions, but leaves them on the record. A letter means that someone has put time and effort into crafting a personal message to you, which does not necessarily hold true with a communication faxed from one person's office to another's, or with a message relayed on someone's telephone answering machine.

When it is well written, a letter accomplishes goals that might not be accomplished otherwise. Since letter-writing is gradually dying out as a means of human communication, today's younger generation will probably be unable to look back with fond remembrance on special letters received that marked the ritual passages of their lives. In the pre-electronic era, the following kinds of letters traditionally were sent to you during childhood, and also as you grew up and finally took your place in the adult world. You would receive a very special letter

- From a relative upon your graduation from eighth grade and high school
- From a grandparent when you finished college
- Perhaps from a close friend who could not be there for your wedding

566

- o Even from a boss who found something exceptional in your work and wanted to praise you
- o Or from your baby's godmother on the occasion of your child's birth
- o Or simply from someone close to you who just felt like "talking to you in a letter" at that particular moment

A verbal compliment or vote of thanks is heard appreciatively but then disappears like a footprint in the wet sand, whereas a written sentiment may be savored again and again, and saved to be enjoyed at still other times.

A beautiful letter is a work of art that lasts.
- These are the kinds of letters it is helpful to know how to write:

- o Business letters (even if they are becoming extinct in the era of new technology)
- o Thank-you letters (for nice gestures like gifts, favors, lunches, dinners, and weekends)
- o Letters of complaint (about a product, service, or an individual)
- o Notes—short letters used to pass on a piece of information or to serve as a reminder
- o Catch-up letters—newsy epistles sent to family members or close friends
- o Letters of reference, written to

    Introduce a person
    Vouch for a person's character or fiscal responsibility
    Help a person get a job
    Help someone become a member of a private club or purchase an apartment in a co-op

- o Letters of congratulation for any good news concerning a relative, associate, or close friend
- o Letters to cheer up someone who is ill or feeling depressed
- o Letters of apology to someone you have offended
- o Letters of condolence to the family or a close friend of someone who has just passed away
- o Love letters (in case you are in the courtship stage)

Each kind of letter has a purpose and helps us get along with one another. This is why each of us should try to keep the art of letter-writing alive and well.

HELPFUL HINTS ON LETTER-WRITING

Writing Good Letters

- Pick a time when you're relaxed and feeling up. Use a comfortable desk, chair, and a good light by which to write.
- Use an excellent pen with just the right point for you. Use black or a dark color ink.
- Use good stationery—good quality stock, and in an appropriate color:

  Gray, cream, or white for office stationery
  Ditto for men's personal stationery
  Any pastel, gray, cream, or white for women's personal stationery
- Either write by hand or type a neat letter
- Think before you write. Make an outline of the points you wish to cover, and you will write cohesively—without forgetting any point.
- Edit your letter. Read it carefully and make corrections with white correcting fluid.
- No letter is too brief. One of the best letters I ever received was simply "Dear Tish, that's it!" (meaning I had finally learned a lesson I needed to learn).
- Research the address of your recipient, including the proper title, postal code, and any other necessary particulars.

Negatives to Watch Out For

- Don't write letters when you're tired and disgruntled. Your physical state influences the way you write and the message you convey.
- Don't use a leaking pen or one running out of ink. Don't use a kooky color; it makes your letter look eccentric.
- Don't dash off a note on a piece of legal paper or a sheet torn from a looseleaf notebook. The quality of your communication takes on the quality of the paper upon which it is written.
- Never send a messy, crossed-out, ink-stained letter to anyone, even to someone who "won't mind."
- A rambling discourse—without a beginning, main part of text, or a conclusion—leaves the recipient feeling you did not care enough about him or her, or for the reason for writing, to do a good job.
- Never send out letters with misspellings and grammatical or punctuation errors.

o An overly lengthy, disorganized letter makes the reader feel lost, wandering through the jungle, searching for the long-lost point of the communication.
o Never send a letter through the mails that you have not signed, or that your secretary has not signed for you (with her initials after your name or with the words "signed in his/her absence."

LETTERS THAT FIT THE OCCASION

Business Letters

Always personalize your business letter if you know the recipient, even if you have only met that person once. The personal touch usually fits in most easily as a last paragraph before you sign off. Some samples:

o *To someone you have just met:*
"It was nice to meet you at the sales meeting last week. I'm glad finally to be able to fit the face to the very pleasant telephone voice."
o *To someone you know well:*
"Best wishes to you, but particularly to Betsy and the boys. I hope they'll come with you the next time."
o *To someone you know well, but whom you have been compelled to criticize* or against whom you must take some negative action:
"This has been a difficult letter to write, because we have been friends for a long time" (or "because we have always had such a good business relationship" or whatever).
o *To a good business customer,* you might add a personal touch such as this in your closing:
"Your business means a lot to me personally, so I want to *make sure* that this transaction is carried out perfectly. I also hope that by now you have shaken off that nasty case of bronchitis and are feeling fit again."
o *To a business associate who has had bad news in his or her life.*
If someone has had news such as a death, divorce, or scandal, you don't have to write a soliloquy on the subject, but it might seem odd to the recipient if you make no reference to it whatsoever. You might put a gentle reference to it in your last paragraph or in a P.S.:
"I know you've been having a tough time lately. I've been thinking about you—and pulling for you."

Closing a letter with trite phrases such as the following is better than *nothing:*

"Hope our paths cross soon again."
"I hope life is treating you well."
"Here's wishing you lots of luck in your new venture."
"Hope things are looking up (or going well) for you."
"See you very soon, I hope."

Thank-you Letters

You should send a thank-you note—even one that is very short and informal—every time you are

- Given a present
- Sent flowers
- Asked to lunch or dinner
- Invited for a weekend
- Asked to a concert, the opera, the theater, even a movie
- The recipient of a favor—such as when a person writes a letter of reference to help your child get into college, or refers a client to you, or finds you an apartment, or serves as a matchmaker for you, or does a lot of research for you to help you out

A thank-you letter can be as short as three sentences:

Dear Charlie,
 Lunch today was splendid—from the point of view of the restaurant, the food, the company and the conversation!
 Many thanks. It was nice catching up.

When some people receive a present, they write a trite, blah, nothing note, such as:

Dear Mathilda,
 Thank you for your nice gift. It was very sweet of you, and I appreciate it.

After reading a note like that, Mathilda probably doesn't even remember what she gave as a gift!

Others thankfully enthuse a little and tell the donor how they are using the present:

Dear Mathilda,
 You cannot imagine what pleasure your scarf has given me. The pinks and blues of the paisley print are so lovely; they pick up my tired old winter dresses and make them look fresh again. I receive many compliments on the scarf every time I wear it, and I seem to be wearing it constantly.
 If you had spent weeks trying to find the perfect gift for me, you could not have chosen better. (Perhaps you did spend weeks finding it!)
 Bless you. I really am delighted with your choice.

- A thank-you note from a man to a woman. Sometimes men feel sheepish when women give them presents—such as when a woman gives a man a tie at Christmas (a common business gift, because it is not personal). Here is a sample thank-you from an executive to the woman account executive in his advertising agency:

Dear Jen,

Your inimitable taste has made my old pin-stripes take on a new lease in life. I feel as though I can once again go to lunch at the Four Seasons feeling properly dressed.

My wife thinks I might even develop some taste in ties as a result of being exposed to your excellent choice. I certainly hope so—and I thank you for showing me the way!

Have a great holiday.

- *A thank-you note for a dinner party.* In this example, one spouse writes to one of the hosts but thanks both on behalf of both:

Dear Marian,

You and Harry gave a *beautiful* dinner last Thursday. We enjoyed meeting your guests, your table looked lovely (I will never forget those white gardenias floating in the centerpiece crystal bowl), and your dinner was *superb.* You may have noticed how George and I were not exactly reticent about helping ourselves to that incredible roast veal!

The Wheelers are wonderful hosts, and we thank you for letting us be present at your delightful party.

- *A thank-you note from the dinner host to a guest who sent flowers the day after the party:*

Dear Susan and Bob,

Such beautiful roses! You shouldn't have sent them, but I'm glad you did. We put them on the coffee table, and that delicious coral color has brightened up the living room considerably.

It was a joy having you both with us.

- *A thank-you for a favor:*

Dear Mort,

You really came through for your old friend. It was thanks to your very persuasive letter that our child was accepted for nursery school. I never thought it would be as hard to get a kid into nursery school as it is to get him into the Wharton Business School.

Anyway, your word was obviously the deciding factor. I promise we won't bother you again—at least for another fourteen years, when Maria will probably need some help getting into college!

Letters of Complaint

The best way to go on record with a complaint in a situation where you are justifiably angry and feeling out of control (and I, for one, *always* feel my complaint is justified) is to write three drafts of the letter but mail only the third one.

I find that when I am emotionally upset, I tend to write an over-heated, rambling letter that commands no respect whatsoever on the other end. Also, the recipient usually does not even understand the reason why I am so upset. By the third or fourth try, I have calmed down, make sense, and am in control of my words once again.

When writing a letter of complaint, it's a good idea to

- o Write in a calm, controlled manner. (Your letter will be much more effective that way.)
- o Leave sarcasm out of your writing (a major fault of mine, one that totally clouds the issue and confuses the recipient). Sarcasm, to be understood, requires a human voice, as well as words.
- o Write an outline of all the points you wish to make—before writing the letter. Then subtract the weaker, less compelling points. Make certain your final letter addresses all the major points.

For example, if you write to the owner of a restaurant where you had a bad scene with the waiter, you might write an emotional letter like this:

> He could not have cared less about the shambles of my lunch party. I was humiliated in front of my guests. I just couldn't get over how rude and unfeeling he was, when I was so upset. And he knew it. And didn't care. It was just terrible . . .

Or you could write an in-control letter like this:

> . . . I relayed to this waiter how important these particular guests were and he feigned complete indifference. He was responsible for the following:
> 1. Having to be summoned three times before he finally took the order, even after I had informed him twice of our time problem
> 2. Making a mistake on the orders of three of my five guests
> 3. Throwing up his hands and making faces, as though he were being persecuted, when one guest sent her under-cooked meat back to be cooked some more
> 4. Purposely laying down the dishes in front of each guest in an overly-noisy manner
> 5. Sighing with disdain whenever we addressed him
> 6. Not bringing the check until fifteen minutes after it was called for

I felt badly for the reputation of your fine restaurant, knowing how you pride yourself on your fine service. I knew it would be important to you to know what happened this noon at your restaurant.

Sincerely,

Letters of Reference

If you are asked to give a letter of reference but feel unable to write it enthusiastically, it is far better to make an excuse not to write it. A lukewarm letter smacks of hypocrisy and can harm the person's cause. For example, any member of the membership committee can see through a letter like this one, addressed to a private club's chairman of the membership committee:

Dear Frank:
George Chilton asked me to write a letter on behalf of his application for membership in the Club.

I told him I would—even though I have known him only for a short time and only in a business atmosphere. He is well known in his law firm. I have, however, never known him socially.

Sincerely,

There is no way that George Chilton will get past the membership committee with that kind of letter written about him.

A good letter of reference brims with enthusiasm and praise. However, before launching into the hyperbole, give up front in the letter:

o The reason you're writing it
o The person's full name, address, telephone number
o Any other statistics that are important to the recipient, such as

The individual's spouse's name and position
Any children's names, ages, and schools
The individual's scholastic record
The person's career record
Special talents (skilled in foreign languages, or a musician, for example)
Involvement in civic activities
Any published works
Important political activities
Any important awards or honors
Special skills in sports or hobbies

A good letter of reference is informative, enthusiastic, and well organized. It should be easy for the recipient to read and find specific bits of information to which to refer when necessary.

• *If you send a letter of introduction on anyone's behalf, the following actions should take place:*

○ The recipient should acknowledge receipt of your letter.
○ The recipient should contact the person about whom you have written.
○ The person you are helping should write to inform you about the meeting with the person to whom you wrote—and should thank you very warmly for the trouble you went to on his or her behalf.
○ You should write the recipient of your letter of introduction once again, to thank him or her for having taken action after receipt of your letter.

This is what should happen in the best of all worlds, but unfortunately, it does not always happen. Someone drops the ball, and manners fly out the window!

Letters of Congratulation

It's one thing to pass a friend on the street and say, "Hey, that's great about George's promotion!" or, "I hear your daughter and son-in-law had a son. What wonderful news!" or, "I read in today's sports page that you won the tennis tournament. Congratulations!"

It's quite another to sit down with pen and paper (or word processor or typewriter) and write a warm letter of congratulations. Such a communication is read, reread, passed around to family members or at the office or at school, perhaps copied and sent to relatives and friends all over the world. It may end up in a scrapbook and be handed down to posterity. The telephone call or the words in the street are not permanent. The words in the letter are.

This kind of letter does not have to be long. You may prefer to buy a greeting card and write a message on the back. What matters is that you write it and write it quickly after you hear the news. A letter of congratulations sent three months after an event occurs is like ice cream that has lost its flavor from being left in the freezer too long.

Your congratulatory letter might contain the following:

○ How you heard the good news and how thrilled you were
○ The fact that you are spreading the word far and wide
○ A description of the delighted reactions of people you know in common when they, too, heard the news
○ A statement of how personally proud you are
○ Wishes for continued good luck in the future

To communicate with someone at the time of great good news means so much to that individual. If you know only the spouse, child, or parent of the person to be congratulated, write that person, because anyone close to someone with good news feels parts of it—and *is* part of it.

Catch-up Letters

These are important letters that communicate your news to someone important in your life. It could be your grandmother, a friend who is ill, your sister who is a student in the Soviet Union longing for mail, or the person you are hoping to marry. This kind of letter is very important when you are away from home and is almost always answered with welcome news from the other end. It is much more memorable than the easy way of communicating (a telephone call), because the recipient knows you have taken time out to stop and think of him or her. If you're on a trip to Chicago, for example, you might:

o Tell the recipient of your letter what you're doing, how you're feeling.
o Write your impressions of the city you're visiting and the people you're meeting.
o Give the human side of the news—not just the fact that "we went by bus to the South Side of Chicago on an architectural tour."
o Talk about what you saw—the examples of the different schools of Chicago architecture, for example—and your reactions to walking through one of Frank Lloyd Wright's houses.
o Describe your feelings about the Chicago skyline on the shores of Lake Michigan.
o Don't just write, "And then we had lunch." Talk about what you ate, what the place looked like, how people looked the same or different from people at home.
o Talk about the tempo, the smells, the sounds of the city. All of a sudden, you will find yourself recalling far more than you realized you were collecting as impressions.

We so seldom write letters like this any more, and yet they give so much pleasure. You will remember to write these letters if you leave a box of stationery on a piece of furniture that is always within range of your vision. When you have already stamped and addressed some envelopes inside the box, you will be drawn to it. *And you will write those letters to the people who would so love to hear from you!*

Letters of Apology

When you have hurt someone's feelings, it is time to act. You may have a tart tongue, you may be very clever and witty in making critical remarks about others while they, unbeknownst to you, are standing listening to your group. Whether you make an unkind remark about someone's new beard and it gets back to him or you inadvertently (or on purpose) take a crack at someone's ideas in the conference room in front of your colleagues, you should apologize—verbally, right on the spot, and then in writing, with a personal note hand-delivered within twenty-four hours of the incident.

Apologies never totally make up for something one did, but at least they are better than nothing. When, for example, the person who has wronged you takes no action, your resentment can fester over time and eat away at you, ruining your productivity. Therefore, knowing how you yourself demand some kind of retribution for a wrong done you, remember everyone else's needs, too, when you are at fault.

It helps to send flowers (from a man or a woman, to a man or a woman) with your note of apology. There's something serene and soothing about flowers. Your note can be long and detailed, if you are trying to justify just how this unpleasant experience happened, or it can be as short as this:

> Gerry,
> It shouldn't have happened, but it did. I am a first class lout, and there is no excuse for what I said. I just hope that since I am such bad news, you will show your usual big heart and forgive me. There's a lot to forgive, I know, but I want you to know I am truly, truly sorry. If you forgive me, I shall be forever in your debt. *Please* put me in your debt!

Condolence Letters

If you are close to a family member of someone who dies, you should send a condolence letter by hand the minute you hear the news.

If you read or hear about the death of someone who is connected to you somehow—through a friend or an office colleague—mail a letter of condolence to the person you know the best. For example, if you know the son of a woman who dies better than you know her husband, write to the son and express your condolences to both him and his father.

If you hear about someone's death long after it occurred—such as reading about the death of a classmate in your college alumni magazine months later—it is not too late to write that person's spouse, parent, or child.

In fact, in the matter of a death, at no time is it "too late" to express your condolences.

- *A condolence letter should consist of*

  o An opening statement of how terrible the news is, and how you know how much the family is suffering from the loss.

- o Any special memories of the deceased person—particularly warm, sunny, and amusing recollections. Make them personal and fun to read. (Recall pranks played back in college days, things that happened at the office, jokes you played on each other on the golf course, or whatever.)
- o Words of praise for the deceased and mention of how much the loss means to you personally. ("You cannot imagine how much I am going to miss that wonderful, funny, warm, kind wife of yours. She used to help me whenever I was low. She was always there for me, so I cannot bear to think of her not being around any more. She was, as you know full well, a bright, blithe spirit, shedding warmth wherever she went.")
- o A sincere offer to "be of assistance in any possible way that I can."

Even if you did not know the deceased, it is a nice gesture to write to the bereaved member of the family whom you do know. For example, a young executive would write his much more senior boss this kind of a letter when he learns of the death of the latter's wife:

Dear Mr. Hasker,

I wish to express my condolences to you at this very terrible time. Although I never had the pleasure of meeting Mrs. Hasker, I have heard you mention her with such fondness, and I have also heard from others in the office how close you were, and what a wonderful woman she was.

I am so sorry for you and your family, and hope that Our Lord will send you the strength needed to bear this immense loss.

Love Letters

The main advice to give about love letters is:

- o Send them.
- o Don't put any promises in them that you can't keep.

Love letters are probably the most cherished letters of all. It's sad to contemplate that in our electronic age millions of people will never receive a love letter in their whole lives!

If you are single and in love with someone else who is single, send love letters whenever you can. A note as short as this can make someone's heart take off on a flight of exultation: "You can't possibly imagine how many times I think about you when I'm away from you. I am *utterly* infatuated."

You can recite love poetry in a love letter. You can write—as I saw one happy young woman read from a letter she received—a litany of the loved one's physical and mental qualities. You can just send a short message like this: "You know I'm no good at writing letters. I just LOVE YOU!"

You can write as long or as short a letter as you wish. Just write it. It feels *so good* to receive it.

NOTES

Notes should be short and to the point, and if they can be amusing, so much the better. They should be efficient, because there is always a purpose to be served.

• You send a note, for example, *to remind the recipient of something:*

Dear Harry,

Just to remind you to bring the Chase file when we meet at the commuter terminal on Monday at 5 P.M. You told me to put a string around your finger. I can't do that, but try sticking this note in your buttonhole in the interim. It might help you remember, even if it won't look too great.

Until "Chase file time" Monday,

• You send a note *simply to please someone,* too:

Dear Abby,

I thought these old snapshots of you, Jack, and me taken in Frankfurt thirty years ago would bring back a few good memories. I don't think we look thirty years older today, do you? I think we look thirty years younger today!

• You send a note *to pass on information.* It's a gracious gesture that is really appreciated:

Dear Geoff:

Found the attached article in an in-flight magazine on my way to Chicago today. Since it mentions your firm, I knew you'd be interested.

or

Dear Ruth:

I remember your great interest in scrimshaw, so when I saw the enclosed booklet on the subject in a mall bookstore the other day, I thought of you.

• *A note or a studio card with a handwritten note on it wishing the person well* are communications that mean a great deal to someone who is ill, recovering in the hospital, or depressed and feeling blue. Sometimes a well-written letter can bring the recipient right out of a minor depression—make a person laugh and forget, at least temporarily, the pain or sorrow he or she feels.

Of course, if a male friend is dying, you would not send a humorous card about his flirting with the pretty nurses. You would send him instead a letter or a card of a beautiful scene or perhaps of cartoon characters in an amusing situation.

If a female friend is having an operation in the hospital, you would not send her a tasteless card with a sex joke on it, but you would send her a happy, bright, funny card.

To anyone who is ill, written words of good cheer like these will help:

> The office has simply ceased to function without you. I always knew you were important, but you don't have to be *that* important! You had better hurry up, get well, and get back to us—or the office will close down. That's how we all feel!

To someone who's alone and feeling depressed:

> I'm waiting to hear from you when I can take you to a great movie I heard about, and we'll go to that nifty pasta restaurant afterward. You are very much missed around here. I know you're having a tough time, but life is full of great things ahead for all of us. So buck up, give me a call, and we'll make that movie date.

Where there is a monogram, printed or engraved, do not write on this top side. When there is no monogram, you would start writing your letter on the top side as side one.

The fold-over note, lying open, showing how a letter would be written on the inside. The top and bottom inside portions would be sides one and two if the note paper had a printed monogram on its top side. If the notepaper had an *engraved* monogram on the top side, you would start writing on the bottom half of the inside as side one. (The top half would bear an indentation from the engraving on the front, so it would be difficult to write on it.)

The underside of the foldover note is the last page for writing.

GREETING CARDS AND HOLIDAY MESSAGES

Sending a greeting card is a thoughtful gesture that gladdens the heart of the recipient, whether its purpose is

- o To commemorate and reinforce a joyous occasion, such as a birth, first communion, Bar or Bat Mitzvah, graduation, birthday, engagement, wedding, or anniversary
- o To mark a special holiday, such as Thanksgiving, Easter, Passover, Halloween, Valentine's Day
- o To show you are thinking of someone at a tough time, such as when someone is in the hospital
- o To send your condolences at the time of someone's death
- o To say "Thank you," whether for a gift, a dinner party, or whatever

- *A little taste is called for.*

There are simply fabulous studio cards to buy in every card shop—attractive, witty, beautiful, sometimes roaringly funny. However, remember that a card you stood and roared over in the shop—for example, one with unexpurgated sexual connotations—may go over like a lead balloon with the recipient of your gesture. After all, you don't know who is going to see the studio card that you sent to someone as a joke—perhaps the young woman's mother, or your old buddy's wife, or the young child of the person to whom you have sent the card.

Send a card that represents you—that is tasteful, that you wouldn't mind anyone attaching your name to if they picked it up. It does not have to be a syrupy, sentimental one (although there many older people who love those). There are clever, funny ones out there that are in complete good taste. Send *that* kind.

Christmas Cards

The most important card season is Christmas and New Year, and here is some advice:

- o Send religious (Nativity scenes, Madonna and child) or Christmas motif cards (Santa and his sleigh, Christmas trees, wreaths, holly and bells) to Christian friends.
- o Send "Seasons Greetings," Hanukkah cards, or New Year cards to Jewish friends at the appropriate season.
- o For a Christian-Jewish couple, send a "Seasons Greetings" card.
- o To Arabs, Moslems, and friends of the Buddhist religion, send "Seasons Greetings" or "Happy New Year" cards.
- o To *everyone,* write a message by hand with black or dark blue ink, and sign your name. The message is the most important part

of the card—it personalizes it and communicates your love and affection for the recipient in a way no printed message can.

- *This is the kind of message you might write on holiday cards:*

We hope you have a great holiday season.

Lots of love to you and yours from all of us.

Hope you have fun this holiday season!

Hope your holidays are wonderful—and that the New Year will be the best ever!

If you have time to write a personal comment about some good news in that family, please do, because it means a lot.

- *To a Christian you might write:*

May you have a holy and happy Christmas—and we're delighted about the news of a baby about to appear!

May the Star of Bethlehem guide you through the New Year and keep you safe, and may you all come visit us again next summer at the lake!

A blessed, holy, joyous Christmas season to you all! We'll miss you this Christmas, but we'll be thinking about you!

- *Update your list of holiday card recipients.*

It is wasteful, thoughtless, and sometimes infuriating to be sent a holiday greeting card full of good cheer addressed to a couple who are divorced or one of whom is now dead. Cull and correct your list carefully. There must be some you can even drop from the list, and perhaps an equal number of new faces to add to the list. Correct all addresses of people who have moved and the names of women who have changed their names and marital status. Make a fresh, accurate list each year, and you will be running a tight, no-waste operation.

- *Always sign your Christmas cards, even if they are printed with your names.* As part of the important personalization of Christmas and other holiday greeting cards, sign each card with a dark-colored ink, even if your name is right there in glorious print. Put a diagonal slash through your name (or names) and sign beneath it.

If you, a woman, know the couple to whom you are sending a particular card much better than your husband does, sign it "Barb and Joe Michaels." If you, the husband, know them better, sign it "Joe and Barb Michaels." It does not matter which name comes first—husband's or wife's—but it makes sense to put the most recognizable name first for a couple who knows only one of you. (A woman in business should sign all her cards with just her own name to people who know nothing about her personal life; a man in business would do the same.)

It goes without saying, of course, that you do not send cards printed with the couple's two names to people in business—unless, of course, they are part of your circle of friends and know you as a couple. It does not matter whether a wife signs all the cards or a husband signs all the cards. (If one has a much better handwriting than the other, the answer as to who should sign lies right there.)

• You may hand-address your envelopes or type them. Be sure to put your return address on the upper left-hand corner of the front of the envelope (not on the back flap), because the people in the post office are too busy to flip over envelopes to return improperly addressed ones to the sender. If your return address is on the front of the envelope, all a post person has to do is draw an arrow from the addressee's name to your return address.

RAISED EMBOSSED CARDS WITH A CHRISTMAS MOTIF

Some people eschew greeting cards and purchase instead rather formal thick white or cream-colored stock cards, bordered in red or green, with a raised embossed motif at the top center—for example, a wreath, a striped stocking, a bunch of holly, or a small decorated tree. These can be ordered from a good stationer like Tiffany or Cartier. They are either engraved with a message such as "The So-and-so Family sends you warmest greetings of love and good cheer for the holiday season," or they are left blank and the person sending them writes a short note on each card by hand. They are expensive—and very chic-looking.

CARDS WITH FAMILY PHOTOS

Recipients usually enjoy the photographic cards send to them by good friends who either have had a family photo printed on each card or slip a color snapshot into each greeting card. (Please don't send an inferior snapshot, like the overexposed one we received last Christmas of what could have been a baby, but then again, it could have been a puppy!)

The photo may be of any part of the three generations of the family or of all three grouped together at a family reunion. The photo may also be of the sender's new house, dog or cat, horse, or boat.

I have also seen Christmas cards devoted to someone's new car, but perhaps that is going too far! I personally feel it is egocentric to send one's own portrait as a Christmas card—or a photograph of yourself traveling in some foreign land or during your summer vacation—but many people do it. It's not very holiday-oriented!

Every year for almost thirty years the Kenyon Bolton family of Cleveland sent a large, wonderful Christmas photo card showing the immensely attractive family of seven all in a row, all dressed alike in a costume, often in a winter scene. That was the card that everyone put in the center of the mantel!

Holiday Letters

Many people laboriously prepare a catch-up letter with all the family news in a typed one- or two-page single-spaced letter that has been reproduced in as many copies as there are holiday cards. I find these great fun to read and enjoy them thoroughly—except for those that go into detail on what little Susie's milk formula is and how Fido had worms last spring but is all better now. A friend who gushes a lot called me up recently and said, "Tish, I need help. I have written a four-page letter about the family activities this past year. It took me three weeks of work. What do you advise me to do about reproducing it? Should I have the type shrunk in size?"

"Give it to an English professor at your university, Carol," I advised her, "someone who doesn't know you. Pay him or her to edit it down mercilessly to one page—or even a half a page. Then it will be wonderful!" (I'm waiting to see if she did that or if I have lost her as a friend.)

THE PERSONAL STATIONERY YOU USE

Your personal stationery says a lot about you. If a handsome-looking pale gray envelope arrives in your mail, holding a letter inside that is written on fine gray paper, with the name engraved across the top in royal blue, you cannot help but be curious and delighted to open it. If you receive a letter on lined scraps and sheets from a yellow legal pad, which are then stuffed into an anonymous envelope, that letter says to you, "I don't care much about you." Of course, there are times when you don't have anything else to write on and must get something into the mail quickly, in which case you can apologize in the letter for the "non-stationery on which this note is being written."

There are many kinds of letter paper and notepaper available for purchase—all sizes and shapes—but if you are looking for a must-have wardrobe of personal stationery, I would advise the following for a man or a woman:

- Quality engraved or plain correspondence cards and matching envelopes. (An alternative to the correspondence card is the fold-over note—see below.)
- Quality engraved or plain letter-paper half sheets (that fold in half) with matching envelopes.

o Lesser-quality letter-paper sheets and matching envelopes printed with the person's name, address, and telephone number for everyday use.

Letter-Paper Half Sheets

Men's and women's good-quality personal letter paper differs in size. The traditional man's size is about 7¼ inches by 10½ inches. The traditional woman's size paper is around 5¾ inches by 7¾ inches. However, there are many women today who choose the larger men's paper, because there is more room to write on.

Men traditionally used only white, cream, or gray stationery; now they are using pale blue, tan, and pale green as well, with black, dark gray, dark blue, maroon, dark brown, and dark green engraving and printing colors. Women use any color stock of their choice, including the palest of pastels, with darker lettering (for example, dark red on pink or dark brown on yellow).

You are supposed to use second plain sheets if your letter is longer than one page (don't use the back of your first sheet unless the stock is very heavy). The letter is folded in half—with bottom edge of the paper brought up to the top edge and inserted into the envelope, as you face the back flap, with the fold on the bottom and the two edges held together at the top.

You may have your name, address, and telephone number put at the top of your stationery. The return address on the envelope should be on the upper left-hand portion of the front, *not* on the back flap, where stationers often like to put it. (Because the Post Office will not promise to return undelivered letters if the return address is not on the front of the envelope, we are going to have to make our stationers shake off their old-fashioned ideas and help us out by putting the return address in the proper place.)

Correspondence Cards

These may be 4¼ inches by 6½ inches or slightly smaller. They may be plain with an engraved (or embossed or printed) name or monogram in the top center or on the upper left side of the card. Options include a colored border to match the lettering, as well as matching tissue-lined envelopes. The cards are usually made of a heavy stock, in a white, ecru, or gray color. (Women also use pastels in their cards.) You may write on both sides and may use the cards for writing notes or invitations.

A fold-over note is inserted into its envelope in this fashion.

Letter Paper for Everyday Use

This is a lesser-quality paper, printed with your name and address (and telephone number, if you wish), to use for writing about things you have ordered, questions about your bills, requests for information, and the like. In other words, use this kind of less expensive stationery to communicate matters of your personal business life. It may be ordered from any stationer, department store, paper goods store, many office supply stores, or through countless mail order catalogues.

Very Nice to Have

There are other items in a stationery wardrobe, one or two of which might be useful to you, to keep in stock in your desk at home.

MONOGRAMMED (OR PLAIN) FOLD-OVER NOTES

These measure approximately 3¾ inches by 5¾ inches and are used as a substitute for correspondence cards (mainly by women). They are very handsome, whether plain or edged in color, with a monogram engraved or printed in the center, or with a monogram in the center plus a narrow matching colored border.

When writing on a fold-over note:

• Don't write on the top side of a monogrammed note (or on the underside, either, if it's engraved—because of the indentation made by the engraving on the paper). Start writing your letter on the bottom inside half of this kind of note, which would be page 1. Page 2 would be the underside of page 1, which you flip up and write on from the top of the edge of the paper, down to the bottom fold line.

• If, however, your fold-over note is plain, the top side (side 1), would be used for the beginning of your note; the underside of the top page would be side 2, the bottom inside half would be side 3, and the underside of side 3 would be side 4. These notes are used for writing short letters or extending invitations. The written invitation would go on the inside bottom half of the fold-over note.

LINED ENVELOPES

It's rather chic to have envelopes that are lined—perhaps in the same color as the engraved monogram. It's nice for the Christmas holidays to use stationery with envelopes lined in red or green for writing your thank-you notes. However, it is an added expense that you can easily ignore.

INFORMALS

These small fold-over notes with a person or a couple's name formally engraved in the front center are not used much any more; they used to be one of the first things a woman ordered when she was married. ("Formally engraved" means that a woman would have "Mrs. Anthony Leigh Brownstone" as her engraved name—never "Barbara Brownstone"; they would have gasped at the thought, before 1960.)

POSTCARDS

Postcards are a convenient way of communicating. They're suitable for personal business matters and as "reminders" for a social event; they are too informal, however, to use as invitations.

You can order yours (from a stationer or office supply store, for example) with your name and address printed at the top—and with a colored border to match the printing, if you wish. Remember to be careful of what you write on postcards, since many pairs of eyes read them. (I learned this the hard way when, in my youth, I got a friend in real trouble at her office. She was job-hunting in secret, and I referred to this fact in a postcard to her from abroad. The matter came to the attention of her boss, who was, to say the least, displeased.)

VISITING/BUSINESS CARDS

Before the women's movement, "ladies" had their own small, engraved calling or visiting cards, with their married name (or single name) engraved in the center. A lady would use this as a gift enclosure, as a reminder to someone to come to lunch or tea, and to leave at someone's house if she called and the person she came to see was not there. Today, women use only their business cards. If a woman is not in business, she should have her own cards made anyway—with her full name, address, and telephone number. These cards have a purpose: to leave with people so they know how to get in touch with her. She may either use her husband's name on her cards ("Mrs. John Templeton Gardner") or her own name ("Mary McAdoo Gardner") or, yet another option, a combination of her own name and her husband's, which is the most informative of all:

Mary McAdoo Gardner
(Mrs. John Templeton Gardner)

Your Monogram

When you are a single woman (or man), you would use the first letter of your given, middle, and family surname to create a monogram. Or a woman might make her surname initial oversized and use it in the middle, flanked by her given and middle names. (In that case, Virginia Hampton Biddle's monogram would be VBH or, used less often, vBh.)

When a woman marries, she drops her middle name and adds her husband's surname. Therefore, when Virginia marries Gil Thurston, her monogram changes to VBT (or vTb). If she were to divorce and become known by her maiden name again, she would return to VHB. If she were to become a widow and then marry a Mr. Smith, she would keep her first husband's surname to use as a middle initial, instead of her own middle name. In other words, she would become VTS in her monogram.

A man is lucky; he just keeps his same three initials throughout his life—unless his wife and he share a monogram on certain wedding gifts (not stationery, however). For example, as a "married" monogram on engraved silver, etched crystal, or embroidered linens, Virginia and Gil Thurston might use vTg as their joint monogram.

23

Addressing
People Properly

People like—and have the right—to be addressed by their proper names and titles. It jars the psyche to be called by an improper name or to see one's name misspelled. If the person you are addressing has a very unusual name (as, for example, did the Hogg sisters of Texas—Ima and Eura), check the spelling before writing. My brother Bob Baldridge, who many years ago decided to spell his surname with a second "d" (because everyone has always misspelled our family name) does not like it now when the second "d" is left out, whereas the rest of the family bristles when the second "d" is included.

A major in the army does not like being addressed as "Captain"; a bishop does not like being referred to as a priest; a former ambassador does not like receiving mail without the "The Honorable" in front of his or her name; and a United States senator is justifiably miffed when he or she receives a piece of mail addressed to just plain "Mr." or "Mrs."

It is difficult to keep up with it all, but it's important to do so. Each of us has a responsibility to care about addressing other people properly.

HOW SHOULD YOU BE ADDRESSED?

A long with your right to be addressed, referred to, and introduced correctly, you also have a responsibility to let other people know how you should be addressed, referred to, and introduced correctly. If you have a difficult name or title, or there's been a change in your name or title, it's your job to educate those with whom you correspond on a regular basis. You should, for example:

- *Always put a telephone number on your letterhead,* so that someone's secretary, or the person him- or herself, will know how to call you easily to find information that may be lacking in your letter.
- *Always keep your biography updated* if you are well-known and distribute your biography before a personal appearance, or if you are included in one of the *Who's Who* publications. Lecture agencies, for example, often send out very out-of-date bios of their speakers, with the result that the speaker is inaccurately introduced, but it's no one's fault other than the speaker's.
- Always send out *a change of address* (or change of telephone, fax, and telex numbers) card to everyone with whom you communicate.
- Always send out a card announcing a change of name to your friends and people with whom you do business.

When You Change Your Name

- *A newly married woman* communicates the change of her name in

- Her wedding invitations
- Her new stationery
- A note to her clubs, associations, and school alumni magazines for their class notes
- Newly printed checks with her new name and address
- Newly printed or engraved business cards

She also obtains a new driver's license, passport, and credit cards with her new name.

- *A bride who retains her maiden name after marriage* communicates it on the "at home" card in the wedding invitation or announcement (when she puts her maiden name and her husband's together with a joint address), and also when her name stays the same on her stationery after the wedding.

When she is known by her maiden name, she must be careful on social occasions to introduce her husband by his name—something I have had to do always. It means speaking very slowly and deliberately, "This is my husband, Bob Holl-en-stein-er." (Woe unto the man or woman who thereafter calls my husband "Bob Baldrige.")

• *A divorced woman* would send a printed card to her friends, business associates, her lawyer, doctors, her children's school administration office, the alumni office of her former schools, all the stores where she has charge accounts, her clubs and associations, house of worship, and the like, announcing:

> **Mrs. Barbara Tucker has resumed her maiden name, and is now known as Ms. Barbara Anderson.**

The announcement should include her present address and telephone number. She would also apply for new credit cards, driver's license, and passport and order new checks printed once again with her maiden name.

WHEN WRITING LETTERS OR SPEAKING TO SOMEONE

• *In letters always use a title with a name.* To mail out letters that are addressed simply to "John Jones" or "Mary Williams" instead of to "Mr. John Jones" or "Ms. Mary Williams" is inexcusable. Unfortunately, this bad habit is ingrained in the mail procedures of many companies today. It's a cop-out. It's lazy and sloppy and should be discouraged at all costs.

• *If you are writing to someone you don't know and do not even know the sex of the person*—because the name could be either masculine or feminine—call the person's company or home to find out. "Excuse me, I'm calling to find out if it is a 'Mr. Cameron Clark' or a 'Ms. Cameron Clark' to whom this letter is being addressed." The recipient of your letter will be appreciative that you cared enough to do some research. (Most people don't bother—they just send the letter addressed to the wrong sex!)

When you have no way of determining the sex of a person with a name that could belong to a man or woman (for example: "Clair," "Morgan," or a family name such as "Caldwell" or "Berkeley" used for a person's given name), it is better not to guess the sex. In this case, send the letter without a title in front of the name.

If you are a person with such a name, always include a title in your return address or in your signature block when you write to someone who doesn't know you. In this way, the recipient of your letter will know how to address you. For example, Morgan Elliott would sign her letter in this way: "(Ms.) Morgan G. Elliott." If Morgan Elliott were writing a letter to someone who knows her husband but whom she hasn't met, she would end her letter with her husband's given name beneath hers, so that the recipient of the letter can readily identify her:

> Sincerely,
> Morgan Elliott (signature)
> (Mrs. Robert)

Writing to People with Professional Titles

You do not use a "Mr." or "Ms." when you use a person's professional title after his or her surname. For example, it is correct to write:

Duane O'Donaghue, M.D. (*not* Dr. Duane O'Donaghue, M.D.)
Agnes Toda, R.N. (*not* Ms. Agnes Toda, R.N.)
Janet Oenslager, Ph.D. (*not* Dr. Janet Oenslager, Ph.D.)
Timothy Winthrop, Esq. (*not* Mr. Timothy Winthrop, Esq.)

When a person uses the initials of his professional organization after his surname, once again you do not use a title before his name. For example, if a man identifies himself as "George O'Hara, A.I.A." (which means he is a member of the American Institute of Architects), it is incorrect to write to him as "Mr. George O'Hara, A.I.A."

Using "Ms."

The use of "Ms." is no longer controversial. It's here to stay and is in common usage. Today "Miss" seems old-fashioned and slightly archaic, except when addressing girls up to the age of eighteen. "Miss" is still used in addressing adult single women on formal invitations, but it is no longer necessary even there.

I applaud the increased use of "Ms." for every written communication. Why should a woman's marital status be known by everyone because there's a "Miss" or a "Mrs." in front of her given name? ("Miss" means she's never been married; "Mrs." in front of her husband's name means she is married; "Mrs." in front of her given name means she's divorced.) Men do not have this marital branding with their title of "Mr."

USING "MISS" IN SPEAKING

Let's face it, for some people it's easier to pronounce "Miss Reynolds" than "Ms. Reynolds" when making an introduction, because "Ms." almost sounds like a bee buzzing around. "Ms." is easy to write, but difficult to say, so if you find yourself saying "Miss" in conversation, you're like everyone else!

When a Man Is a Jr., Sr., 2nd, 3rd, or 4th

When father and son live in the same city and share the same name, the father uses "Sr." after his surname and the son uses "Jr." after his. When the father dies, the son usually drops the "Jr." within two years' time, since there is no longer a confusion between the two men—unless, of course, the man is the son of a very famous man (like the late Franklin D. Roosevelt, Jr., who, all during his life felt the need to use the "Jr." to distinguish him from his late father).

When a son is named "the 2nd," he is the nephew or grandson of a man of the same name. In other words, he is not named after his father. If he were, he would be "Junior."

When a boy is named "the 3rd," he is named after his great-grandfather or great-uncle of the same name.

A suffix may be given in a numerical or Roman numeral form—that is, either "2nd" or "II" after the surname.

The numbers are supposed to make a distinction among living men of the same name. When Lawrence Baugh II dies, for example, Lawrence Baugh III would do well to drop the "III" and become "II" within a year or two. If there were a Lawrence Baugh IV, he would similarly move up to "III" after the death of Lawrence Baugh II.

Using "Messrs."

"Messrs." (an abbreviation for the French word "messieurs") is used as a title for two or more brothers. For example, if you were sending an invitation to George and Edward Wasserberger, two brothers who manage the Mark Cross leather stores, you would address the envelope to "The Messrs. Wasserberger."

Addressing Envelopes for Invitations

(*See also* "Addressing Wedding Invitations" in chapter 12.)

o To a married couple:

Mr. and Mrs. Philip Geyelin
Their address

o To a married couple, if she has kept her own name:

Mr. Philip Geyelin and Ms. Sherry Parker
Their address

> o To a married couple whose combined two names are too long to put on one line:

Mr. Richardson Henry Pratt III
and Ms. Antonia Dellarosa Quantobella
Their address

(Indent three spaces for the second line and write "and" followed by the spouse's name.)

> o To a couple who are living together but are not married:

Mr. Richard Anderburg
Ms. Cynthia K. Talbott
Their address

(Unmarried live-togethers receive one invitation. They are listed on separate lines in alphabetical order, and there is no "and" joining their names. The "and" is reserved for married couples.)

> o When both have military rank, the higher ranked person is listed first:

Major Gregory Swanson and Lieutenant Deborah Swanson
Address

> o When the woman is higher-ranked than the man, her name comes first on the envelope:

Judge Diana Renshaw and Mr. Mark Renshaw
Address

> o When both are doctors:

The Doctors Branton, *or*
Dr. August C. Branton and Dr. Susan G. Branton

> o When inviting a young boy (nine or under):

Master William Berkeley

> o When inviting a young girl (up to the age of eighteen):

Miss Agatha Primton

When You Don't Have a Clue as to Whom You Are Writing

When you don't have a name and must write a letter to a store, company, or institution, you may do it in any of several ways. My two preferred ways are as follows:

• Use "Ladies and Gentlemen" for a salutation, which makes the recipient of either sex feel good upon opening the letter.

• Use a memo form, such as this letter of complaint to the Armshaw Plumbing Company:

> Writer's address
> Writer's telephone number
> August 5, 1993

to: Armshaw Plumbing Company
     Company's address
re: <u>Improperly executed repairs of furnace at 311 South Fair-mont</u>

The statement of complaint would follow, without a salutation, and would be signed by the writer without a complimentary closing above his or her name.

The Southern Use of "Sir" or "Ma'am"

Down south, well-mannered children are trained to say "sir" and "ma'am" repeatedly as a mark of respect to almost anyone older than themselves. When they are out of college and working in another part of the country, they should try to drop the usage of the "sir" and "ma'am," which, although very polite, are slightly reminiscent of an attitude of servitude to many people who are not from the South and often make the non-Southerner feel embarrassed. Instead of using "Yes, sir" and "No, ma'am" all the time, a polite young person from the South could substitute the older person's name: "Good morning, Mr. Peters"; "Thank you, Ms. Reynolds"; "Good night, Dr. Jenkins."

Calling People by Their First or Last Names

We are a very informal country, and many people feel that the informality has gone too far in many respects, resulting in inefficiency, a lack of respect for senior authority, and a total misunderstanding of proper deference. I'm with them, so forgive me if I sound a little starchy about this.

• When you are in your twenties and you meet someone in his or her forties or older, call that person by a last name until told not to.

• When you have met someone and chatted for a few minutes and then you write him or her a letter, write using the person's surname in the salutation, instead of the given name. If you feel the person is much older and more important than you, sign your own full name; to use your given name only would be too informal.

If you had a really lengthy chat during your first meeting with this person, but you still feel a bit uneasy about using the person's first name only in the letter salutation, use both names (i.e., Dear Mary Thurston, or Dear Henry Pelham). Or, if you feel you both got on very well the one time you met, you might write as a salutation: "Dear Mary (if I may):" This holds true for personal or business letters.

• *When you first meet someone and you write or call him (or her), don't use that person's nickname* when it is used only by his good friends. If you meet a man named Wilson Nollon, for example, and you hear a couple of people who are obviously his good friends call him "Roly," address him or write him as "Wilson." My blood chills when young people I don't know well at all call me by my very familiar name "Tish" instead of "Letitia," and I think most people over the age of forty feel that way. (Of course, what I like best of all is to be called "Ms. Baldrige" until I know the other younger person well.)

If you are called by a nickname most of the time, something like "Slim" or "Red," for example, be sure to have your real name included on your stationery letterhead and on your business cards. You may always put your nickname in parentheses after your given name, but it is very uncomfortable for a person who has never even met you to have to address an envelope to "Mr. Shorty McLean" or "Ms. Peaches Cornwall."

HOW TO ADDRESS SPECIFIC GROUPS

The charts that follow, showing how to properly address people in official life, cover most forms of address that you are likely to encounter. Since many forms of address are conventional, there is some overlap between the charts that follow and those that appear in my *Complete Guide to Executive Manners* (Rawson Associates, 1985). Because of limited room on the page in these charts, names and titles are run in columns and hyphenated to fit into the space. For example, please remember that

o You write husband's and wife's names on one line on an invitation, unless they are too long. In the latter case, you would write their names on two lines, indenting the spouse's name three spaces:

The Honorable Scott Kilduff McLean
and Mrs. McLean

o If you are writing a letter to a foreign ambassador, you would write:

His Excellency
Joseph Hardwick (*or, if he is titled,* **Sir Joseph Hardwick**)
Ambassador of Great Britain
(Embassy address)

Dear Ambassador Hardwick (*or* **Dear Sir Joseph**):

Please remember the proper line spacing when you read the charts.

United States Officials

Any executive who deals with government officials should have a copy of the latest United States official ranking in his or her office, in order to know how to address them properly and how to seat them at a meal. Each President of the United States makes a few changes to suit him in the precedence of the officials he addresses or sees. The chart that follows, the precedence as of August 1989 in the Bush administration, will obviously undergo small changes in the years to come.

THE OFFICIAL RANKING FOR UNITED STATES OFFICIALS

The President of the United States
The Vice President of the United States
The Speaker of the House of Representatives
The Chief Justice of the United States
Former Presidents of the United States
The Secretary of State
The Secretary General of the United Nations
Ambassadors of foreign powers
Widows of former Presidents of the United States
Associate Justices of the Supreme Court of the United States
Cabinet members
    The Secretary of the Treasury
    The Secretary of Defense
    The Attorney General
    The Secretary of the Interior
    The Secretary of Agriculture
    The Secretary of Commerce
    The Secretary of Labor
    The Secretary of Health and Human Services
    The Secretary of Housing and Urban Development
    The Secretary of Transportation
    The Secretary of Energy
    The Secretary of Education
    The Secretary of Veterans' Affairs
Director, Office of Management and Budget
The United States Trade Representative
The Senate (Senators are ranked with each other according to length of continuous service)
Governors of States
Former Vice Presidents of the United States
The House of Representatives (ranked according to their state's date of admission to the Union)
Governor of Puerto Rico

Chief of Staff for the President
Assistants to the President
National Security Advisor
Chargés d'Affaires of foreign powers
The Under Secretaries and Deputy Secretaries of the Executive Departments
Director of the Central Intelligence Agency
Administrator, Agency for International Development
Director, U.S. Arms Control and Disarmament Agency
Secretaries of the Army, Navy, and Air Force
Chairman, Board of Governors of the Federal Reserve System
Chairman, Council on Environmental Quality
Chairman, Joint Chiefs of Staff
Chiefs of Staff of the Army, Navy, and Air Force (ranked according to date of appointment)
Commandant of the Marine Corps
(5-star) Generals of the Army and Fleet Admirals
The Secretary General, Organization of American States
Representatives to the Organization of American States
Director, United States Information Agency
Administrator, General Services Administration
Administrator, National Aeronautics and Space Administration
Chairman, Civil Service Commission
Director, Defense Research and Engineering
Director of ACTION
Administrator, Environmental Protection Agency
Deputy Under Secretary of State
Commandant of the Coast Guard
Assistant Secretaries of the Executive Departments
Chief of Protocol
Members of the Council of Economic Advisers
Active or Designate U.S. Ambassadors and Ministers (career rank, when in the United States; when they are in their foreign country posts, they are given much higher rank)
The Mayor of the District of Columbia
Under Secretaries of the Army, Navy, and Air Force
(4-star) Generals and Admirals
Assistant Secretaries of the Army, Navy, and Air Force
(3-star) Lieutenant Generals and Vice Admirals
Former U.S. Ambassadors and Ministers to Foreign Countries
Ministers of Foreign Powers (serving in embassies, not accredited)
Deputy Assistant Secretaries of the Executive Departments
Deputy Chief of Protocol
Counselors of embassies or legations of foreign powers

(2-star) Major Generals and Rear Admirals
(1-star) Brigadier Generals and Commodores
Assistant Chiefs of Protocol

ADDRESSING GOVERNMENT OFFICIALS: A SAMPLING

Personage	Introduction and Addressing Envelopes	Letter Salutation	Speaking To	Place Card
The President	The President The White House Address (Abroad he is introduced as "The President of the United States of America.")	Dear Mr. President:	Mr. President	The President
The First Lady	Mrs. Madison (She is the only official woman always addressed out of respect as "Mrs. Madison," without a given name.) *A social invitation would be addressed to:* The President and Mrs. Madison	Dear Mrs. Madison:	Mrs. Madison	Mrs. Madison
The Vice President	The Vice President The White House Address *A social invitation would be addressed to:* The Vice President and Mrs. Adams	Dear Mr. Vice President:	Mr. Vice President	The Vice President

• When a president is no longer in office, he retains the title as a courtesy, but there are variations in the way in which he is addressed. Instead of writing him simply as "The President, The White House," you would address him as "President Reagan" and use his office address.

Instead of writing simply to "Mrs. Reagan, The White House," as before, after the end of the administration, you would write to "Mrs. Ronald Reagan," care of her office address.

The salutation in a letter to the president in office is simply "Dear Mr. President." Once he has left the office, the salutation is "Dear President Reagan."

These are small nuances, but they matter in the scheme of things.

Personage	Introduction and Addressing Envelopes	Letter Salutation	Speaking To	Place Card
Vice President's Wife	Mrs. John Adams Address	Dear Mrs. Adams:	Mrs. Adams	Mrs. Adams
Speaker of the House	The Honorable Michael Duncan Speaker of the House *or, socially:* The Speaker of the House and Mrs. Duncan	Dear Mr. Speaker:	Mr. Speaker	The Speaker of the House
Chief Justice	The Chief Justice The Supreme Court Address *or, socially:* The Chief Justice and Mrs. Warner	Dear Mr. Chief Justice:	Mr. Chief Justice	The Chief Justice
Associate Justice	Justice Zissu The Supreme Court *or, socially:* Justice Zissu and Mrs. Zissu	Dear Justice: *or* Dear Justice Zissu	Justice *or* Justice Zissu	Justice Zissu
Cabinet Member	The Honorable Desmond Palmer Secretary of Labor Address *or, socially:* The Secretary of Labor and Mrs. Palmer	Dear Mr. Secretary	Mr. Secretary *or* Secretary Palmer	The Secretary of Labor
Under Secretary of Labor	The Honorable Otto Norgren Under Secretary of Labor *or, socially:* The Undersecretary of Labor and Mrs. Norgren	Dear Mr. Under Secretary:	Mr. Under Secretary *(subsequently* Sir)	The Under Secretary of Labor
Attorney General	The Honorable Edward R. Warden Attorney General of the United States *or, socially:* The Attorney General and Mrs. Warden	Dear Mr. Attorney General:	Mr. Attorney General *(subsequently* Sir)	The Attorney General

Personage	*Introduction and Addressing Envelopes*	*Letter Salutation*	*Speaking To*	*Place Card*
Director of Central Intelligence	The Honorable Agnes L. Schmidt Director of Central Intelligence Address *or, socially:* The Director of Central Intelligence and Mr. Helmut Schmidt	Dear Director:	Madam Director	The Director of Central Intelligence
U.S. Senator	The Honorable Frederick H. Lee United States Senate Address *or, socially:* Senator and Mrs. Frederick H. Lee	Dear Senator Lee:	Senator *or* Senator Lee	Senator Lee
U.S. Representative	The Honorable Sarah Thune House of Representatives Address *or, socially:* The Honorable Sarah Thune and Mr. Christopher Thune	Dear Ms. Thune:	Ms. Thune	The Honorable Sarah Thune *or* Ms. Thune
American Ambassador Abroad	The Honorable David R. Luce American Embassy Address *or, socially:* The Honorable David R. Luce and Mrs. Luce	Dear Ambassador Luce: *or* Dear Mr. Ambassador:	Ambassador Luce	Ambassador Luce
Governor	The Honorable Francis L. Fine Governor of Florida Address *or, socially:* Governor and Mrs. Francis L. Fine	Dear Governor: *or* Dear Governor Fine:	Governor *or* Governor Fine	The Governor of Florida
State Senator	The Honorable Jorge Morales *or, socially:* State Senator Jorge Morales and Mrs. Morales	Dear Senator Morales	Senator Morales	The Honorable Jorge Morales

Personage	Introduction and Addressing Envelopes	Letter Salutation	Speaking To	Place Card
Mayor	The Honorable Stanley Breck, Jr. Mayor of Providence *or, socially:* Mayor and Mrs. Stanley Breck, Jr.	Dear Mr. Mayor: *or* Dear Mayor Breck:	Mayor Breck	The Mayor of Providence
Judge	The Honorable Robert Quinlan Judge, Appellate Division Supreme Court of the State of New York *or, socially:* Judge and Mrs. Robert Quinlan	Dear Judge Quinlan:	Judge Quinlan	Judge Quinlan

- It's important to note that a U.S. Senator's and a U.S. Representative's place cards are not done identically. For the Senator use "Senator Lawson," but if the person is a Representative, his card should read "Mr. Lawson" or, preferably, "The Honorable William Lawson."

- A person of rank should either have his or her place card written according to his or her position (e.g., "The Secretary of Labor" or "The Ambassador of Great Britain") or the place card should contain his or her title and surname ("Judge Atkins"; "Major Jones"; "Dr. Clark"). See the charts given in this chapter for the correct forms of address.

- If you are in doubt as to someone's title, or as to whether or not you should put "The Honorable" or the guest's position on the card, use "The Honorable." With the exception of medical doctors, judges, and the military, you can always flatter a person who holds or has held an official job by putting on the place card "The Honorable David Atwater" or "The Honorable Susan Walters." It's a safety valve—like calling a woman from another country "Madam" when you can't remember her name.

ADDRESSING OFFICIALS BY THEIR TITLES IN CONVERSATION

It is customary to address a very important official by his or her title and not by name. For example:

"Mr. President" (or "Madam President") when speaking to him (or her)
"Mr. Secretary" or "Madam Secretary," for a cabinet position
"Mr. Under Secretary" or "Madam Under Secretary"
"Mr. Ambassador" or "Madam Ambassador"
"Mr. Mayor" or "Madam Mayor"

Note that we say "Governor" when talking to a governor, not "Mr. Governor." We say "Mr. Ambassador," not "Mr. Special Representative to the United Nations." The only definitive statement we can make concerning American protocol is that there is no rule without an exception.

Addressing Women

ADDRESSING THE SPOUSES OF OFFICIALLY RANKED PEOPLE

	Introducing/ Addressing an Envelope	Letter Salutations	Speaking To	Place Card
When an official's wife uses her husband's name	The Secretary of Commerce and Mrs. Roe	Dear Mrs. Roe	Mrs. Roe	Mrs. Roe
When an official's wife goes by her own name	The Secretary of Commerce Mr. Ralph Baldwin and Ms. Marian Smith	Dear Ms. Smith	Ms. Smith	Ms. Smith
Spouse of high-ranking woman	Senator Ann Green and Mr. David Green	Dear Mr. Green	Mr. Green	Mr. Green
When both husband and wife have rank	The Honorable David Green and The Honorable Ann Green	Dear Senator Green	Senator Green	Senator Green
	Commander Jerome Tate and Lieutenant Tate	Dear Lieutenant Tate	Lieutenant Tate	Lieutenant Tate

The wife of an official goes by her husband's name in official life— i.e., *Mrs. Theodore Wells* (rather than Mrs. Elise Wells) in the United States; *Signora Antonio Carici* in Italy; *Madame Henri Blanche* in France, Belgium, and the French part of Switzerland (as well as French-speaking African countries); *Frau Hans Kauffmann* in Germany, Austria, and the German part of Switzerland; *Señora Miguel Flores* in Spain and Spanish-speaking Latin America.

In the United States, women who work under their own names are addressed by their own names, but rarely does that work for the American woman who accompanies her official husband abroad. She should not try to use her own name when she is with her husband on a trip involved with his work, not hers. It creates protocol problems for the officials of a host country that does not have many, if any, women in top positions.

Of course, if it is the woman official who is the senior ranked person and her husband is accompanying *her* on her mission, she would use her own title and name, not his.

USE "MADAME" WHEN ADDRESSING A WOMAN FROM A FOREIGN COUNTRY

We call women in this country "Mrs.," "Miss," or "Ms.," followed by a surname. When we meet a woman from another country, we often have trouble catching a complicated name, and we don't know whether to call her "Miss" or "Mrs." The solution is to call her simply "Madame." French is the language of diplomacy throughout the world, and "Madame" is almost as catch-all as "Ms." in the American idiom.

Use "Madame" for a woman who is out of her teens or if you know for a fact that she is married. It makes life very simple. You don't have to say "Madame Abdourahmane" when you're talking with her. Just "Madame" will do.

"The Honorable"—A Title of Respect in America

"The Honorable" in front of a person's name is a title held for life by a person who holds or has held high office at the federal, state, or city levels. However, there is a nuance that must be remembered: A person who is addressed by others as "The Honorable" should not put the title on his or her own business cards, a personal letterhead, or on the invitations he or she extends. If, for example, an ex-official is now a partner in a law firm, on the firm's stationery his name would be listed with the other partners with "The Honorable" before it, but if it is his stationery alone, his name should not bear that honorific. In other words, it is a distinction bestowed by someone else on a person, not by the person on him or herself.

The following are among those who carry "The Honorable" title:

The President and the Vice President
Cabinet members, Deputy Secretaries, Under Secretaries, and Assistant Secretaries
Presidential assistants
American career and appointed ambassadors
American representatives (including alternates and deputies) to international organizations
The Chief Justice of the Supreme Court, Associate Justices, judges of other courts
All members of Congress
The Secretary of the Senate; the Clerk of the House
The Sergeants at Arms of the Senate and House
Librarian of Congress

Comptroller General (General Accounting Office)

Heads, assistant heads, and commissioners of U.S. government
   agencies

Governor and Lieutenant Governor of a state

Secretary of State, Chief Justice, and Attorney General of a state

State Treasurer, Comptroller, or Auditor

State Senator, Representative, Assemblyman, or Delegate

Mayor

Members of the City Council, Commissioners, etc.

In addressing an invitation to a married woman who is in office and
whose husband has no rank, her name precedes his:

> The Honorable Julia Rosen and Mr. Geoffrey Rosen
> Address

or, if you prefer:

> The Honorable Julia Rosen
>   and Mr. Geoffrey Rosen
> Address

When she is no longer in office, she still retains "The Honorable," but
her name returns to its place after her husband's:

> Mr. Geoffrey Rosen and The Honorable Julia Rosen
> Address

The British: Our Friends with Many Titles

Since we do much business with Great Britain, it is important for
those having a great deal of contact with the country to understand its
layers of leadership: the Crown, the government, and the peers of the
realm.

Protocol for the Royal Family is carefully prescribed, and even
though philosophically we Americans do not adhere to the principles of
a monarchy, we should respect our British friends' admiration for it. It is
impossible to please the British in their own country and to please
British business people visiting her if we are completely unknowledge-
able about their country's history or the Crown.

Some pretty silly, petty storms have raged in past years over such
questions as whether or not an American ambassador's wife should
make a formal curtsey in greeting the Queen. When the Queen is in the
United States an American woman's slight bow, made while shaking
hands with Her Majesty, would appropriately replace a curtsey. However,
in the presence of the Queen in England, I believe one should do as the
British do. If all the British women curtsey to the Queen, why should the
wife of the American ambassador be any different? Or for that matter, an

American business woman in England on a business trip who is fortunate enough to meet her?

It is quite logical that Americans are not as formal as the British are with their own officials and the peerage. The following charts on English officials and the titled peerage represent what is proper for an American business person to do when speaking to, introducing, or writing to them.

Members of the British Commonwealth outside of England are not as formal as the English; certainly the Canadians are informal by comparison.

THE ROYAL FAMILY

• One does not write directly to a member of the Royal Family, but to "The Private Secretary to . . ." One writes, for example, to the secretary of the following:

Her Majesty the Queen
His Royal Highness, Prince Philip, The Duke of Edinburgh
Her Majesty Queen Elizabeth, the Queen Mother
His Royal Highness, The Prince Charles, Prince of Wales
Her Royal Highness, The Princess of Wales
His Royal Highness, The Duke of York
Her Royal Highness, The Duchess of York
His Royal Highness, The Prince Edward
Her Royal Highness, The Princess Anne (Mrs. Mark Phillips)
Her Royal Highness, The Princess Margaret, Countess of Snowden

• Introductions are made and place cards are written exactly as the titles above.

• Except for the Queen and the Queen Mother (both of whom are addressed as "Your Majesty"), all family members are addressed as "Your Royal Highness," and all are subsequently addressed as "Sir" or "Ma'am."

• If you are presented to the Queen, you do not speak first. You wait for the royal personage to speak first. Your conversation will be limited at best. For example, at Wimbledon the Queen might praise the American players' performances, to which you would reply, "Thank you for those kind words, Your Majesty."

• If you are fortunate enough to be invited by Her Majesty the Queen to tea, your invitation will come from her Master of the Household, and it might read something like this:

The Master of the Household
is Commanded by Her Majesty to invite
(your name written here)
to an Afternoon Party at Buckingham Palace
on Tuesday, February 4th from 4 to 6:00 o'clock

THE BRITISH GOVERNMENT

Official	Introducing and Addressing Envelope	Letter Salutation	Speaking To	Place Card
The Prime Minister	The Rt. Hon. Mary Smith, M.P. The Prime Minister (M.P. means Member of Parliament) *or, socially:* The Prime Minister and Mr. Ivan Smith	Dear Prime Minister:	Madam Prime Minister	The Prime Minister
The Home Secretary (Equivalent of our Secretary of State)	The Rt. Hon. Ronald Coates, P.C., M.P. Home Secretary *or, socially:* The Rt. Hon. Ronald and Mrs. Coates	Dear Mr. Coates: *or, if titled:* Dear Sir Ronald: *or* Dear Lord Coates:	Mr. Coates *or, if he is titled, it might be:* Sir Ronald *or* Lord Coates	The Home Secretary

(Other cabinet posts would be addressed in a similar manner.)

Official	Introducing and Addressing Envelope	Letter Salutation	Speaking To	Place Card
A British Ambassador to the United States	His Excellency David Leeds Ambassador of Great Britain *or, if he is titled, it might be:* His Excellency Sir David Leeds et cetera	Dear Ambassador Leeds: *or, if titled:* Dear Sir David:	Mr. Ambassador *or* Sir David	The Ambassador of Great Britain

NOTE: The British would close a letter to one of their officials with "Yours sincerely," which an American may use in a letter to a British official; "Sincerely yours" is also proper.

Many British officials and peers have initials after their surnames, standing for orders, honors, and knighthoods. You should always write to such a person in the same manner he writes his name to you—with or without the initials. For example, a titled knight might be addressed as: Sir George Creighton, G.C.M.G.

THE PEERAGE

Peer	Introducing; also Addressing Envelope	Letter Salutation	Speaking To	Place Card
A nonroyal duke	The Duke of Oakford *or* The Duke and Duchess of Oakford	Dear Duke: Dear Duchess:	Duke Duchess	The Duke of Oakford The Duchess of Oakford
	(The English often address a duke and duchess as "Your Grace" and speak of them as "His Grace the Duke of . . ." but Americans are not expected to follow this procedure.)			
Duke's eldest son and daughter-in-law	Marquess of Chester *or, socially:* The Marquess and Marchioness of Chester	Dear Lord Chester: Dear Lady Chester:	Lord Chester Lady Chester	Lord Chester Lady Chester
Marquess's eldest son; Earl's wife, a countess	Earl of Meads *or, socially:* Earl and Countess of Meads	Dear Lord Meads: Dear Lady Meads:	Lord Meads Lady Meads	Lord Meads Lady Meads
Viscount, eldest son of an earl	Viscount Brentwood *or, socially:* Viscount and Viscountess Brentwood	Dear Viscount Brentwood: Dear Lady Brentwood:	Lord Brentwood Lady Brentwood	Viscount Brentwood Viscountess Brentwood
Baron Baroness	The Lord Lyndhurst *or, socially:* Lord and Lady Lyndhurst	Dear Lord Lyndhurst: Dear Lady Lyndhurst:	Lord Lyndhurst Lady Lyndhurst	Lord Lyndhurst Lady Lyndhurst
Baronet	Sir Albert Northrop, Bt. *or, socially:* Sir Albert and Lady Northrop	Dear Sir Albert: Dear Lady Northrop:	Sir Albert Northrop Lady Northrop	Sir Albert Northrop Lady Northrop

Canadian Officials

	Introducing and Address on Envelope	Letter Salutation	Speaking To	Place Card
Governor General	His Excellency Eric C. Johnson *or, socially:* Their Excellencies Governor General and Mrs. Johnson	Dear Governor General:	Governor General	The Governor General of Canada
Lieutenant Governor of Canada	His Honour The Honourable Gerald L. Dowd Lieutenant Governor *or, socially:* Lieutenant Governor and Mrs. Dowd	Dear Lieutenant Governor:	Lieutenant Governor Dowd	The Lieutenant Governor of Canada
Prime Minister of Canada	The Right Honourable Andrew C. Fitch, P.C., M.P. Prime Minister of Canada *or, socially:* The Prime Minister and Mrs. Fitch	Dear Mr. Prime Minister:	Prime Minister Fitch	The Prime Minister of Canada
Premier of a province of Canada	The Honourable Carolyn Cadré Premier of the Province of Quebec *or, socially:* The Honourable Carolyn Cadré and Mr. Jacques Cadré	Dear Madame Premier:	Premier Cadré	The Premier of Quebec
Member of Senate	The Honourable Laura Flynn The Senate, Ottawa *or, socially:* The Honourable Laura Flynn and Mr. Lesley Flynn	Dear Senator Flynn:	Senator	The Honourable Laura Flynn
Member of House of Commons	Samuel Morris, Esq., M.P. House of Commons *or, socially:* Mr. and Mrs. Samuel Morris	Dear Mr. Morris:	Mr. Morris	Samuel Morris, Esq., M.P.

	Introducing and Address on Envelope	Letter Salutation	Speaking To	Place Card
Mayor of a city or town	His Worship Mayor Kenneth Woods City Hall *or, socially:* His Worship Mayor Kenneth Woods and Mrs. Woods	Dear Mr. Mayor:	Mr. Mayor	The Mayor of Toronto
Chief Justice	The Right Honourable Roger C. Bolton, Chief Justice of Canada *or, socially:* The Right Honourable Roger C. Bolton and Mrs. Bolton	Dear Mr. Chief Justice:	Chief Justice Bolton	The Chief Justice of Canada

NOTE: Since people in Great Britain and the Commonwealth spell in *Honourable,* with the *u,* it is a nice touch to address them with their own spelling.

Diplomatic Protocol with Other Nations

WRITING TO OFFICIALS OF FOREIGN REPUBLICS

When you write to officials of a foreign republic, follow the style given in this chart of the country of France:

Official	Introducing; also Name on Envelope	Letter Salutation	Speaking To	Place Card
President of the Republic	His Excellency Henri Vaudoyer President of the Republic of France Address *or, socially:* The President of France and Madame Vaudoyer	Dear Mr. President:	Mr. President	The President of the Republic of France
Prime Minister of the Republic of France	His Excellency Jean de l'Abeille Prime Minister of the Republic of France *or, socially:* The Prime Minister of France and Madame de l'Abeille	Dear Mr. Prime Minister:	Mr. Prime Minister	The Prime Minister of the Republic of France

Official	Introducing and Addressing Envelope	Letter Salutation	Speaking To	Place Card
Minister of Foreign Affairs of the Republic of France	Her Excellency Jeanne d'Arcy Minister of Foreign Affairs *or, socially:* The Minister of Foreign Affairs and Monsieur Pierre d'Arcy	Dear Madame Minister:	Madame Minister	The Minister of Foreign Affairs of the Republic of France

"His Excellency" or "Her Excellency" for Foreign Officials

Americans use "The Honorable" as a title in front of a person's given name and surname to note the importance of the person's present or former position. For the heads of state, ambassadors, cabinet officers, etc., of other countries (as well as for high-ranking members of the clergy), it is proper to use "His Excellency" (or "Her Excellency") before the given name and surname. For example, an envelope is addressed:

> His Excellency
> Giovanni Nanni
> Ambassador of the Republic of Italy

We would introduce the dignitary to an assemblage in the same manner. In most cases, we address the envelope in the way we formally introduce the person. (Note, however, that the Commonwealth nations do not use "His Excellency," but rather "The Right Honourable.")

What is confusing is that what we properly call a foreign official in the United States may not be the way he is properly addressed in his own country. For example, we address a foreign ambassador to this country as "His Excellency" on the envelope and letter address as well as in an introduction, but we call him "Mr. Ambassador" to his face. In many foreign countries, he is called "Your Excellency" to his face. The nuances are subtle but important. It is important to learn how to address foreign officials in this country. If you have business abroad, you should also learn the protocol in whatever country or countries you are doing business.

Western European Titles

The king or queen of any foreign country is addressed as "Your Majesty," and referred to as "His Majesty" or "Her Majesty" respectively.

The prince consort to the queen is referred to as "His Royal Highness" and is addressed as "Your Royal Highness."

When royal titles still exist in a country that is not a monarchy, even though these titles are meaningless, they are still treated with respect by the people in that country. Western Europe has a long history and a love of tradition, and therefore people who have inherited defunct but legitimate titles may use the royal crest on their stationery, engraved on their silver flatware, etc.

In order of rank, the titles are these:

- Prince and princess. (You call them by their title and surname, not their given names, when introducing them; in conversation call them "Prince" and "Princess.")
- Duke and duchess. (You call them by their title and surname, not their given name, when introducing them; in conversation, call them "Duke" or "Duchess.")
- Marquess and marchioness (*marquis* and *marquise* in France, *marchese* and *marchesa* in Italy, *marques* and *marquesa* in Spain)
- Viscount and viscountess
- Count and countess
- Baron and baroness

You would write an invitation to them in this manner: "Count and Countess Philippe de Beaumont." If one of the couple is titled and the other is not, use the title for the one who holds it: "Signor Emmanuele Capriccio and Contessa Eleanora Capriccio."

Many Western Europeans do not use their titles when doing business in the United States, but when you write to them in their country and when you are visiting in their country, you should use their titles.

The United Nations

Unlike the diplomatic corps accredited to Washington, D.C., the United Nations diplomats change in rank and precedence on a rotating basis (which means that length of service in the job or importance of the country has little to do with who outranks whom).

Official	Introducing and Addressing Envelope	Letter Salutation	Speaking To	Place Card
The Secretary General	Her Excellency Françoise d'Estain Secretary General of the United Nations	Dear Madame Secretary General:	Madame Secretary General (Madame d'Estain, *subsequently*)	The Secretary General of the United Nations

Official	Introducing and Addressing Envelope	Letter Salutation	Speaking To	Place Card
A foreign UN ambassador	His Excellency Koto Matsumada Ambassador of Japan Permanent Mission of Japan to the United Nations	Dear Mr. Ambassador:	Mr. Ambassador (Sir, *subsequently*)	Ambassador Matsumada
The United States Representative to the United Nations	The Honorable Henry Gregory United States Representative to the United Nations	Dear Mr. Ambassador:	Mr. Ambassador (Sir, *subsequently*)	Ambassador Gregory

Invitations to UN ambassadors and their spouses are addressed to their residences as follows:

His Excellency Koto Matsumada and Madame Matsumada

or

Her Excellency Françoise d'Estain and Monsieur Eric d'Estain

Military Rank

• *The Army, Air Force, and Marine Corps* have the following commissioned officers according to rank:

General
Lieutenant General
Major General
Brigadier General
Colonel
Lieutenant Colonel
Major
Captain
First Lieutenant
Second Lieutenant

• *The Navy and Coast Guard* have the following:

Admiral
Vice Admiral
Rear Admiral
Captain
Commander
Lieutenant Commander
Lieutenant

Lieutenant, junior grade
Ensign

NOTE: All officers in the Navy and Coast Guard are addressed as "Mr." up through the rank of lieutenant commander. A woman officer is addressed "Ms." or "Miss," never "Mrs."

A captain in the Navy or Coast Guard has a higher rank than a captain in the Army, Air Force, or Marine Corps.

A warrant officer's rank lies between that of a commissioned and a noncommissioned officer.

HOW TO ADDRESS A MILITARY MAN OR WOMAN

Examples of Military Rank	Making Introductions/ Addressing Envelopes	Letter Salutation	When Speaking To	Place Card
First lieutenant	First Lieutenant Richard Dix, USMC *or, socially:* First Lieutenant and Mrs. Richard Dix	Dear Lieutenant Dix:	Lieutenant Dix, *or,* Lieutenant	Lieutenant Dix
Captain in the Navy	Captain Joseph Piteo, USN *or, socially:* Captain and Mrs. Joseph Piteo	Dear Captain Piteo:	Captain Piteo, *or* Captain	Captain Piteo
Lieutenant colonel	Lieutenant Colonel Frank Haig, USMC *or, socially:* Lieutenant Colonel and Mrs. Frank Haig	Dear Colonel Haig:	Colonel Haig, *or,* Colonel	Colonel Haig
Chief warrant officer	Chief Warrant Officer Jane Turner *or, socially:* Chief Warrant Officer Jane Turner and Mr. Anthony Turner	Dear Chief Warrant Officer Turner: *or, informally:* Dear Ms. Turner:	Chief Warrant Officer Turner *or, informally:* Ms. Turner	Ms. Turner
Noncommissioned officers in Army, Air Force, and Marine Corps	Master Sergeant Tony Tatum *or, socially:* Master Sergeant and Mrs. Tony Tatum	Dear Sergeant Tatum:	Sergeant Tatum	Mr. Tatum

(Follow same form for any rating, including Sergeant Major, Sergeant First Class, Platoon Sergeant, Corporal, Specialist (classes 4 to 9), Private First Class, etc.)

Examples of Military Rank	Making Introductions/ Addressing Envelopes	Letter Salutation	When Speaking To	Place Card
Enlisted person in Navy	SN Robert Peltz Address of his command *or, socially:* Seaman and Mrs. Robert Peltz	Dear Seaman Peltz:	Seaman Peltz	Seaman Peltz
Retired officer in Army or Air Force	Major Robert Orr, USAF Retired Address *or, socially:* Major and Mrs. Robert Orr	Dear Major Orr:	Major Orr	Major Orr
Retired officer in Navy or Coast Guard*	Rear Admiral Spencer Davis, USN Retired Address *or, socially:* Rear Admiral and Mrs. Spencer Davis	Dear Admiral Davis:	Admiral Davis	Admiral Davis
Cadet at West Point (same for Air Force Academy, with address change)	Cadet Mark Boland, U.S. Army Company ___, Corps of Cadets United States Military Academy West Point, NY 10996	Dear Mr. Boland: *or,* Dear Cadet Boland:	Mr. Boland	Mr. Boland
Midshipman at U.S. Naval Academy; Cadet at U.S. Coast Guard Academy	Midshipman Joan Doan U.S. Naval Academy *or* Cadet Stephen Cole United States Coast Guard Academy	Dear Ms. (*or* Miss) Doan: Dear Mr. Cole:	Ms. *or* Miss Doan Mr. Cole	Ms. Doan

*Only Navy and Coast Guard officers with rank of commander and above retain their titles after retirement; officers in the Reserve do not.)

Religious Officials

In closing a letter to a very high religious official, use "Respectfully yours" or use "Sincerely" or "Sincerely yours."

PROTESTANT CLERGY

Official	Making Introductions/ Addressing Envelopes	Letter Salutation	Speaking To/ Place Card
Clergyman with Doctor's degree	The Reverend Dr. Amos E. Long *or, socially:* The Reverend Dr. Amos E. Long and Mrs. Long	Dear Dr. Long:	Dr. Long
Clergywoman without Doctor's degree	The Reverend Anne Smith *or, socially:* The Reverend Anne Smith and Mr. Peter Smith	Dear Ms. *or* Miss Smith:	Ms. *or* Miss Smith
Presiding Bishop of the Episcopal Church in the United States	The Right Reverend James Gard, Presiding Bishop *or, socially:* The Right Reverend James Gard and Mrs. Gard	Dear Bishop Gard:	Bishop Gard
Bishop of the Episcopal Church	The Right Reverend David Webb Bishop of Washington *or, socially:* The Right Reverend David Webb and Mrs. Webb	Dear Bishop Webb:	Bishop Webb
Methodist Bishop	The Reverend Michael Forest Methodist Bishop *or, socially:* The Reverend Michael Forest and Mrs. Forest	Dear Bishop Forest:	Bishop Forest
Dean	The Very Reverend Angus Dunn *or,* The Very Reverend Angus Dunn, Dean of St. John's *or, socially:* The Very Reverend Angus Dunn and Mrs. Dunn	Dear Dean Dunn:	Dean Dunn
Archdeacon	The Venerable Stewart G. Dodd Archdeacon of Boston *or, socially:* The Venerable Stewart G. Dodd and Mrs. Dodd	Dear Archdeacon Dodd:	Archdeacon Dodd
Canon	The Reverend Randolph Tate Canon of St. Andrew's *or, socially:* The Reverend Randolph Tate and Mrs. Tate	Dear Canon Tate:	Canon Tate

• The highest officials of the Episcopal Church, the Archbishops of Canterbury and York, are Privy Counsellors and have seats in the House of Lords. You would address the envelope to "The Most Reverend and Right Honourable Archbishop of Canterbury (or York)." The salutation would read: "Dear Archbishop."

• Clergy with degrees optionally use their degree initials after their names: "The Right Reverend James Gard" or "The Right Reverend James Gard, D.D., Ll.D."

• An Episcopal cleric who is not in a religious order may call himself "Father." In writing him, use his surname, rather than his Christian name—for example, "The Reverend Father Smith."

• A Protestant minister who retires remains "The Reverend So-and-so." If he or she resigns, that person normally becomes "Mr." or "Ms."

MORMON CLERGY

Official	Making Introductions/ Addressing Envelopes	Letter Salutation	Speaking To/ Place Card
Mormon Bishop	Mr. Timothy Blake Church of Jesus Christ of Latter-day Saints *or, socially:* Mr. and Mrs. Timothy Blake	Dear Mr. Blake:	Mr. Blake

ROMAN CATHOLIC HIERARCHY

Official	Making Introductions/ Addressing Envelopes	Letter Salutation	Speaking To/ Place Card
The Pope	His Holiness, the Pope *or* His Holiness, Pope Augustus III	Your Holiness:	*Speaking to:* Your Holiness
The Apostolic Delegate in Washington (the Pope's representative)	His Excellency The Most Reverend Bishop of (City) The Apostolic Delegate Address	Your Excellency:	Your Excellency/His Excellency the Apostolic Delegate
Cardinal	His Eminence, Joseph Cardinal Sheehan Archbishop of St. Louis	Your Eminence: *or,* Dear Cardinal Sheehan:	Your Eminence/Cardinal Sheehan
Bishop and Archbishop	The Most Reverend Paul Murphy, Bishop (Archbishop) of Chicago	Your Excellency: *or,* Dear Bishop Murphy:	Excellency/ Bishop Murphy

Official	Making Introductions/ Addressing Envelopes	Letter Salutation	Speaking To/ Place Card
Monsignor	The Right Reverend Julius Cuneo	Dear Monsignor Cuneo:	Monsignor Cuneo
Priest	The Reverend Father James Orr Church rectory address	Dear Father Orr:	Father Orr
Brother	Brother David Maxwell	Dear Brother David: *or,* Dear Brother Maxwell:	Brother David *or* Brother Maxwell
Nun	Joan Reynolds, R.S.C.J. *or,* Sister Mary Annunciata	Dear Sister:	Sister Reynolds *or* Sister Mary Annunciata

EASTERN ORTHODOX COMMUNION

Official	Making Introductions/ Addressing Envelopes	Salutation	Speaking To
Patriarch	His Holiness, the Ecumenical Patriarch of Constantinople	Your Holiness:	Your Holiness
Bishop and priest	*Same as Roman Catholic Church*		
Archimandrite	The Very Reverend Gregory Costos	Reverend Sir:	Father Costos

JEWISH FAITH

Official	Making Introductions/ Addressing Envelopes	Letter Salutation	Speaking To	Place Card
Rabbi	Rabbi Melvin Schwartz Address *or, socially:* Rabbi and Mrs. Melvin Schwartz	Dear Rabbi Schwartz:	Rabbi *or* Rabbi Schwartz	Rabbi Schwartz
Cantor	Cantor Samuel Stein Address *or, socially:* Cantor and Mrs. Samuel Stein	Dear Cantor Stein:	Cantor Stein	Cantor Stein

MILITARY CHAPLAINS

Making Introductions/ Addressing Envelopes	Letter Salutation	Speaking To	Place Card
Major John Martin, Chaplain Address	Dear Major Martin: or, Dear Chaplain: or, for a Catholic chaplain: Dear Father Martin: or, for a Jewish chaplain, Dear Rabbi Martin:	Chaplain or Major Martin	Major Martin or, for Catholic, Father Martin or, for Jewish, Rabbi Martin

Foreign Professionals

We should accord foreign professionals their titles when addressing them. For example, in Italy, if you have finished university and earned your degree, you are called "Dottore" (for a man) or "Dottoressa" (for a woman) as the title before your surname for the rest of your life. In writing a letter, you may abbreviate the title to "Dott." in front of either his or her surname—"Dott. Cavalchini." We Americans should use this title if we have any correspondence on personal or business matters with an Italian who merits this honorific.

In many countries a man or woman who has earned a professional degree is thereafter addressed by the title of that profession (and not necessarily by his or her name) for the rest of that person's life. For example, in France, in speaking to a person, you would address a lawyer formally as "Monsieur l'Avocat" (Mr. Lawyer) or a woman ambassador as "Madame l'Ambassadeur." In Italy you would say "Signor Avvocato," and you would call your architect "Signor Architetto." In Germany, instead of calling the CEO of the company "Herr Schmidt," you'd call him "Herr Direktor"; an engineer would be addressed as "Herr Ingenieur," and so on. (It makes life very easy for people who can't remember names; all they have to remember is a professional title!)

Once an American becomes involved at length with a foreigner in a country where a professional title is important—whether it's a business or a social matter—the polite thing to do is to use his or her title in addressing that person. Learn the foreign pronunciation, learn how to write the title in the foreign tongue. Your foreign colleague will be pleased and respect you more because of it.

For Questions Relating to Protocol

When you're in a protocol quandary, here's where to go for help. (Be sure you have first checked the charts contained in this book.)

- For further information on titles and precedence of U.S. Government officials, and for listings and addresses of the Washington diplomatic corps:

  o Call The Department of State, Office of Protocol, Ceremonial Section (202/647-1735).
  o Consult *The Social List of Washington, D.C., and Social Precedence in Washington* (published by Thomas J. Murray, 10335 Kensington Parkway, Kensington, MD 20895).

- For information on British government officials and the peerage, consult *Debrett's Peerage and Baronetages* (published by Debrett's Peerage, 73-77 Britannia Road, London S.W. 6 2JR, England).

- For information on the United Nations precedence, call the United Nations, Office of Protocol in New York (212/963-7176).

- For information on protocol questions in your state government, call the Governor's Office in the State Capitol; for city government, call the Mayor's Office. For questions of military rank, call the nearest military establishment.

Afterword

I wish to thank very warmly those who use this book to look up solutions to specific dilemmas, and I throw myself in gratitude at the feet of those who have the stamina and interest to read the book all the way through! In becoming immersed in this review of exemplary human behavior, the reader has also received a big dose of my personal philosophy. Like it or not, I can't keep my philosophy out of my writing, because I feel it so strongly, even passionately.

No matter how dark the horizon may seem at any given time, we must remember that life is a precious gift. It is to be *enjoyed,* not complained about, for however long we are privileged to have it. I look on manners simply as taking good care of this precious, immensely valuable gift. There's a joy in being decent to other people and receiving their thanks in return. Even when our efforts are not appreciated by those who benefit from them, we should keep moving ahead—with positive, considerate attitudes firmly in mind—remembering all those sunny days and happy times when human beings *do* interact beautifully with one another.

It's a great feeling to know that we're doing the right thing. It's a secure, comfortable, even cozy feeling. When we know all the rules, then we have the license to be intelligent mavericks and rebel, adapting them tastefully when it is appropriate to do so. When we don't know the rules in the first place, our behavior may be judged poorly.

If we don't consciously teach our children the rules, we might very well be helping our society move toward social anarchy. We therefore have the enormous responsibility to bring our own and everyone else's children into the next decade—and the century to come—trained in self-discipline and armed with ethics, values, and morals. And we must certainly must not allow the nation's supply of the "milk of human kindness" to dry up!

The world that lies ahead is full of promise, excitement, and hope for peace and the betterment of mankind. We may not be in the forefront of the technological advances personally, but we certainly can be in the forefront of good human relations. I'll take a nice, warm, compassionate human being over a shiny new technological marvel any day.

Actually, why not have both—the warm human being *and* the innovative new machine? There's no reason they can't operate harmoniously together!

623

AN ADDITIONAL
NOTE OF
THANKS

I would like to add a note of thanks to the following people and organizations who patiently fed me information and helped in many ways: Patricia Keogh, who worked so hard on research as my assistant in New York; Eileen Kamara of Brewood Stationers; Petrossian Caviar; Tiffany & Co.; Molly Baldrige and Buddy Kring; Megan and Craig Murray; Alice and Walker Wainwright; Jean Bilus; Gail and Hiram Guttierrez; Ted Kleisner and Sharon Rowe of The Greenbriar; Hickey Freeman Suits; K & D Liquors; Joel Schreiber of A. T. Harris (Traditional Men's Formalwear); Sherry-Lehmann Inc. of New York; Phoenix House; William Davis, R.N., M.S., Mount Sinai Hospital; Page Kjellstrom; Nana Greller; Nancy Baldridge; Midge Baldrige; Elise Moore-Searson, Social Secretary to the British Ambassador; Protocol Office, Department of State; The White House Social Office.

INDEX

H

Y